Clinical Specialties

medical student revision guide

"This book is what I would have wished for in my medical student days"

From the Foreword by Stella Vig, National Clinical Director for Elective Care

Feedback, errors and omissions
We are always pleased to receive feedback (good and bad) about our books – if you would like to comment on any of our books, please email info@scionpublishing.com.

We've worked really hard with the authors to ensure that everything in the book is correct. However, errors and ambiguities can still slip through in books as complex as this. If you spot anything you think might be wrong, please email us and we will look into it straight away. If an error has occurred, we will correct it for future printings and post a note about it on our website so that other readers of the book are alerted to this.

Thank you for your help.

Clinical Specialties

medical student revision guide

Rebecca Richardson

BMBS, BMedSci
Junior Doctor, Royal Derby Hospital, Derby

Ricky Ellis

PhD, MRCS, MBChB, BSc, DPD, MFSTEd, FHEA
Urology Specialist Registrar, Royal Derby
Hospital, Derby

Community medicine

Geriatrics

Gynaecology

Obstetrics

Paediatrics

Psychiatry

Dermatology

Ear, Nose & Throat

Ophthalmology

Anaesthetics

Palliative care

Scion

Scion Publishing Limited

The Old Hayloft, Vantage Business Park, Bloxham Road, Banbury OX16 9UX, UK

www.scionpublishing.com

Important Note from the Publisher

The information contained within this book was obtained by Scion Publishing Ltd from sources believed by us to be reliable. However, while every effort has been made to ensure its accuracy, no responsibility for loss or injury whatsoever occasioned to any person acting or refraining from action as a result of information contained herein can be accepted by the authors or publishers.

Readers are reminded that medicine is a constantly evolving science and while the authors and publishers have ensured that all dosages, applications and practices are based on current indications, there may be specific practices which differ between communities. You should always follow the guidelines laid down by the manufacturers of specific products and the relevant authorities in the country in which you are practising.

Although every effort has been made to ensure that all owners of copyright material have been acknowledged in this publication, we would be pleased to acknowledge in subsequent reprints or editions any omissions brought to our attention.

Registered names, trademarks, etc. used in this book, even when not marked as such, are not to be considered unprotected by law.

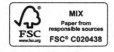
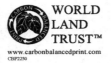

www.carbonbalancedprint.com
CBP2250

Typeset by Medlar Publishing Solutions Pvt Ltd, India

Printed in the UK

Last digit is the print number: 10 9 8 7 6 5 4

Contents

Foreword

I think back to my medical student days fondly. They were packed full of excitement, learning, demanding work schedules and fun. I learnt how to translate heavy, almost unreadable tomes into my revision notes (personalised with colourful annotations), and how to pass exams. Ensuring that the basic facts were clearly structured in my memory was important and allowed me to add in experiential learning through patient and other clinical interactions.

I continue to employ these practices in my everyday work as a Consultant Surgeon, as in this profession **we never stop learning**. This is the magic and attraction of medicine! I enjoy my time as a trainer and encourage my medical students to understand the basics first, and then **create their own way of learning** by annotating and adding to these.

This book is simple to use and concise despite the breadth and depth of what it covers. It entices the reader to use it as a personal board, to add newly learnt facts or clinical experiences. It has already completed the arduous work of **summarising key points and highlighting co-dependencies or important life-changing facts**. Rebecca and Ricky have used a broad group of reviewers to ensure that this book does what it sets out to do; to support learning and revision in a way that fits modern life and act as **a scaffold that provides safe and proper practice**, with signposts for an individual to pursue their interests with more detail.

The world is becoming ever busier, and the medical curriculum even larger as our medical knowledge develops. **This book is what I would have wished for in my medical student days**. It would have saved me time, a precious commodity when everyone is tired. If we can support our medical students to learn and enjoy life, we can look forward to a rejuvenated NHS workforce crucial to delivering the excellent care we wish for in the NHS.

Stella Vig
Consultant Surgeon and Trainer
National Clinical Director for Elective Care

Preface

I remember it well. Countless evenings sat at my desk, desperately trying to work out what I needed to know, and how I was going to know it. Hours spent trudging through textbooks, soaking up line after line of information, only to be left certain that after a week on my new placement, it would all be forgotten. **Medical school is tough**. The vast volume of knowledge that must be acquired and retained, to achieve the standards expected of a safe and successful doctor, is a daunting task. But as you will find at every stage in your medical career, **help is always available if you know where to look**. For you, I hope this book can be your help. I present it as your trusted companion, a loyal friend that will stand by your side through good times and bad, something to turn to when you need **guidance, reassurance, or simply just a place to start!**

There is no end of resources available for medical students, all designed to make the journey from student to doctor that little bit easier. For me, I found this wealth of information to be just as much of a curse as it was a blessing. Not only was I faced with the overwhelming task of learning it all, but I first had to find and dissect the parts that were relevant to me. **Wouldn't it be easier if everything I needed to know was in the same place?** The simple answer – yes. And that is how I started to write this book.

My first goal when creating the *Medical Student Revision Guides* was to bring together **all the key topics needed for medical school exams and life as a junior doctor** in one readily available place. I did this through summarising a variety of recognised resources, including textbooks, articles and clinical guidelines. This has been **supplemented by the expert knowledge of specialists** in each field, who have reviewed each chapter to ensure it is accurate and reflects the most up-to-date guidance.

My second goal was to do everything I could to help you remember this information. I appreciate everyone is unique in the way they learn, but with most of us relying on **vision as our dominant sense**, it seemed illogical not to utilise its power. As such, I have specifically designed this book with an **extensive use of colour, diagrams and summary tables**, to create a resource that is visually striking and a refreshing change from your current textbooks. The informal 'notes-style' layout and dedicated column that allows for your own annotations on each page, are features that I hope make the content feel **more accessible and easier to engage with**.

It is my sincere hope that you find this book useful, whether it be as your comprehensive revision resource, or a quick reminder of a condition that you come across on the ward. **I am forever grateful for any feedback** that can help me to better help you, so please do leave a review with your honest thoughts.

I wish you luck with your exams, and all the best for your future careers.

Rebecca Richardson

Disclaimer

It is important to note that this book is designed as a revision tool and aide-memoire. It is not intended to give an in-depth understanding of each condition, but rather to focus on the key points that often appear in undergraduate exams. It should not be solely relied upon in clinical situations; please always check the most current and local guidelines before implementing management or administering any treatment.

Every attempt has been made to ensure that the most up-to-date information has been included at the time of writing this book. However, due to the continuously evolving nature of the medical profession, and with variations in clinical practice between hospital Trusts, this cannot be guaranteed. It is therefore advised that you correlate these notes to other resources, and supplement them with your own clinical encounters, to ensure a complete learning experience. Readers should also ensure that they learn all elements of their own medical school curriculum, regardless of whether they are covered in this book.

Acknowledgements

I must firstly say a huge thank you to the team at Scion Publishing for making this book a reality. A special mention to Jonathan and Clare, for your tireless work overcoming layout issues and design problems, to ensure the end product was everything I had hoped it would be.

Secondly, I would like to thank my co-author, Ricky. Your advice and guidance have been invaluable in this process. Your wealth of experience in the field of medical education has undoubtedly benefited the book and its readers, and remains an inspiration for my future work.

My thanks are extended to all those who have contributed time and expertise as a chapter reviewer. I will be eternally grateful that you could see the potential in my work in its early stages and gave up your own time to help me achieve it. The abundance of knowledge and experience you have brought is priceless and will underpin the learning of many future doctors.

Finally, to my loved ones. To Mum and Dad, for the years of selflessness and sacrifice that allowed me the opportunities to achieve all that I have today. To my brother, Chris, whose artistic talent never fails to amaze me, and has inspired the covers and diagrams of both my books. To Nana, Gran, Grandad and Margaret, for the timeless wisdom and unconditional love that only grandparents can provide. And to Martin, for your endless patience, support and encouragement in all that I do.

Thank you.

About the authors

Rebecca Richardson is a junior doctor currently working in the East Midlands. After graduating from the University of Nottingham as one of the top students in her year, with first class honours, she became passionate about helping others to follow in her footsteps. Her revision notes have already helped hundreds of medical students across the UK prepare for their exams. Rebecca has continued her mission to support students and trainees through creating content for a variety of medical education platforms, as well as running regular virtual teaching sessions to help students practise for their clinical examinations.

Ricky Ellis is a Urology Specialist Registrar, Honorary Clinical Senior Lecturer and Research Associate for the Intercollegiate Committee for Basic Surgical Examinations (ICBSE). Ricky is an award-winning trainer and regularly organises teaching courses including the internationally delivered 'Urology Boot Camp for Medical Students'. He is passionate about improving training for medical students and junior doctors and was awarded the prestigious Association of Surgeons in Training and Faculty of Surgical Trainers Silver Suture Award for contributions to and excellence in surgical training.

Peer reviewers

Section	Peer reviewer
Anaesthetics	**Dr Richard Telford** Retired Consultant Anaesthetist, Royal Devon and Exeter Foundation NHS Trust
Community-based medicine	**Dr Juanita Amin** General Practitioner, Sandwell and West Birmingham NHS Trust
	Dr Misha Patel GP Trainee, Nottinghamshire Healthcare NHS Foundation Trust, University Hospitals of Derby and Burton NHS Trust
Dermatology	**Dr Beenish Afzal** Specialty Registrar Dermatology, Sheffield Teaching Hospitals NHS Foundation Trust
Ear, nose & throat	**Mr Thomas Stubington** ENT Specialist Registrar, East Midlands
Geriatric medicine	**Dr Rosemary Arnott** Registrar in Geriatric Medicine, Sherwood Forest Hospitals NHS Foundation Trust
Gynaecology	**Mr Ben Peyton-Jones** Consultant Obstetrician and Gynaecologist, Royal Devon and Exeter Foundation NHS Trust
Obstetrics	**Mr Ben Peyton-Jones** Consultant Obstetrician and Gynaecologist, Royal Devon and Exeter Foundation NHS Trust
Old age psychiatry	**Dr Sandar Kyaw** Higher Training Specialist Registrar, Older Adult Psychiatry, Sherwood Forest Hospitals NHS Foundation Trust
Ophthalmology	**Dr Di Zou** Senior Ophthalmology Registrar, Queens Medical Centre, Nottingham
Paediatric oncology	**Dr Eleanor Bea McLaren** Paediatric Registrar, Royal Devon and Exeter Foundation NHS Trust
Paediatrics	**Dr Katherine Jones** Paediatric Registrar, Royal Devon & Exeter Foundation NHS Trust
Palliative care	**Dr Jennifer Walker** ST4 Palliative Medicine Higher Trainee, East Midlands
Psychiatry	**Dr Laura Davis** Consultant in Old Age Psychiatry, Nottinghamshire Healthcare NHS Foundation Trust
	Dr Divyanish Specialist Registrar General Adult Psychiatry, Derbyshire Healthcare NHS Foundation Trusts

General abbreviations

Each chapter begins with a set of abbreviations specific to that chapter.

2ww – 2 week wait
a. – Arterial
ABCDE – Airways, Breathing, Circulation, Disability, Exposure
ABG – Arterial blood gas
ABX – Antibiotics
AXR – Abdominal X-ray
BB – Beta-blocker
BD – Twice a day
BG – Blood glucose
BMI – Body mass index
BP – Blood pressure
Ca – Calcium
CBT – Cognitive behavioural therapy
CCB – Calcium channel blocker
CCF – Congestive cardiac failure
CF – Cystic fibrosis
CHF – Chronic heart failure
CI – Contraindication
CK – Creatine kinase
CKD – Chronic kidney disease
CMV – Cytomegalovirus
CN – Cranial nerve
CNS – Central nervous system
CPAP – Continuous positive airway pressure
CPR – Cardiopulmonary resuscitation
Cr – Creatinine
CRP – C-reactive protein
CRT – Capillary refill time
CSF – Cerebrospinal fluid
CT – Computed tomography
CV – Cardiovascular
CVA – Cerebrovascular accident
CVD – Cardiovascular disease
CXR – Chest X-ray
D&V – Diarrhoea and vomiting
d – Day
DBP – Diastolic blood pressure
DDx – Differential diagnosis
DM – Diabetes mellitus
DOAC – Direct oral anticoagulant
DRE – Digital rectal examination
DVLA – Driver and Vehicle Licensing Agency
Dx – Diagnosis
ECG – Electrocardiogram
ECT – Electroconvulsive therapy
EEG – Electroencephalogram

eGFR – Estimated GFR
ENT – Ear, nose and throat
EPO – Erythropoeitin
ESR – Erythrocyte sedimentation rate
FBC – Full blood count
FHx – Family history
G&S – Group & save
GA – General anaesthetic
GCS – Glasgow Coma Score/Scale
GFR – Glomerular filtration rate
GI – Gastrointestinal
GP – General practitioner
h – Hour
Hb – Haemoglobin
HF – Heart failure
HIV – Human immunodeficiency virus
HR – Heart rate
HTN – Hypertension
ICP – Intracranial pressure
Ig – Immunoglobulin
IHD – Ischaemic heart disease
IM – Intramuscular
inc. – Including
IV – Intravenous
IVDU – Intravenous drug user
Ix – Investigation
LFT – Liver function test
LHS – Left-hand side
LMWH – Low molecular weight heparin
LOC – Loss of consciousness
m – Month
mcg – Microgram
MCS – Microscopy, culture and sensitivity
MDT – Multidisciplinary team
MI – Myocardial infarction
min – Minute
MND – Motor neurone disease
MRI – Magnetic resonance imaging
Mx – Management
NBM – Nil by mouth
NSAID – Non-steroidal anti-inflammatory drug
N&V – Nausea & vomiting
OCD – Obsessive–compulsive disorder
OD – Once a day
OT – Occupational therapist
PCR – Polymerase chain reaction

PE – Pulmonary embolism
PET – Positron emission tomography
PHx – Past history
PNS – Peripheral nervous system
PO – Per ora (orally)
PR – Per rectum
PRN – Pro re nata (as required)
pulm. – Pulmonary
RA – Rheumatoid arthritis
RBC – Red blood cell
RFT – Renal function test
RHS – Right-hand side
r/o – Risk of
R/V – Review
re – Regarding
RF – Risk factor
RR – Respiration rate
s – Second
SALT – Speech and language therapy
SBP – Systolic blood pressure
SC – Subcutaneous
SD – Standard deviation
SE – Side-effect
SL – Sublingual
SLE – Systemic lupus erythematosus
SOB – Shortness of breath
SSRI – Selective serotonin reuptake inhibitor
Sx – Symptoms
TB – Tuberculosis
TCA – Tricyclic antidepressant
TDS – Three times a day
TFT – Thyroid function test
TIA – Transient ischaemic attack
TNM – Tumour, nodes, metastases
Tx – Treatment
U&Es – Urea & electrolytes
USS – Ultrasound scan
UTI – Urinary tract infection
VBG – Venous blood gas
vit – Vitamin
VTE – Venous thromboembolism
W – Week
WBC – White blood cell
WCC – White cell count
WHO – World Health Organization
y – Year

How to use this book

The underlying principle of this book is to present information in a way that is **eye-catching, clear and easy to remember.** This page will explain some of the **key layout features** that have been used to achieve this.

1. Notes column – each page is divided into a main text section, and a tinted notes column. The notes column is used to house additional information, and to provide space for your own notes, should you wish to make any.

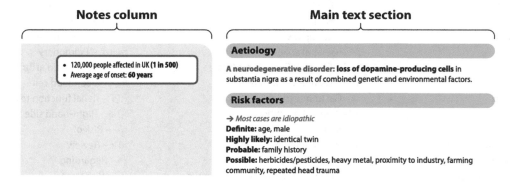

Notes column

- 120,000 people affected in UK **(1 in 500)**
- Average age of onset: **60 years**

Main text section

Aetiology

A neurodegenerative disorder: **loss of dopamine-producing cells** in substantia nigra as a result of combined genetic and environmental factors.

Risk factors

→ *Most cases are idiopathic*
Definite: age, male
Highly likely: identical twin
Probable: family history
Possible: herbicides/pesticides, heavy metal, proximity to industry, farming community, repeated head trauma

2. Text colour
- chapter coloured text – used to expand on a point / provide extra information
- grey text – used for less important information
- red text – used for red flags and emergency points
- blue text – used for extra points / annotations

3. Highlighting – words/phrases that have been highlighted are linked to extra information. Look for another highlight of the same colour on the page to find this information. *The below example uses yellow highlighting to link 'ABX' to the additional information 'use CENTOR score to assess need for ABX'.*

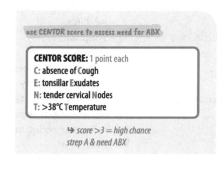

use CENTOR score to assess need for ABX

CENTOR SCORE: 1 point each
C: absence of Cough
E: tonsillar Exudates
N: tender cervical Nodes
T: >38°C Temperature

↳ *score >3 = high chance strep A & need ABX*

Tonsillitis²

→ *acute bacterial infection (Strep. pyogenes, staphs, M. catarrhalis)*

SYMPTOMS
- **Sore throat** + odynophagia ± pus on tonsils
- Pyrexia, malaise etc.
- Lymphadenopathy

MANAGEMENT: if **unilateral Sx** → ENT referral
- Analgesia, fluids, soft food
- **ABX:** PO phenoxymethylpenicillin (or clarithromycin) 5–10d

4. Box colours – a variety of different boxes are used to display information.
- **Yellow tinted box** – for triggers / risk factors, complications & prognosis
- **Blue tinted box** – for differential diagnoses
- **Red box** – for red flags / emergency points
- **Chapter coloured box** – for all other types of information

Risk factors for severe GORD
- **Neuro disorders** e.g. cerebral palsy
- **Preterm** especially if bronchopulmonary dysplasia
- **Post-surgery** (for oesophageal atresia / diaphragmatic hernia)

Yellow-tinted

DDx microcytic anaemia: 'TAILS'
- **Thalassaemia** (α- or β-thalassaemia trait)
- **Anaemia of chronic disease** e.g. renal failure
- **Iron-deficiency anaemia**
- **Lead poisoning**
- **Sideroblastic anaemia**

Blue-tinted

Red flags of head injuries
- LOC >5min
- Seizure
- GCS <15 2h post-injury
- Focal neurological deficit
- Amnesia >5min
- Signs of fracture
- High risk trauma
- ≥3× vomiting

Red

COMMUNITY-BASED MEDICINE

01

ABBREVIATIONS

AAA – Abdominal aortic aneurysm
ABPM – Ambulatory blood pressure monitoring
ACEi – Angiotensin-converting enzyme inhibitor
ACh – Acetylcholine
ACR – Albumin creatinine ratio
ACTH – Adrenocorticotrophic hormone
ADH – Antidiuretic hormone
AED – Anti-epileptic drug
AF – Atrial fibrillation
AI – Aluminium
ARB – Angiotensin receptor blocker
BB – Beta-blocker
BDR – Bronchodilator reversibility
BiPAP – Bilevel positive airway pressure
BNP – B-type natriuretic peptide
BZD – Benzodiazepine
CAP – Community-acquired pneumonia
CBT – Cognitive behavioural therapy
(RL) CCB – (Rate-limiting) Calcium channel blocker
CF – Cystic fibrosis
CFTR – Cystic fibrosis transmembrane conductance regulator
COPD – Chronic obstructive pulmonary disease
CPAP – Continuous positive airway pressure
CPA – Costophrenic angle
Cr – Creatinine
CTD – Connective tissue disorder
DCC – Direct current cardioversion

DHP – Dihydropyridine
FeNO – Fraction of expired nitrous oxide
FEV_1 – Forced expiratory volume in 1 second
FVC – Forced vital capacity
GH – Growth hormone
GOJ – Gastro-oesophageal junction
GORD – Gastro-oesophageal reflux disease
H_2RA – Histamine H_2 receptor antagonist
HAP – Hospital-acquired pneumonia
HBPM – Home blood pressure monitoring
IAP – Intra-abdominal pressure
IBD – Inflammatory bowel disease
IBS – Irritable bowel syndrome
ICS – Inhaled corticosteroid
IDA – Iron-deficiency anaemia
ILD – Interstitial lung disease
LA – Long-acting
LABA – Long-acting beta agonist
LAMA – Long-acting muscarinic antagonist
LDH – Lactate dehydrogenase
LRTI – Lower respiratory tract infection
LTRA – Leukotriene receptor antagonist
LTs – Leukotrienes
LV – Left ventricle
LVH – Left ventricular hypertrophy
Mg – Magnesium
$MgSO_4$ – Magnesium sulphate
MRC – Medical Research Council
Neb – Nebuliser
NIV – Non-invasive ventilation
NMD – Neuromuscular disorder

NO – Nitrous oxide
OCP – Oral contraceptive pill
OGTT – Oral glucose tolerance test
PCKD – Polycystic kidney disease
PCOS – Polycystic ovary syndrome
PCV – Packed cell volume
PE – Pulmonary embolism
PEF – Peak expiratory flow
PG – Prostaglandin
PLA_2 – Phospholipase A_2 receptor
PPI – Proton pump inhibitor
PUD – Peptic ulcer disease
RF – Respiratory failure
RSV – Respiratory syncytial virus
SA – Short-acting
SABA – Short-acting beta agonist
SAMA – Short-acting muscarinic antagonist
SJW – St John's wort
SOB – Shortness of breath
SSRI – Selective serotonin reuptake inhibitor
T1RF – Type 1 respiratory failure
T2RF – Type 2 respiratory failure
TB – Tuberculosis
Tg(Ab) – Thyroglobulin (antibody)
TLC – Total lung capacity
TPO(Ab) – Thyroid peroxidase (antibody)
TR(Ab) – Thyroid receptor (antibody)
TSH – Thyroid-stimulating hormone
VZV – Varicella zoster virus

Asthma

Chronic, reversible increases in airway resistance due to **bronchospasm, inflammation** & **mucus production**

Pathophysiology

Triggers activate mast cells to release spasmogens & chemotaxins:

1. Early phase: **bronchospasm** (**spasmogens:** histamine, PGs, leukotrienes)
2. Late phase: **inflammation** (**chemotaxins:** attract eosinophils/monocytes)

Types

1. **Extrinsic:** type 1 hypersensitivity reaction ($\uparrow$ IgE ± other atopies)
   - early onset/younger patients (may improve with age)
   - in adults = OCCUPATIONAL ASTHMA: chemicals, enzymes in flour, animal substances
2. **Intrinsic:** non-immune mechanisms (often no cause identified)
   - late onset/middle-aged patients

Symptoms

- Wheeze, SOB, cough – worse at night / early morning / on exercise
- Chest tightness

Investigations

- **Hx:** FHx/PHx of atopies, typical Sx with diurnal variation, identifiable trigger
- **Auscultation:** expiratory polyphonic wheeze
- **Atopy tests:** skin prick / serum IgE
- **Spirometry + bronchodilator reversibility test (BDR)**
- **FeNO test (fraction of expired NO)** – if still unsure of Dx in kids **or** if >17y
- **PEF:** monitor variability over 2–4w
- **Direct bronchial challenge:** last resort

Management of acute asthma (adults)[1]

Triggers

- allergens: pets, pollen, dust mites
- cold air
- emotion
- smoking
- viral infection
- pollution
- drugs: NSAIDs/BBs

Diagnostic test results

- **FEV$_1$:FVC** <70%
- **PEF** >20% variability
- **BDR:** FEV$_1$ ≥12% improvement or ≥200ml volume increase
- **FeNO** >40ppb

Key elements of diagnosis

1. **History** – variable symptoms, triggers, PHx or FHx of atopy
2. **Examination** – wheeze
3. **Spirometry** – bronchodilator reversibility
4. **Response to trial of Tx**

NO = produced in response to inflammation

Severe attack	Life-threatening attack
• incomplete sentences • accessory muscles • hyperinflated chest • pulsus paradoxus*	• exhaustion/confusion • silent chest • cyanosis
• **PEF 33–50% of best** • RR ≥25 • HR ≥110	• **PEF <33% of best** • spO$_2$ <92% • $\downarrow$HR & $\downarrow$BP
*$\downarrow$SBP with inspiration	ABG: $\uparrow$CO$_2$, O$_2$ <8, low pH

Parasympathetic action: ACh → M$_3$ receptors = bronchoconstriction & $\uparrow$mucus
Sympathetic action: adrenaline → β$_2$ receptors = bronchodilation & $\downarrow$mucus

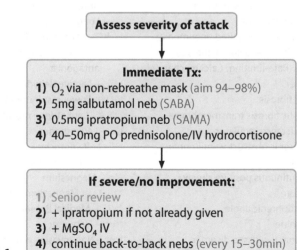

Assess severity of attack

Immediate Tx:
1) O$_2$ via non-rebreathe mask (aim 94–98%)
2) 5mg salbutamol neb (SABA)
3) 0.5mg ipratropium neb (SAMA)
4) 40–50mg PO prednisolone/IV hydrocortisone

If severe/no improvement:
1) Senior review
2) + ipratropium if not already given
3) + MgSO$_4$ IV
4) continue back-to-back nebs (every 15–30min)

Fig. 1.1

[1] NICE (2021) CKS – Scenario: Acute exacerbation of asthma

Management of chronic asthma[2]

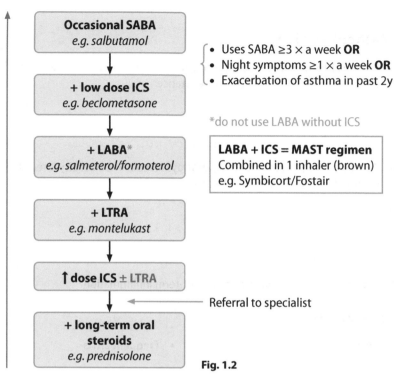

Consider stepping down if Sx controlled for 3 months

Occasional SABA
e.g. salbutamol

+ low dose ICS
e.g. beclometasone

+ LABA*
e.g. salmeterol/formoterol

+ LTRA
e.g. montelukast

↑ **dose ICS ± LTRA**

+ long-term oral steroids
e.g. prednisolone

- Uses SABA ≥3 × a week **OR**
- Night symptoms ≥1 × a week **OR**
- Exacerbation of asthma in past 2y

*do not use LABA without ICS

LABA + ICS = MAST regimen
Combined in 1 inhaler (brown)
e.g. Symbicort/Fostair

Referral to specialist

Fig. 1.2

OTHER FACTORS TO CONSIDER:

1. **Lifestyle:** smoking, weight loss, breathing exercises
2. **Inhaler technique:** spacer, add-ons
3. **Safety-net:** including signs & Mx of acute attack
4. **Follow-up appointment:** annual review with practice nurse

Safety-netting

SEEK MEDICAL ATTENTION IF:
- Symptoms are getting worse/interfere with daily life
- Waking up at night

SIGNS OF AN ACUTE ATTACK:
- Reliever inhaler isn't helping
- Too breathless to speak/eat/sleep
- Very tight chest / coughing a lot
- RR increasing / feel like can't get enough air

Medications

1. **Beta-2 agonists (SABA/LABA)**
   - Beta-2 selective → relaxes smooth muscle in lungs
   SE = tachycardia, muscle cramps/tremors

2. **Inhaled corticosteroids**
   - ↑ lipocortin → inhibits PLA_2
   - reduced arachidonic acid conversion to LTs/PGs
   - ↓ inflammation
   *SE = oral candidiasis (**rinse mouth**)*

3. **Leukotriene receptor antagonists (LTRAs)**
   - ↓ bronchoconstriction & mucus
   - ↓ eosinophils & inflammation
   SE = GI upset, headache, hepatic disorder, Churg–Strauss syndrome (vessel inflammation)

4. **Long-term oral steroids**
   - same mechanism as ICS
   - more systemic SEs
   SE: acne, hair, ↑ weight, HTN, cataracts, osteoporosis, immunosuppression/infections → cause adrenal suppression so ↓ dose gradually

Components of an asthma review

- Level of control – poor control suggested if:
  ‣ using SABA >3× per week
  ‣ night symptoms
  ‣ interfering with activities
  ‣ chest tightness, wheeze
- Any exacerbations
- Compliance/technique
- Side-effects of medications

What to do in an asthma attack

- Sit up straight
- Puff of PRN inhaler – up to 10 times
- If no improvement call 999

Chronic obstructive pulmonary disease

Chronic, progressive, **poorly reversible** airway obstruction including **chronic bronchitis & emphysema**

Risk factors for COPD
- Smoking
- Occupational dust
- Childhood infections
- α1 antitrypsin deficiency

↳ Consider if young / no other risk factors

Pathophysiology

1. **Chronic bronchitis:** ↑ mucus production & inflammatory cells → scarred/ thickened epithelium → ↑ airway resistance

'Blue-bloaters':
- *Chronic productive cough (lasting ≥3m in 2 successive years)*
- *Poor alveolar ventilation = T2RF: $\downarrow O_2$ & $\uparrow CO_2$ (LOSE HYPOXIC DRIVE)*

2. **Emphysema:** ↑ protease activity destroys alveoli → ↓ elasticity & recoil, enlarged air spaces (↓ surface area)

'Pink-puffers':
- *↑ RR & HR (compensate for ↓ gas exchange)*
- *Cachexia (high energy demand for respiration)*
- *Poor gas exchange = T1RF: $\downarrow O_2$ & normal CO_2*

3. **Bronchiolitis/acute bronchitis:** short-term inflammation (usually viral)

Symptoms

- Productive cough – clear, white sputum
- Progressive dyspnoea + wheeze
- Frequent LRTIs

Signs

Inspection: ↑ RR, flapping tremor, cyanosis, barrel chest, pursed lips
Palpation/percussion: reduced chest expansion, hyperresonance
Auscultation: polyphonic expiratory wheeze, ↓ breath sounds

Investigations

- **Hx & examination:** suspect if symptoms in >35y with a risk factor
- → **Ask about RED FLAGS (cancer):** weight loss, fatigue, chest pain, haemoptysis
- → **Ask about heart failure Sx:** PND, ankle swelling, ↓ exercise tolerance
- **Spirometry + BDR:** assess severity with **Gold criteria**
  - ▸ **FEV$_1$** <80%   **FEV$_1$:FVC** <0.7   ▸ **PEF:** little variation
  - ▸ **BDR:** no improvement
- **CXR:** hyperinflation, flat diaphragms, ↓ peripheral markings
- **Other:**
  - ▸ **FBC:** Hb, PCV, (↑CRP if infection)
  - ▸ **ABG:** $\downarrow O_2 \pm \uparrow CO_2$
  - ▸ **ECG/ECHO:** cor pulmonale / RV hypertrophy
  - ▸ **sputum culture:** r/o infection

MRC Dyspnoea Scale	
1	Only SOB on strenuous exercise
2	SOB if hurrying/walking up hill
3	SOB on flat
4	Stop for breath after 100m
5	SOB with dressing, etc.

Gold criteria	
Mild	FEV$_1$ >80%
Moderate	FEV$_1$ 50–79%
Severe	FEV$_1$ 30–49%
V. severe	FEV$_1$ <30%

Interpreting spirometry	Obstructive	Restrictive
FEV$_1$	<80%	<80%
FVC	Normal	<80%
FEV$_1$:FVC	<0.7	Normal
Examples	Asthma, COPD, bronchiectasis, CF	ILD, NMD, scoliosis, pulmonary oedema, obesity

Management of COPD[3]

SMOKING CESSATION: only intervention that reduces mortality
- Nicotine replacement: patches, gum
- Varenicline: nicotine receptor partial agonist
- Bupropion: noradrenaline/dopamine reuptake inhibitor
- E-cigarettes: lack long-term evidence but thought to be **90% safer**
→ Patient can self-refer to smoking cessation clinics

VACCINATIONS: pneumococcal & flu vaccine

PULMONARY REHAB: 3× a week for 6w
- Exercises to improve SOB
- Educate and promote self-management

MUCOLYTICS: e.g. carbocisteine
- May help chronic productive cough
- Review after 4 weeks → stop if no benefit

OPTIMISE WEIGHT: dietitian referral
- BMI too high: exercise/healthy diet
- BMI too low: nutritional supplements

INHALED THERAPY: only if lifestyle interventions have been offered & still SOB

Fig. 1.3 Inhaled therapy.

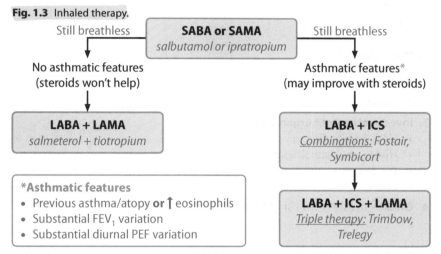

Still breathless ← **SABA or SAMA** *salbutamol or ipratropium* → Still breathless

No asthmatic features (steroids won't help)

Asthmatic features* (may improve with steroids)

LABA + LAMA *salmeterol + tiotropium*

LABA + ICS *Combinations: Fostair, Symbicort*

***Asthmatic features**
- Previous asthma/atopy **or** ↑ eosinophils
- Substantial FEV_1 variation
- Substantial diurnal PEF variation

LABA + ICS + LAMA *Triple therapy: Trimbow, Trelegy*

** May consider theophylline after trialling SABA/LABA or if unsuitable for inhaled therapy

Management of acute exacerbations

SIGNS
1. ↑ sputum volume/purulence
2. ↓ exercise tolerance/SOB on exertion
3. Worsening wheeze

INVESTIGATIONS
- Sputum sample if purulent
- ABG, FBC, U&Es
- CXR, ECG

MANAGEMENT
1. **Nebulised bronchodilators:** SABA & SAMA (back-to-back)
   + theophylline if insufficient response
2. **Oral corticosteroids:** 30mg OD prednisolone for 5d
3. **Oxygen:** 88–92% via Venturi mask
4. **Antibiotics:** e.g. doxycycline
   If ≥2 of ↑ sputum, ↑ purulence, ↑dyspnoea

SABA/SAMA: relieve acute bronchospasm
LABA/LAMA: ↑FEV_1, TLC & improve SOB

Antimuscarinic side-effects:
- Constipation (can't poo)
- Urinary retention (can't wee)
- Dry mouth (can't speak)
- Blurred vision (can't see)
- Confusion (can't remember)

Side-effects of other medications:
- **Theophylline:** headache, insomnia, tachycardia, N&V, arrhythmia, hypokalaemia
- **Varenicline/bupropion:** GI upset, dry mouth, taste disturbance, anxiety/depression, insomnia

Safety-netting: may give **rescue pack** (steroid + ABX)

Warn of ↑ risk of pneumonia & signs of exacerbation
- ↑ sputum volume/purulence
- ↓ exercise tolerance / ↑ SOB on exertion
- Worsening wheeze

Warn of ↑ risk of pneumothorax
- Sudden onset SOB
- Chest pain
- Cyanosis

COPD complications
- Acute exacerbations
- Polycythaemia
- Respiratory failure
- Cor pulmonale
- Pneumothorax
- Lung carcinoma

Follow-up
- At least once a year
- Measure FEV_1 & FVC
- Assess on MRC Dyspnoea Scale (see previous page)
- Review need for referral to specialist services

---

[3]NICE (2018, updated 2019) *COPD in over 16s* [NG115]

Hypertension

Hypertension = a major cause of premature death

> **Risk factors**
> - age >65y
> - male
> - FHx
> - obese
> - sedentary
> - **salty diet**
> - alcohol/caffeine
> - DM
> - renal disease

> **Refer <40y with HTN for Ix of underlying cause:**
>
> 1. **RAS:** MRI, CT angiography, Doppler
> 2. **CKD:** urinalysis, CCs, U&E, eGFR
> 3. **Aortic coarctation:** radio-femoral delay, MRI
> 4. **Endocrine cause:** renin, aldosterone, TFT

Normal BP		<120/80
High BP		<140/90
Hypertension	Stage 1	clinic BP >140/90 **and** ABPM >135/85
	Stage 2	clinic BP >160/100 **and** ABPM >150/95
	Stage 3	clinic systolic >180 **or** diastolic >110

ABPM: 2 readings per hour for 1 day
— use average
HBPM: 4 readings (2× am & 2× pm) for 7 days
— use average

> **Aims of Tx:**
>
> <80y: BP <140/90
> >80y: BP <150/90

> **Follow-up: annual review**
>
> - of BP
> - of risk factors: smoking, alcohol, BMI, HbA1c
> - of medications & symptoms

Classification

1. **Primary hypertension** (95%)
   - Cause unknown
2. **Secondary hypertension** (5%) → **suspect in younger patients**
   - Renal disease (80%) – glomerulonephritis, CKD, renal artery stenosis, PCKD
   - Endocrine – Conn's (↑ aldosterone), Cushing's (↑ cortisol), acromegaly (↑ GH), hyperthyroidism
   - Drugs – steroids, NSAIDs, OCP, liquorice
   - Other – pregnancy, aortic coarctation, phaeochromocytoma

Symptoms

1. **Essential HTN** (gradual ↑ BP over years) = ASYMPTOMATIC
2. **Malignant HTN** (rapid, sustained ↑ BP) = HEADACHES, VISUAL DISTURBANCES, RENAL DYSFUNCTION
   → Diagnosed if SBP >200 **or** DBP >120 **AND** bilateral retinal haemorrhages/exudates ± papilloedema

Complications/consequences

- **Heart** – LVH → dilation & eventual failure
- **Aorta** – AAA & aortic dissection
- **Brain** – intracranial haemorrhage & stroke
- **Kidney** – CKD (glomerular destruction & nephron ischaemia)
- **Eyes** – hypertensive retinopathy

Investigations

1. **Clinic BP** – 2 readings >140/90mmHg
2. **24h ABPM** (or HBPM)
3. **Investigate target organ damage**
   - U&Es & urine dip (for proteinuria)
   - HbA1c, cholesterol, lipids
   - Fundoscopy
   - ECG
4. **QRISK** – to assess 10y risk of CVD
→ based on age, sex, ethnicity, BMI, DM, CKD, AF, FHx

Management[4]

1. **LIFESTYLE:**
   - **Diet:** <1tsp salt daily, fruit & veg, low fat dairy, low saturated fats
   - **Exercise:** >30min 4/5× a week
   - **Weight loss:** BMI 18–25 target
   - **Smoking cessation & alcohol reduction:** <14 units spread over week

2. **MEDICATION IF:**
   - Stage 1 if <80y AND ≥1 of:
     - CVD/renal disease
     - end organ damage
     - QRISK ≥20%
     - DM
   - All stage 2 or 3

3. **IF TX-RESISTANT HTN** (with 3 medications) → refer for Ix of 2° cause

---

[4] NICE (2019, updated 2022) *Hypertension in adults* [NG136]

PHARMACOLOGICAL TREATMENT

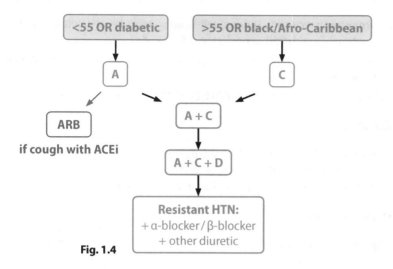

Fig. 1.4

A = **ACEi**, e.g. ramipril, lisinopril

ARB = angiotensin receptor blocker, e.g. losartan

C = Ca channel blocker (DHP), e.g. amlodipine, lercanidipine

D = diuretic (thiazide-like), e.g. indapamide

α-blocker = doxazosin, prazosin

β-blocker = atenolol, bisoprolol

other diuretic = spironolactone only if K⁺ ≤4.5

(K⁺-sparing diuretic & aldosterone antagonist)

SIDE-EFFECTS OF TREATMENT

ACEis

Side-effects:	Monitor:
• Dry cough (common)	• U&Es
• Hyperkalaemia	**Contraindications:**
• Angioedema	• Renovascular disease
• ↓ renal function if already poor*	• Caution with spironolactone
*nephroprotective if adequate renal perfusion (good for diabetics)	*only stop if ↑creatinine by >30% or ↓eGFR by >25%

ARBs

Side-effects:	Monitor:
• Hyperkalaemia	• U&Es
• ↓ renal function	**Contraindications:**
	• Renovascular disease

Thiazide-like diuretics

Side-effects:	Monitor:
• Hypokalaemia	• U&Es
• Impaired glucose control	• BP
• Exacerbate gout	**Contraindications:**
*rely on renal excretion	• Renal impairment
	• Gout
	• DM

Spironolactone

Side-effects:	Monitor:
• Hyperkalaemia	• U&Es
• Gynaecomastia	**Contraindications:**
	• Renovascular disease
	• Caution + ACEi

Calcium channel blockers

Side-effects:	Monitor:
• Headache	• BP
• Flushing	• HR
• Ankle oedema	**Contraindications:**
	• Avoid rate limiting in CHF

Others

α-blocker	• Postural hypotension
β-blocker	• Bronchospasm (avoid in asthma)

Atrial fibrillation

Rapid, irregular heart rhythm due to uncoordinated contraction of the atria

1. **Paroxysmal:** recurrent, sudden, self-limiting episodes of palpitations → sometimes Tx with **'pill in pocket'** e.g. flecainide
2. **Persistent:** AF >7 days → needs **beta-blocker** to rate control & **cardioversion** to 'reset' rhythm
3. **Permanent:** long-term AF → **RATE CONTROL** vs. rhythm control

Causes

- **Cardiac:** HTN, heart failure, IHD, valve disease
- **Respiratory:** PE, chest infection, lung cancer
- **Systemic:** sepsis, thyrotoxicosis, ↑ alcohol/caffeine, ↓ electrolytes

> **Causes:** Mrs **SMITH** has AF
> **S**epsis
> **M**itral valve stenosis
> **I**HD
> **T**hyrotoxicosis
> **H**ypertension

Investigations*

1. **Systems examination:**
   - Irregularly irregular pulse
   - Signs of underlying disease, e.g. murmur/HF
2. **12-lead ECG:** if normal do 24h ambulatory ECG

   Fig. 1.5

   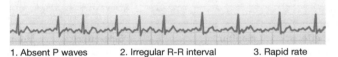

   1. Absent P waves   2. Irregular R-R interval   3. Rapid rate

3. **Bloods:**
   - FBC, TFTs, U&Es, LFTs, glucose
   - Alcohol levels (if suspicious)

4. **CXR/ECHO:** investigate cause

*Consider app on mobile phone, to enable rhythm recording by patient during symptoms

Management[5]

A) RATE & RHYTHM CONTROL

DO NOT COMBINE BB + RL CCB

* NOT digoxin as monotherapy unless immobile

1. Rate control: target HR **60–80** → beta-blocker (**or** RL CCB if BB contraindicated) (often combined with digoxin*)
2. Rhythm control: if **new onset** <48h, **reversible cause, HF** → flecainide/amiodarone or DCCV (direct current cardioversion)

Long-term side-effects: hepatotoxic, phototoxic, thyrotoxic, lung fibrosis

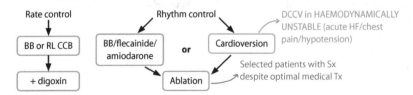

DCCV in HAEMODYNAMICALLY UNSTABLE (acute HF/chest pain/hypotension)

Selected patients with Sx despite optimal medical Tx

Rate control → BB or RL CCB → + digoxin

Rhythm control → BB/flecainide/amiodarone **or** Cardioversion → Ablation

B) STROKE PREVENTION (ANTICOAGULATION)

1. Assess risk with CHA$_2$DS$_2$-VASc score: anticoagulate females if score ≥2 or men if ≥1

→ **DOAC** (rivaroxaban, apixaban, edoxaban, dabigatran) = more predictable & ↓ ICH risk

→ **Warfarin** (if mechanical valve/mitral stenosis or low eGFR) = **needs close monitoring**

2. Assess bleeding risk with ORBIT* score: ≥3 needs closer anticoag. monitoring

C) LIFESTYLE

- Weight loss, diet, exercise
- ↓ alcohol, caffeine, smoking
- Optimise RFs: BP, renal function, etc.

[5] NICE (2021) *Atrial fibrillation* [NG196]

Complications
- **STROKE**
- ↓ LV function
- Peripheral embolism
- Vascular dementia
- ↓ quality of life

Symptoms
- SOB
- Syncope
- Palpitations
- Chest pain

Warfarin: vit K antagonist (reversible)
↑ INR: NSAIDs, cranberry juice, SSRIs, ABX
↓ INR: AEDs, rifampicin, barbiturates, SJW, smoking

NB: warfarin = teratogenic   **INR aim: 2–3**

CHADSVaSc score

C	Congestive HF	1
H	HTN	1
A$_2$	Age >74y	2
	Age 65–74y	1
D	Diabetes	1
S$_2$	Previous stroke/TIA	2
Va	Vascular disease	1
Sc	Sex category = female	1

5 Predictors of ORBIT score

Age ≥75y	1
eGFR <60	1
Treatment with antiplatelet	1
Bleeding history	2
Hb <130 (females) <140 (males), ↓ haematocrit or Hx of anaemia	2

*****ORBIT score** now recommended by NICE over HASBLED score to calculate bleeding risk for those with AF

Follow-up
- In 1y to check for Sx of AF
- Annual R/V of stroke & bleed risk

Safety-net
- Signs of MI/stroke (LOC, severe chest pain/SOB, dizzy)
- If HR >150 or SBP <90
Advise may need to inform DVLA (if symptomatic)

For **elective electrical cardioversion** (not emergency): ANTICOAGULATE before with LMWH or 3 weeks other agent

Gastro-oesophageal reflux disease

20% of adults experience heartburn. M:F = 3:1

Symptoms

- Retrosternal pain
  - ▶ **worse lying/bending** down & with hot liquid/alcohol
  - ▶ **relieved by antacids**
- Regurgitation/water brash – sudden filling of mouth with saliva
- Odynophagia
- Atypical chest pain
- Nocturnal wheeze/cough
- Tooth decay

Causes

1. **Anatomical:** sphincter dysfunction / hiatus hernia (sliding/rolling)
2. **Physiological:**
   - smoking/alcohol
   - spicy/fatty food, large meals late at night
   - drugs (anticholinergics, nitrates, TCAs, CCBs)
   - ↑ IAP (pregnancy/obesity)

Investigations

- **History** – diagnosis made on clinical symptoms
- **FBC** – check for anaemia
- **Ambulatory 24h pH testing** – press record when getting symptoms → use to calculate **DeMeester Score**
- **Barium swallow** – identify anatomical causes of GORD
- **High resolution manometry (HRM)** – measures oesophageal pressure / sphincter function
- **OGD (oesophagogastroduodenoscopy)** – DONE IF ALARM SYMPTOMS via **urgent 2ww referral**

Initial management[6]

1. **LIFESTYLE**
   - Weight loss, ↓ smoking & alcohol, ↓ stress
   - Smaller meals >3h before bed, avoid spicy food
   - Raise head of bed/sleep in a more upright position
   - **Medication review:** anticholinergics, nitrates, TCAs, CCBs, NSAIDs

2. **MEDICAL TREATMENT**
   - Antacid/alginates
   - Full dose PPI (4–8w) e.g. omeprazole 20mg OD
   - H_2 receptor antagonist (2nd line / PPI contraindicated)

3. **SURGICAL TREATMENT:** restore anatomical position of stomach & GOJ, repair herniae & recreate anti-reflux valve
   - NISSEN FUNDOPLICATION = 360° wrap of fundus around lower GOJ
     (SE of surgery = dysphagia)

Indications for surgery → Failure of medical Tx
→ Do not want lifelong PPI → Extra-oesophageal Sx
(wheeze, hoarse, cough, chest pain, aspiration)
} + GOOD EVIDENCE OF REFLUX ON pH/ MANOMETRY TESTING

[6]NICE Clinical Guideline: *Gastro-oesophageal reflux disease and dyspepsia in adults* [CG184]

Dyspepsia (indigestion)

Symptoms: abdo pain, bloating, N&V, heartburn, food/acid regurgitation

DDx:
- GORD
- Gastric cancer
- PUD (gastric/duodenal)
- Oesophageal cancer

Sliding: GOJ + part of fundus above diaphragm
Rolling: Only part of fundus above diaphragm
(↑ risk strangulation)

Complications of GORD
In adults: oesophagitis/ulcers → Barrett's → adenocarcinoma
In children: aspiration pneumonia, frequent otitis media
In infants: feeding difficulties, ↓ growth, distressed behaviour

ALARM Symptoms

Anaemia (iron-deficient)
Lost weight
Anorexia
Recent onset & progressive
Melaena or haematemesis
Swallowing difficulties (dysphagia)
55 years or older (+ one of above)

Barrett's oesophagus:

stratified epithelium → columnar

Sx: similar to GORD or asymptomatic

Ix: same as for GORD **PLUS BIOPSY**

Mx: treat GORD
- **No dysplasia:** repeat OGD in 2–5y
- **Low grade:** repeat 6 months + ablation
- **High grade:** repeat OGD + resection

Biopsy assessed with Prague criteria based on height & circumference of epithelium affected

Risk of adenocarcinoma in 1y:
Low grade = 0.7%
High grade = 7%

Peptic ulcer disease

Complications

1. **Acute bleed** – endoscopic coagulation/ clipping
   – interventional radiology (embolisation)
2. **Perforation** – urgent surgical repair (Graham patch)
3. **Stricture** – endoscopic dilation & stenting
   – OR bypass via gastrojejunostomy

H. pylori test & treat

TEST: ^{13}C urease breath test or *H. pylori* faecal antigen
TREAT: triple therapy = PPI + 2 × ABX
(metronidazole, amoxicillin, clarithromycin)

Medications

1. **ANTACIDS:** Na, Mg, Al salts
   ► react with acid to ↑ pH
2. **ALGINATES:** Gaviscon Advance
   ► react with acid to form raft
3. **H$_2$RAs:** famotidine/cimetidine
   ► block histamine = ↓ H$^+$ release
   SE: diarrhoea, rash
4. **PPIs:** omeprazole, lansoprazole
   ► irreversible proton pump inhibition
   *SE: hyponatraemia, **osteoporosis**, CKD, hypomagnesaemia, C. difficile*

Safety-netting: for suspicion of GI cancer

- Return immediately if develop any ALARM symptoms

NICE STATES 2WW REFERRAL IF ANY OF:
- dysphagia
- >55y with weight loss **PLUS**
  ► reflux **OR**
  ► dyspepsia **OR**
  ► upper abdominal pain

Signs of oesophageal malignancy
- Progressive dysphagia (solids → liquids → saliva)
- Weight loss & anorexia
- Retrosternal chest pain
- Lymphadenopathy
- Cough/aspiration
- Raised platelets

Investigations:
- FBC (microcytic anaemia)
- 2ww for endoscopy + biopsy
- Barium swallow

Causes

- *H. pylori* – causes **PUD** or **gastric cancer**
- NSAIDs (+ steroids & SSRIs)
- Zollinger–Ellison syndrome (ZES)
- Smoking/caffeine

ZES – rare condition where tumours (gastrinomas) of the pancreas & duodenum secrete gastrin, causing excess stomach acid production

DUODENAL near pylorus	GASTRIC lesser curve
• **pain relief on eating**/milk • no anorexia/vomiting 90% caused by *H. pylori*	• **pain worse on eating** • anorexia & vomiting

Symptoms

- Dyspepsia – retrosternal heartburn
- Burning epigastric pain – related to food/hunger
- ± haematemesis/melaena

Investigations

<55y & no ALARM Sx: clinical Dx
>55y or ALARM Sx: 2ww for endoscopy

Management[7]

1. **LIFESTYLE:** weight loss, ↓ smoking & alcohol, ↓ stress, smaller meals

2. **MEDICATION REVIEW:** stop NSAIDs if possible

3. **MEDICAL THERAPY:**
→ **1st line:** full dose PPI (4–8w) omeprazole 20mg OD
→ **2nd line:** *H. pylori* 'Test & Treat' = triple therapy **(7 days)** then PPI

Summary of dyspepsia management

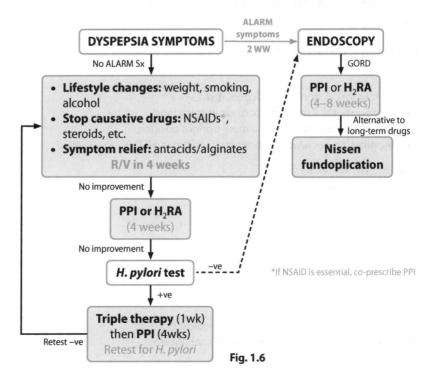

Fig. 1.6

---

[7] NICE (2014, updated 2019) *Gastro-oesophageal reflux disease and dyspepsia in adults* [CG184]

Irritable bowel syndrome

- A group of abdominal symptoms for which no organic cause is found
- Affects up to 20% of the population (F>M; peak onset 20–30y)

Diagnostic criteria

≥6 months of abdominal pain/discomfort
→ relieved on defecation **OR**
→ associated with altered bowel frequency / stool form
AND

≥2 of the following:
- bloating/distension
- passage of mucus
- incomplete evacuation/straining/urgency
- symptoms worsened by eating

± non-intestinal symptoms, e.g. urinary, headache, fatigue, back pain, dysmenorrhoea

Investigations

- Careful history and physical examination
- FBC, ESR/CRP – r/o IBD
- Faecal calprotectin – r/o IBD
- **Coeliac screen** – endomysial antibodies (EMA) / tissue transglutaminase (tTG) antibodies
- CA 125 – for older women to r/o ovarian cancer

Management[8]

1. DIET/LIFESTYLE   Signpost to online resources/leaflets
- **Low FODMAPs diet** – limit insoluble fibres & sugars that trigger bloating
  → encourage a food diary to monitor triggers
- **Regular meals**, without long gaps between
- At least 8 cups of **fluid per day but avoid caffeine**/fizzy drinks
- **Regular exercise** + weight loss

2. PSYCHOLOGICAL
- CBT
- **Encourage self-care**

3. PHARMACOLOGICAL
- **Constipation:** laxatives (avoid lactulose as worsens bloating)
- **Diarrhoea:** anti-diarrhoeals (loperamide)
- **Abdominal pain/cramps:** antispasmodics (mebeverine / hyoscine butylbromide)
- **Chronic/resistant pain:** low dose amitriptyline (SSRIs = 2nd line)

Follow-up

- Agreed between clinician & patient dependent on symptoms/response to treatment, etc.
- SAFETY-NET FOR RED FLAGS OF BOWEL CANCER

Abdo pain/discomfort
Bloating
Changed bowel habits

Must screen for cancer red flags

- Weight loss
- Fresh red PR bleed
- Altered bowel habit >60y
- FHx colon cancer <50y
- Abdo or rectal mass
- IDA in >60y

Need 2ww referral for colonoscopy

Risk factors/causes
- **Stress, anxiety, depression** – MOST COMMON
- **Gastroenteritis** – precedes up to 30% of cases
- Antibiotics
- Eating disorders
- Trauma/surgery

Prognosis
- Not associated with any serious long-term disease
- Symptoms may fluctuate in severity

FODMAPs diet (avoid in IBS)

Fermentable	– wheat/rye
Oligosaccharides	– legumes
Disaccharides	– fruit & veg
Monosaccharides	– milk, yoghurt
And	– soft cheese
Polyols	– sweeteners

---

[8]NICE (2008, updated 2017) *Irritable bowel syndrome in adults* [CG61]

Hyperthyroidism

Raised circulating thyroid hormones T_3 & T_4 (= thyrotoxicosis); F>M

General symptoms

- Anxious, irritable, insomnia
- Fatigue/weakness
- Hot/sweaty, tremor/palpitations
- Menorrhagia/diarrhoea
- ↓ weight (but ↑ appetite)

General signs

- ↑ HR/arrhythmia
- ↑ SBP
- Hyperreflexia
- ± goitre

Causes

1. **Autoimmune/Graves' disease (70%)** Risk factor: P/FHx autoimmune disorders
   - autoimmune stimulation of thyroid follicular cells
   - IgG autoantibodies (TRAb & TPOAb)
2. **Toxic multinodular goitre (15%)** Risk factor: elderly/I_2 deficient
   - T_3/T_4-secreting nodules irresponsive to –ve feedback
3. **Solitary toxic adenoma (5%)**
   - benign T_3/T_4-secreting nodule (avg. 3mm) irresponsive to –ve feedback
4. **Drug-induced:** iodine, amiodarone, lithium
5. **Secondary causes (rare):** TSH-secreting pituitary adenoma, pregnancy

Management[9]: need specialist input!

1. SYMPTOMATIC RELIEF: β-blockers
e.g. propranolol 20–40mg tds

2. ANTI-THYROID DRUGS: carbimazole/propylthiouracil
Titration regimen: high dose then titrate down to euthyroid
Block & replace: maintain high dose + levothyroxine replacement

3. RADIOACTIVE IODINE (^{131}I): Contraindications: pregnancy/lactation, <16y

4. THYROIDECTOMY: if compression Sx, malignant nodule, Tx-resistant
Post-op complications: hypothyroidism, hypocalcaemia, vocal cord paresis/hoarseness

Specific to autoimmune hyperthyroidism

- Goitre
- Pretibial myxoedema
- Acropachy – swollen hands & clubbing
- **Graves' ophthalmology:**
  - ► exophthalmos – bulging eyes
  - ► lagophthalmos – cannot close eyes
  - ► periorbital oedema

Investigations

- **Hx & examination** – obs, reflexes, etc.
- **TFTs** (TSH, free T_3 & T_4)
- **Autoantibodies** (TRAb, TPOAb)
- **Technetium uptake scan**
  - ► if no autoantibodies
  - ► patchy uptake in nodules
  - ► diffuse uptake in Graves'
- **Assess eye disease (Graves')**
  - ► visual fields / eye movements
  - ► CT/MRI of orbit

TFTs in hyperthyroidism

PRIMARY: ↑T_3/T_4, ↓TSH
SECONDARY: ↑TSH, ↑T_3/T_4
SUBCLINICAL: normal T_3/T_4, ↓TSH

Raised TSH & T_3/T_4 often due to poor compliance or assay interference

not if pregnant

Medication side-effects

ANTITHYROID DRUGS:
- Rash/cholestatic jaundice
- Agranulocytosis: infection & bleeding risk
→ FBC before Tx and **monitor closely**

RADIOACTIVE IODINE:
= risk of hypothyroidism

Safety-netting/follow-up

1. **Signs of agranulocytosis:**
   = sore throat, mouth ulcer, bruising
2. **Signs of thyroid crisis:**
   = severe ↑HR & temp, confusion
   Triggers: illness, stress, surgery
3. **Signs of tracheal compression:**
   = SOB/stridor/dysphagia

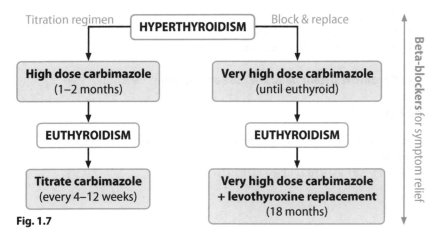

Fig. 1.7

[9]NICE (2021) CKS – *Hyperthyroidism*

Hypothyroidism

Low circulating thyroid hormones T_3 & T_4; F>M

General symptoms

- Depression/psychosis
- Slowed intellectual activity
- Fatigue/weakness
- Cold
- Amenorrhoea/constipation
- ↑ weight
- ↓ libido

General signs

- ↓ HR
- Anaemia
- Hyporeflexia
- Dry skin
- Hair loss (outer 1/3 eyebrow)
- ± non-pitting oedema
- ± goitre

Causes

1. **Autoimmune/Hashimoto's thyroiditis:** Risk factor: autoimmune disorders, 60–70y
   - autoantibodies against TPO (TPOAb)
   - gradual gland destruction: lymphocyte infiltration & fibrosis → **may have goitre**
   - initial hyperthyroid state: damage releases T_3/T_4
2. **Primary atrophic thyroiditis:**
   - autoimmune gland destruction
   - extensive lymphocyte infiltrate atrophies gland → **no goitre**
3. **Previous hyperthyroidism treatment**
   - Post thyroidectomy or radioactive iodine
4. **Iodine deficiency** (most common cause worldwide)
5. **Drug-induced:** amiodarone, lithium, carbimazole, excess iodine
6. **Congenital:** absence/underdevelopment of thyroid gland or enzyme deficiency
7. **Postpartum thyroiditis:** development within 1 year of giving birth (lasts 4–6m)
8. **Secondary causes (very rare):** hypopituitarism

Investigations

- **Hx & examination** – obs, reflexes, appearance, systems review
- **TFTs** (TSH, free T_3 & T_4)
- **FBC** – for anaemia
- **Autoantibodies** (TPOAb)

Management[10]

Thyroid hormone replacement therapy: levothyroxine (T_4)
- Low dose & titrate up until desired TSH levels reached
  - ▸ r/v dose monthly initially, then every 3–4m
  - ▸ r/v dose annually once stable
- LIFELONG THERAPY
↳ *Patients with goitre, suspected malignancy, cardiac disease, treatment-resistant or planning a pregnancy need referral to endocrinologist in 2° care*

---

[10]NICE (2019) CKS – *Thyroid disease*

DDx
- Diabetes mellitus
- Adrenal insufficiency
- Coeliac disease
- Anxiety/depression
- Dementia

most common cause in UK

TFTs in hypothyroidism

PRIMARY: ↓ T_3/T_4, ↑ TSH
SECONDARY: ↓ TSH, ↓ T_3/T_4
SUBCLINICAL: ↑ TSH but T_3/T_4 normal

Sick euthyroid syndrome: temporary ↓ TSH during illness

Starting doses of levothyroxine:

18–49y: 50–100mcg
≥50y or CVD: 25–50mcg

Complications of hypothyroidism
- CVD/stroke
- Dyslipidaemia
- Heart failure
- **Myxoedema coma**

Myxoedema coma

- hypothermia, coma & seizures
Precipitated by another problem, e.g. heart failure, sepsis, stroke

GP FOLLOW-UP: annual TFTs & assess CVD risk: lipids, HbA1c, BP, weight

Type 2 diabetes mellitus

Combination of **insulin resistance & deficiency**, resulting in **persistent hyperglycaemia** & **beta cell decline**.

Epidemiology

>3.5 million people in the UK (T2DM = majority of cases)

Pathophysiology

= combination of genetic & environmental factors

Risk factors

- Genetics: FHx, south Asian/Afro-Caribbean, male
- ↑ age
- Metabolic syndrome: central obesity, ↑ BP, ↑ lipids/cholesterol, ↑ glucose
- Obesity, sedentary lifestyle, poor diet, smoking/alcohol

2° T2DM: CF, chronic pancreatitis, Cushing's, acromegaly, PCOS, drugs (steroids, thiazides, antipsychotics)

Symptoms

- Polyuria, polydipsia
- Fatigue } gradual onset
- Recurrent infections

Management[11]

LIFESTYLE
HbA1c 42–48 = pre-diabetes → referral to national prevention programme + annual HbA1c checks

1. **Diet:**
   - Low glycaemic index carbs (wholegrains, cereals, legumes, lentils)
   - Fat <35%, saturated fat <10% (e.g. veg. oil not butter, lean meats)
   - High fibre – vegetables (+ fruit)

2. **Weight loss:** calorie restriction AND exercise (20–30min/day)

3. **Reduce smoking/alcohol**
   Education to enable self-management is key

PHARMACOLOGICAL: aim for HbA1c <48 (6.5%)

OGTT = 75g glucose & wait 2h

Diagnostic criteria:	Normal	Impaired	Diabetes
FASTING mmol/L	<6.1	6.1–6.9	≥7.0
OGTT mmol/L	<7.8	7.8–11.0	≥11.1
HbA1c mmol/mol	<42	42–48	>48

↪ Symptomatic + 1 positive test OR
Asymptomatic + 2 positive tests

Complications: often 1st presentation
Microvascular
- Retinopathy (visual blurring)
- Polyneuropathy (pain/numbness)
- Nephropathy

Macrovascular
- Erectile dysfunction
- Cardiovascular disease (MI)
- Cerebrovascular disease (stroke)

Monitoring diabetes control

1. **HbA1c** – over 3m
2. **Finger-prick** – if on insulin
3. **Urine dip** – glucose, ketones, protein

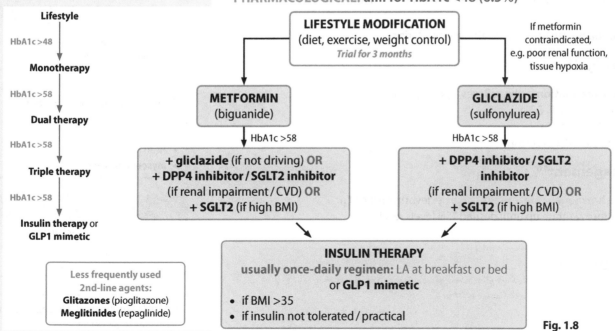

Lifestyle
HbA1c >48 ↓
Monotherapy
HbA1c >58 ↓
Dual therapy
HbA1c >58 ↓
Triple therapy
HbA1c >58 ↓
Insulin therapy or GLP1 mimetic

LIFESTYLE MODIFICATION
(diet, exercise, weight control)
Trial for 3 months

If metformin contraindicated, e.g. poor renal function, tissue hypoxia

METFORMIN (biguanide)
HbA1c >58 ↓
+ **gliclazide** (if not driving) OR
+ **DPP4 inhibitor / SGLT2 inhibitor** (if renal impairment / CVD) OR
+ **SGLT2** (if high BMI)

GLICLAZIDE (sulfonylurea)
HbA1c >58 ↓
+ **DPP4 inhibitor / SGLT2 inhibitor** (if renal impairment / CVD) OR
+ **SGLT2** (if high BMI)

INSULIN THERAPY
usually once-daily regimen: LA at breakfast or bed
or **GLP1 mimetic**
- if BMI >35
- if insulin not tolerated / practical

Less frequently used 2nd-line agents:
Glitazones (pioglitazone)
Meglitinides (repaglinide)

Fig. 1.8

[11] NICE (2021) CKS – Type 2 diabetes

MEDICATION SIDE-EFFECTS

Hypoglycaemic	Advantages	Disadvantages	
METFORMIN (biguanides) ↓gluconeogenesis & ↑glucose utilisation	↓CV risk no weight gain	GI upset (bloating/diarrhoea) not if eGFR <35	**Stop metformin if** eGFR <30 or Cr >150
GLICLAZIDE (sulfonylurea) ↑insulin secretion via K⁺ channel closure	rapid effect cheap	hypos **weight gain**	
GLITAZONES ↓insulin resistance via PPARa	low risk of hypos improve lipid profile ↓CVD risk	**weight gain** bone fractures ↑risk fluid retention	**Contraindicated in:** CCF, elderly, bladder cancer
SGLT 2 INHIBITORS ↓glucose reabsorption in kidneys	**weight loss** reduce SBP & ↓CVD risk good in renal disease	UTIs/candidiasis euglycaemic ketoacidosis	
SITAGLIPTIN (DDP4 inhibitors) ↑insulin release	low risk of hypos	nausea & acute pancreatitis	
GLP1 MIMETICS ↑insulin release	**weight loss** ↓CV risk if CVD	nausea & acute pancreatitis S/C injections only	

Reasons for non-compliance

- Prefer their usual diet
- Forget to take medication
- Don't like needles (monitoring/insulin)
- Medication side-effects
- Cannot see chronic complications / importance of Mx

Follow-up/review: (at least once a year)

- **Review glucose control**
  - HbA1c: every 3m, then every 6m if well controlled
  - review medication
- **Screen for complications:** fundoscopy, foot check, urine dip
- **Reduce CVD risk:** BP <140/80, QRISK
- **ENSURE ACCESS TO SUFFICIENT EDUCATION:**
  - DIETITIAN, diabetes.org.uk, local support groups
  - ensure they understand risk of long-term complications

Safety-netting

1. **Signs of hypos***
   - Lethargy, confusion, aggression
   - Sweaty/pale/shaking   *Mx: glucose PO 10–20g
2. **Driving safety**
   - Inform DVLA
   - Test blood glucose within the 2h prior to driving

> **Risk of complications**
> - ↑risk MIs (×4), stroke (×2)
> - ↑risk infection & ulcers
> - risk of blindness
> - risk of kidney failure

Infectious disease in the community

Differentials
- Tick bite allergy
- Cellulitis
- Erythema multiforme
- Chronic fatigue syndrome

Risk factors for Lyme disease
- Temperate climate
- Endemic area
- Outdoor activity
- Tick *in situ* >48h

Prophylactic antibiotics (doxycycline) if in endemic area / high risk tick bite attached for ≥36h
→ must be started within 72h of bite

Complications of shingles
- Post-herpetic neuralgia
- Ocular disease
- Motor neuropathy

Ramsay Hunt syndrome

= VZV infection of **geniculate ganglion of facial nerve**

Symptoms:
- Facial palsy + painful vesicles of ear/soft palate
- Sensorineural hearing loss & vertigo

Herpes zoster ophthalmicus

= VZV infection of **ophthalmic division of trigeminal nerve**

Symptoms: Hutchinson's sign (vesicles on nose)
Management: urgent referral to ophthalmology

Lyme disease

AETIOLOGY: bacterial infection (*Borrelia* species) transmitted to humans via tick bites

SYMPTOMS
1. ACUTE
   - **Erythema migrans:** characteristic circular/target sign rash (1–4w after bite)
   - **Systemic symptoms:** fever, malaise, headache, fatigue, lymphadenopathy
2. COMPLICATIONS
   - **Musculoskeletal symptoms:** arthralgia, arthritis
   - **Neurological symptoms:** facial nerve palsy, radiculopathy, mononeuritis multiplex, meningitis/encephalitis
   - **Cardiovascular symptoms:** pericarditis, heart block

INVESTIGATION
1. **Careful Hx & examination:** for risk factors, tick bite, rash
2. **Serology (ELISA = enzyme immunoassay):** IgM and IgG antibodies for Lyme disease
3. **Lumbar puncture:** in neuroborreliosis, CSF shows ↑WCC, ↑protein, oligoclonal IgG band

MANAGEMENT[12]: urgent specialist referral if CNS/cardiac involvement
1. **Antibiotics:** PO doxycycline 100mg BD for 21 days (IV ceftriaxone if CNS or cardiac involvement)
2. **Follow-up & management of ongoing symptoms:** fatigue, pain, depression

Shingles

EPIDEMIOLOGY: most commonly seen in elderly/immunosuppressed

PATHOGENESIS: reactivation of VZV infection within the dorsal nerve root

SYMPTOMS: lasts several days
→ **PAINFUL blistering vesicular rash** (dermatomal & unilateral)
→ Often preceded by tingling/numbness

INVESTIGATIONS: Dx usually on clinical Sx

MANAGEMENT
1. **Antiviral Tx:** aciclovir/valaciclovir (5–7 d)
2. **Analgesia:** paracetamol/amitriptyline
3. **Avoid vulnerable people:** immunocompromised, elderly, pregnant women, neonates

[12] NICE (2018) *Lyme disease* [NG95]

Notifiable diseases[13]

DEFINITION: diseases which must be reported to local health protection team if a case is suspected

LIST OF DISEASES INCLUDED:

Acute encephalitis
Acute infectious hepatitis
Acute meningitis
Acute poliomyelitis
Anthrax
Botulism
Brucellosis
Cholera
Covid-19
Diphtheria
Enteric fever (typhoid or paratyphoid fever)
Food poisoning
Haemolytic uraemic syndrome (HUS)
Infectious bloody diarrhoea
Invasive group A streptococcal disease
Legionnaires' disease
Leprosy
Malaria
Measles
Meningococcal septicaemia
Mumps
Plague
Rabies
Rubella
Severe acute respiratory syndrome (SARS)
Scarlet fever
Smallpox
Tetanus
Tuberculosis
Typhus
Viral haemorrhagic fever (VHF)
Whooping cough
Yellow fever

[13] www.gov.uk (updated 2021) *Notifiable diseases and causative organisms*

Miscellaneous community-based medicine

> Note that patients benefit physically & mentally from regular work, so be wary of repeated sick notes

Fit Notes

What are Fit Notes?
- Evidence of a patient's ability to work
- They can be written by any doctor, including GPs
- They are not job-specific, but give general advice on a patient's functional status & how this may impact work
- A patient can be deemed as 'not fit for work' or 'may be fit for work' (could do some altered form of work)

Things to consider: mobility, stamina, mental state, sensory disturbances (hearing, sight, touch)

Patients can self-certify for 7 days

Disease prevention & screening

LEVELS OF DISEASE PREVENTION

1. **Primary prevention:** preventing disease before it happens

e.g. education on healthy eating, exercise, smoking cessation, immunisation programmes

2. **Secondary prevention:** reducing the impact of disease which has already happened

e.g. screening programmes (mammograms for breast cancer, FIT test for colorectal cancer)

3. **Tertiary prevention:** reduce the impact of ongoing disease

e.g. stroke rehabilitation programmes, diabetes management programmes

NHS health checks

DEFINITION: 5-yearly check between ages 40 and 74 to assess for early signs of disease
→ *Diseases assessed for:* CVD, CKD, stroke, T2DM, dementia

FEATURES ASSESSED
- Family history of illness
- Smoking, alcohol, diet, exercise habits
- Weight & height
- Blood pressure
- Blood tests (cholesterol, HbA1c, U&Es)

MANAGEMENT

1. **Education:** on diet, exercise, weight loss, smoking & alcohol cessation, signs of dementia
2. **Statin:** if QRISK >10%
3. **Anti-hypertensives & oral hypoglycaemics:** if indicated for HTN or T2DM

RESULTS
- **QRISK score** – gives 10-year risk of CVD
- **HbA1c** – categorises any diabetes/pre-diabetes
- **Cholesterol level** – risk of hypercholesterolaemia
- **eGFR** – risk of CKD
- **BP** – categorises stage of HTN

GERIATRIC MEDICINE 02

ABBREVIATIONS

ACEi – Angiotensin-converting enzyme inhibitor
AChE – Acetylcholinesterase
ADLs – Activities of daily living
ADRT – Advanced decision to refuse treatment
AMD – Age-related macular degeneration
AMT – Abbreviated mental test
BMD – Bone mineral density
BPH – Benign prostatic hyperplasia
CCB – Calcium channel blocker
CCF – Congestive cardiac failure
CGA – Comprehensive geriatric assessment
CNS – Central nervous system
COMT – Catechol-O-methyltransferase
COPD – Chronic obstructive pulmonary disease
CPR – Cardiopulmonary resuscitation
CVD – Cardiovascular disease
DA – Dopamine

DM – Diabetes mellitus
DNACPR – Do not attempt cardiopulmonary resuscitation
FTD – Fronto-temporal dementia
GI – Gastrointestinal
IAP – Intra-abdominal pressure
ICD-10 – International Classification of Diseases version 10
IPC – Intermittent pneumatic compression
LBD – Lewy body dementia
L-dopa – Levodopa
LOC – Loss of consciousness
LPA – Lasting power of attorney
MDT – Multidisciplinary team
MMSE – Mini-Mental State Exam
MOAB – Monoamine oxidase B
MoCA – Montreal Cognitive Assessment
MS – Multiple sclerosis
MSU – Mid-stream urine

MUST – Malnutrition Universal Screening Tool
NA – Noradrenaline
NG – Nasogastric
NMDA – N-methyl-D-aspartate
OT – Occupational therapy
PD – Parkinson's disease
PDD – Parkinson's disease dementia
PEG – Percutaneous endoscopic gastrostomy
PNS – Peripheral nervous system
POC – Package of care
PT – Physiotherapy
RA – Rheumatoid arthritis
REM – Rapid eye movement
RIG – Radiologically inserted gastrostomy
SALT – Speech and language therapy
SNS – Sympathetic nervous system
URTI – Upper respiratory tract infection
UTI – Urinary tract infection

Definitions

ADLs: *Personal ADLs* are activities essential to survival, e.g. washing/dressing/toileting/eating/moving. *Instrumental ADLs* aid a person to function and enjoy life fully, e.g. cooking/cleaning/shopping/using the phone. Knowing these needs helps determine how dependent/independent a person is and so how much support they need.

Confusion screening bloods: blood tests to rule out organic causes of confusion; includes FBC, U&Es, LFTs, TFTs, glucose, calcium, vit B12, folate.

Creutzfeldt–Jakob disease: a very rare condition, often of unknown cause, which presents as a rapidly progressive dementia with ataxia.

CVD risk factors: hypertension, diabetes, hyperlipidaemia, smoker, previous stroke/TIA/MI.

Parkinsonism: having some/all of the motor symptoms of idiopathic Parkinson's disease, but due to a different disease process.

REM sleep disorder: characterised by acting out dreams while sleeping. Seen in idiopathic Parkinson's disease, Lewy body dementia and multiple system atrophy.

TUG test (Timed Up and Go test): used to assess physiological performance. Patient stands up, walks 3 metres, turns around, walks back, sits down. The length of time this takes correlates closely with degree of frailty.

Wernicke–Korsakoff syndrome: from thiamine (B1) deficiency. Wernicke = acute encephalopathy (confusion/ataxia/nystagmus); Korsakoff = chronic memory impairment with confabulation (making stuff up).

Gerontology

The study of social, cultural, psychological, cognitive, and biological aspects of ageing

Geriatric giants: the 6 Is

- **I**atrogenesis
- **I**nstability
- **I**mpaired cognition
- **I**mpaired senses
- **I**ncontinence
- **I**nadequate nutrition

Frailty can be secondary to dementia, where cognitive impairment means support is required for ADLs

Challenges of geriatric medicine

- Multiple diagnoses
- Non-specific symptoms/signs
- Polypharmacy – **use START/STOP TOOL to assess if all medications are needed**
- Increased vulnerability to and reduced recovery from illness
- High prevalence of cognitive dysfunction
- Increased risk of falls
- Complex ethics

AGEING: 'The accumulation of **cellular damage** over time that leads to a **generalised decline** in function and an increased probability of death'[1].

FRAILTY: a state of **increased vulnerability** to illness, and of **not returning to baseline functioning** following a stressor event. **Not all older people are frail**, but prevalence increases with advancing age.
The frail phenotype includes:
- unintentional weight loss/sarcopenia → can test grip strength
- weakness, exhaustion, slow walking speed → TUG test
- low level of physical activity
- falls, immobility, delirium, memory loss, incontinence   **Fig. 2.1**

Clinical frailty scale[2]

Very fit	Robust, active and energetic
Well	**No active disease symptoms**, exercise from time to time
Managing well	**Medical problems are well controlled**, but not regularly active beyond walking
Vulnerable	**Not dependent** on others but **symptoms limit activities**, e.g. being slow / increasingly tired
Mildly frail	Need **help with more involved ADLs** (e.g. transport, shopping, housework)
Moderately frail	Need **help with all outside activities & housework;** difficulties with stairs, bathing, dressing
Severely frail	**Completely dependent for personal care** but not at high risk of dying
Very severely frail	**Approaching end of life** – may not recover from minor illness
Terminally ill	**Life expectancy <6m** but not otherwise evidently frail

International classification of functioning (ICF)[3]

Describes health against domains of:

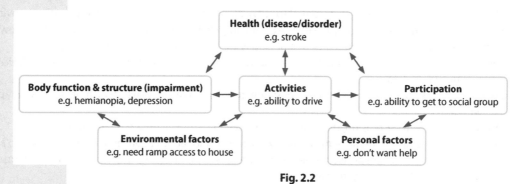

Fig. 2.2

[1] Woodford H (2016) *Essential Geriatrics*, 3rd edition. CRC Press.
[2] Rockwood K, Song X, MacKnight C, *et al.* (2005) A global clinical measure of fitness and frailty in elderly people. *CMAJ*, **173:** 489.
[3] World Health Organization (2001) *International Classification of Functioning, Disability and Health (ICF)*.

Comprehensive geriatric assessment (CGA)

→ *Gold standard for managing frailty*

CGA = A **multidisciplinary** diagnostic process that considers the **medical, psychological & functional** capabilities of a frail older person, to develop a **coordinated and holistic management plan** for acute treatment & long-term follow-up.

5 DOMAINS OF THE CGA: *referenced with colour coordinated management categories throughout the chapter*

Domains	Items to be assessed
Physical health (medical)	Comorbidities New diagnoses Medication review Nutritional status: MUST tool[4] Frailty status
Mental health	Cognition: MoCA, AMT, MMSE Capacity Mood/anxiety Fears
Functional aspects	Basic ADLs: Barthel Index[5] Instrumental ADLs Mobility, gait & balance: Berg Balance[6] Activity participation
Social aspects	Formal/informal carers (family/social services) Social networks/visitors Legal matters (power of attorney, etc.)
Environment	Housing/place of residence Supportive equipment Safety features, e.g. alarms Transport facilities

Assessment scales for mental function

1. **Abbreviated mental test (AMT) = 10 questions** to quickly identify/ monitor cognitive impairment
   → carried out on all patients >65y admitted to hospital
   → score <8 needs further investigation (e.g. MMSE/CAM/MoCA)

2. **Mini-Mental State Exam (MMSE)*** = **standardised quantitative test, examining a variety of domains**
   *Limitation: depends on educational background

   Domains: Orientation, Registration, Calculation, Recall, Language, Attention
   → score <23/30 = dementia (if patient has at least 8y of education)

3. **Montreal Cognitive Assessment (MoCA)** = **more in-depth assessment of cognitive function**
   = 90% sensitivity for **mild cognitive impairment**, 100% sensitivity for diagnosis of **Alzheimer's**
   = good to discriminate between normal and mild cognitive function, but not so much between moderate and severe

---

MUST (Malnutrition Universal Screening Tool)
A scoring system that uses BMI, % weight loss & risk of weight loss to identify adults who are at risk of malnutrition.

Barthel Index: 100-point score that assesses independence level for a number of different ADLs.
Berg Balance Scale: 14-item scale designed to measure balance of the older adult in a clinical setting.

Key MDT members for CGA
- Doctors & nurses
- Physiotherapist
- Occupational therapist (OT)
- Social workers
- Speech & language therapists
- Dietitians, optometrists, podiatrists, etc.
Communication is key!

AMT
1. Age
2. Time
3. Address for recall
4. Year
5. Place
6. Identify 2 people
7. Date of birth
8. Year 1st World War began
9. Current monarch
10. Recall address

Summary of key concepts in geriatric medicine
- **HOLISTIC CARE** – use the CGA framework to address all elements of care, including psychological, physical & social
- **REDUCE POLYPHARMACY** – avoid unnecessary medications & for those which are needed, start at low dose & increase slowly
- **PROBLEM SOLVING** – as well as using CGA framework to help guide management, consider all aspects when investigating issues

---

[4] British Association of Parenteral and Enteral Nutrition (BAPEN) (2011) *Malnutrition Universal Screening Tool* (MUST). Malnutrition Advisory Service.
[5] Mahoney FI & Barthel DW (1965) Functional evaluation: the Barthel Index. *Md State Med J,* **14**:61.
[6] Kreutzer J, DeLuca J & Caplan B (eds) (2011) *Encyclopedia of Clinical Neuropsychology: Berg Balance Scale.* Springer.

Dementia

All healthy older adults have a slowing to cognition and reduced capacity for novel memory formation. A disease process is suspected when brain impairments start impacting on a person's ability to function.

- **In the UK** over **850,000** people live with dementia
- **7.1% of people over 65y** in the UK have dementia
- There is a **F>M predominance**[7]
- Biggest risk factor = **AGE**[7]

Aetiology

- **Neuronal loss:** location in brain determines the symptoms
- Often **temporal lobe** involved = **short-term memory** (amygdala & hippocampus)

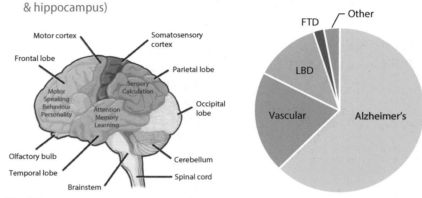

Fig. 2.3

Fig. 2.4 Prevalence of different types of dementia.

Symptoms of dementia

- **Memory loss**
- Difficulties with higher cognitive processes (≥1 of):
  - ▸ **impaired executive function** (e.g. problem solving, emotions)
  - ▸ **apraxia** (difficulty motor planning)
  - ▸ **agnosia** (difficulty recognising objects)
- → symptoms cause **impaired function** with **NO OTHER MEDICAL EXPLANATION**
- → symptoms present for **≥6m**

Types of dementia[7]

All types of dementia = **PROGRESSIVE & IRREVERSIBLE**
- **Alzheimer's disease:** 50–75% ⎤
- **Vascular dementia:** 20% ⎦ often mixed
- **Lewy body dementia (LBD):** 10–15%
- **Fronto-temporal dementia (FTD):** 2%

ALZHEIMER'S DISEASE: most common type of dementia (>500,000 people in UK)
- **Aetiology:** characteristic **beta-amyloid plaques & neurofibrillary tangles**
- **Pathogenesis: brain atrophy**, particularly hippocampus
- **CT brain:** volume loss and enlarged ventricles
- **History of illness:** usually **progressive** decline
- **Cause: unknown**
  - ▸ early onset (<65y) there is some familial link
  - ▸ association with *APO-E* gene
  - ▸ association with CVD risk factors
- → Average life expectancy = 7y

Symptoms of Alzheimer's disease
Progressive memory loss that *affects function*
- forget names, people, places
- repeat themselves
- cannot remember new info
- misplace items in odd places
- confusion about time of day
- getting lost in a familiar environment
- problems finding words ⎤
- mood/behaviour problems ⎦ later on

[7] Alzheimer's Society UK (2019)

VASCULAR DEMENTIA: 2nd most common type of dementia (150,000 people in UK)
- **Aetiology: cardiovascular disease** of cerebral blood vessels
- **Pathogenesis:** diseased blood vessels → multiple small areas of **ischaemia** → brain cell death
- **CT brain:** small vessel ischaemic change
- **History of illness:** usually **stepwise progression** *Often correlates with brain insult, e.g. after stroke*
- **Cause:** strong link with cardiovascular risk factors

LEWY BODY DEMENTIA (LBD): 3rd most common type of dementia: 5%
- **Aetiology:** characterised by **Lewy body protein deposits** in the basal ganglia and thalamus
- **History of illness: parkinsonism** often occurs, but motor symptoms occur **after** or within **one year** of memory problems
- **Cause: unknown**
- **Diagnosis:** based on clinical symptoms

> **DIFFERENTIAL DIAGNOSES OF LBD:**
> - **Parkinson's disease dementia** – patient with idiopathic Parkinson's disease developing cognitive decline **more than one year** after diagnosis
> - **Alzheimer's** – not associated with hallucinations, altered consciousness, sleep disturbance, movement disorder
> - **Schizophrenia** – prominent hallucinations/delusions early on

FRONTO-TEMPORAL DEMENTIA (FTD): rarer (2% of dementias)
- **Aetiology: tau protein deposits** in frontal and temporal lobes
- **Pathogenesis:** protein deposits cause brain cell death
- **History of illness:** earlier age onset (56–61y) and 40% have family history
  - ▸ several different subtypes → behavioural variant = $^2/_3$
  - ▸ slow onset
  - ▸ progressive non-fluent aphasia

Differentials of dementia

- Delirium
- Substance misuse
- Other mental illness, e.g. depression*
- Traumatic brain injury
- Metabolic (hypothyroidism, vitamin B12 deficiency)
- Medications (steroids, antidepressants)

Investigations & diagnosis

1. **Detailed collateral Hx:** onset/duration Sx, cognitive & functional decline, impact on ADLs *diagnosis primarily from clinical presentation so collateral history is KEY*
2. **Cognitive tests:** screen patients for impairment and help confirm diagnosis, e.g. MoCA
3. **Exclude reversible causes**
   - **Physical examination:** CNS/PNS, gait, CVS, thyroid
   - **Confusion screening bloods:** exclude other causes of cognitive impairment ± lumbar puncture if uncertain of Dx
   - **Medication review:** look for correlation of medications & duration of symptoms
   - **CT/MRI:** do not use alone to diagnose dementia BUT to exclude other causes / confirm diagnosis

Symptoms of vascular dementia
Problems with memory, thinking & reasoning
- Problems planning/organising
- Problems decision making / problem solving
- Problems concentrating
- Difficulty following steps/instructions, e.g. a recipe
- Slower thought speed
- Often overlaps with symptoms of Alzheimer's

Symptoms of Lewy body dementia
Early stages
- Fluctuating memory loss
- Hallucinations & delusions
- Parkinsonism
- REM sleep disorder
- Falls
Later stages
- Motor problems (similar to Parkinson's)
- Mood swings / short-tempered
- Speech & swallow problems

Symptoms of behaviour variant of FTD
- Loss of inhibition
  - ► Rude & compulsive
- Personality changes
  - ► Loss of interest in people
  - ► Loss of sympathy/empathy
- Crave food (often sweet/fatty)
  - ► Eat until vomit
- Speech/language difficulties
Cognitive deficit not so obvious

***Depressive pseudodementia**
= dementia-like symptoms (attention and memory deficit) secondary to depression

Other causes of dementia

Deficiencies
- Alcohol-related dementia (including Wernicke–Korsakoff syndrome)
- Hypothyroidism
- B12 deficiency

Neurological disorders
- Down syndrome
- Huntington's
- MS
- MND
- PDD
- CJD
- Pugilistic dementia (repetitive head trauma)

'Confusion screening bloods'
FBC, U&Es, LFT, TFT, glucose, calcium, vit B12, folate

PATIENT-CENTRED CARE IS KEY
- Gather as much info about patient as possible from carers/family/friends
- Create 'This is Me' book
- Patient can become easily distressed
  - ▸ reassure and orientate them
  - ▸ create familiar/friendly environment

MANAGE AS AN MDT

Consider CAPACITY!
Organise ADRT/LPA/DNACPR while patient still has capacity

Management[8]

There is NO CURE – eventually progresses to dependence and palliative care approach due to worsening incontinence, dysphagia, immobility

MEDICAL: (not curative → aim to maintain current cognitive status)
- Cholinesterase inhibitors: donepezil, rivastigmine, galantamine
  → For **mild–moderate** Alzheimer's, LBD or Parkinson's
- NMDA receptor antagonists[9]: memantine
  → For **moderate** Alzheimer's but intolerant of / contraindication to ACh inhibitors **OR**
  → For **severe** Alzheimer's disease
- Manage cardiovascular risk factors: in vascular dementia, e.g. hypertension, diabetes, stop smoking advice
  NB No medical treatment available for fronto-temporal dementia

PSYCHOLOGICAL: interventions to promote cognition, independence and wellbeing
- Group cognitive stimulation therapy
- Group reminiscence therapy
- Occupational therapy / cognitive rehabilitation

SOCIAL
- Social services care plan: home help, equipment, meals on wheels, day care, etc.
- **Offer carer support to those looking after patients with dementia**

Summary of treatment for Alzheimer's

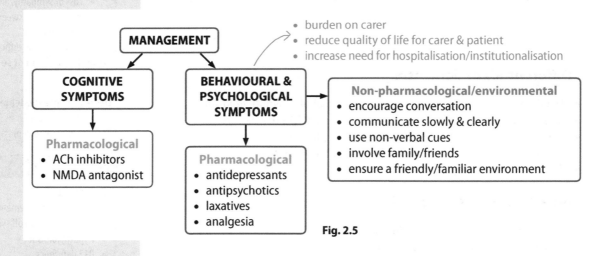

Fig. 2.5

Other points to note:
- Carers of those with dementia may qualify for **financial support**
- **MUST INFORM DVLA:** patients can still drive if deemed safe but eventually cognitive decline will prevent driving
- Consider discussing **LPAs and ADRTs** before too late

---

[8] NICE (2018) *Dementia* [NG97]
[9] NICE (2011, updated 2018) *Donepezil, galantamine, rivastigmine and memantine for the treatment of Alzheimer's disease* [TA217]

Delirium

A common clinical syndrome characterised by **disturbed consciousness/attention, cognitive function** or **perception**, which has an **acute onset** and **fluctuating course**

Epidemiology

→ Occurs in approximately 20% of hospital admissions
→ Causes increased length of stay / mortality post-discharge
→ Symptoms may persist for 6–12m after underlying cause is treated

Wait for patient to regain capacity before making important decisions

Types of delirium

Hyperactive
- agitation, confusion, hallucinations/delusions
- mood disturbance (affective lability)
- disturbed sleep

Hypoactive (more common)
- often unrecognised*: similar to depression
- withdrawn, not eating/drinking, sleeping a lot
- hallucinations/delusions

*must take special care to spot these patients

Causes: 'DELIRIUM'

Drugs/dehydration – withdrawal, new, toxicity
Electrolyte imbalance – e.g. hyponatraemia
Level of pain / lack of analgesia
Infection/inflammation – UTIs, URTI, post-op
Respiratory failure – hypoxia/hypercapnia
Impaction of faeces/Intracranial
Urinary retention
Metabolic/MI – liver/renal, hypoglycaemia

NB 50% of delirium cases occur in patients with prior dementia

Diagnosis

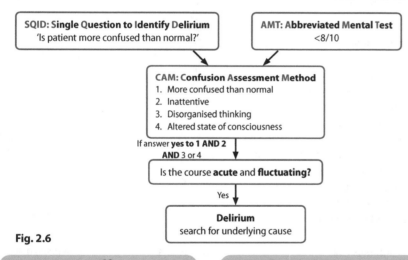

SQID: Single Question to Identify Delirium
'Is patient more confused than normal?'

AMT: Abbreviated Mental Test
<8/10

CAM: Confusion Assessment Method
1. More confused than normal
2. Inattentive
3. Disorganised thinking
4. Altered state of consciousness

If answer **yes to 1 AND 2 AND** 3 or 4

Is the course **acute** and **fluctuating**?

Yes

Delirium
search for underlying cause

Fig. 2.6

Drugs causing delirium:
- opiates
- antihistamines
- benzodiazepines
- antipsychotics
- antimuscarinics

Management[10]

TREAT UNDERLYING CAUSE
→ **if ignored = high mortality**

ENVIRONMENTAL
- Reassure, keep orientated, active, nourished, hydrated

MEDICAL
- Reduce medications (avoid opioids, anticholinergics)
- Only use drugs if other interventions have failed and patient is a risk to themselves or others
  ‣ haloperidol 0.5mg = 1st line
  ‣ lorazepam 0.5mg (if haloperidol contraindicated)

CI in Parkinson's & LBD

Investigations

To find cause:
- Collateral Hx (establish baseline cognition)
- Physical examination (consciousness level, infection)
- Confusion screening bloods
- Urine MCS – only if high suspicion of UTI*
- CXR, ECG, CT / MRI
- Assess nutrition status
- Medication review

Risk factors
- INCREASED AGE
- underlying dementia
- poor hearing/vision
- recent surgery
- previous episodes
- terminal illness

*DO NOT DO URINE DIP IN >65y AS 50% WILL HAVE BACTERIURIA → MCS if symptomatic / no other obvious source of infection

Outcomes of delirium
- Full recovery
- Prolonged hospital stay
- Ongoing functional impairment
- Ongoing cognitive impairment (3× risk of dementia)

---

[10]NICE (2010, updated 2019) *Delirium* [CG103]

Parkinson's disease

- 120,000 people affected in UK **(1 in 500)**
- Average age of onset: **60 years**

Symptoms often don't manifest clinically until **80%** of dopamine-producing cells are lost
Pre-clinical signs:
- Depression
- Anosmia
- Constipation
- REM sleep disorder
- Postural hypotension

NB There is massive fluctuation in motor symptoms with an unpredictable 'ON–OFF' phenomenon
= sudden switch from mobility ('on-phase') to immobility ('off-phase') in seconds or minutes

FALLS IN PARKINSON'S = COMMON DUE TO MULTIPLE RISK FACTORS
- Cognitive impairment (dementia)
- Freezing gait / gait impairment
- Reduced lower extremity strength
- Polypharmacy
- Depression/anxiety
- Postural hypotension
- Dyskinesia
- Postural instability

Aetiology

A **neurodegenerative disorder: loss of dopamine-producing cells** in substantia nigra as a result of combined genetic and environmental factors.

Risk factors

→ *Most cases are idiopathic*
Definite: age, male
Highly likely: identical twin
Probable: family history
Possible: herbicides/pesticides, heavy metal, proximity to industry, farming community, repeated head trauma

Symptoms

Queen's Square Brain Bank Criteria for diagnosis:
Rigidity + bradykinesia
± postural instability
± resting tremor

Motor symptoms
Bradykinesia: slowness of movements
- Hypophonia – soft, monotonous voice
- Micrographia – small handwriting

Rigidity
- Trouble getting up from chair
- Difficulty with fine finger movement
- Mask-like face

Postural instability: difficulty in maintaining balance
- High falls risk

Resting tremor
- Worse if anxious/angry/excited
- Better with action

Non-motor symptoms
- Depression/anxiety (in 40%)
- Psychosis (hallucinations/delusions – usually visual)
- Cognitive impairment (⅓ develop dementia)
- Autonomic dysfunction (constipation, urinary incontinence, postural hypotension, hypersalivation/drooling)

Other
- Anosmia (early symptom)
- Insomnia/REM sleep disorder/restless legs
- Fatigue
- Seborrhoeic dermatitis (oily skin)

A drop in blood pressure >20mmHg SBP or >10mmHg DBP on standing PLUS symptoms (dizziness or LOC)

Possible protective factors

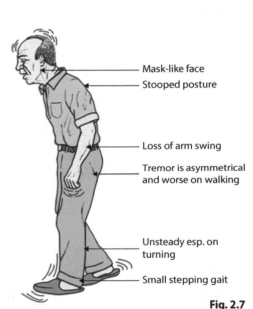

- Smoking
- Caffeine

Mask-like face
Stooped posture
Loss of arm swing
Tremor is asymmetrical and worse on walking
Unsteady esp. on turning
Small stepping gait

Fig. 2.7

Cognitive problems in Parkinson's disease

- **Mild cognitive impairment (MCI)***: in 25% newly diagnosed with PD
- **Parkinson's disease dementia (PDD)**
= a dementia syndrome with **insidious onset** and
slow progression within the context of **established PD**

up to 6× more likely to develop dementia if have PD

*MCI is a risk factor for developing PDD

DDx of parkinsonism

Type of parkinsonism	Suggestive features
Idiopathic PD	**Unilateral** onset & persistent asymmetry **Upper limb** predominance Presents with **bradykinesia** Treatment responsive (to L-dopa)
Vascular PD	**Bilateral** onset **Lower limb** predominance Presents with **falls / gait problems**
Drug-induced parkinsonism	History of antipsychotics (especially 1st generation) or metoclopramide
Lewy body dementia	Prominent **cognitive impairment prior to parkinsonism** **Hallucinations/delusions** *Can also be present in Alzheimer's dementia* Fluctuating level of consciousness
Progressive supranuclear palsy (PSP) rare and poor prognosis	**Eye signs** (vertical gaze palsy) **Cognitive impairment** (frontal disinhibition) Not responsive to dopaminergic treatment
Multi-system atrophy (MSA) rare and poor prognosis	Prominent **autonomic features** (postural hypotension, incontinence, impotence) **Cerebellar signs** Not responsive to dopaminergic treatment

Investigations & diagnosis

- History and examination
- Confusion bloods – rule out acute/reversible causes
- Medication review – check for antipsychotics causing drug-induced parkinsonism
- CT/MRI – rule out differentials, e.g. vascular cause
- L-dopa test – if responsive, suggests idiopathic parkinsonism
- PET/SPECT (DAT) scan – detect ↓ dopaminergic activity in basal ganglia *Only if uncertainty (PD is a CLINICAL DIAGNOSIS)*

> Diagnosis is made by **clinical presentation**, therefore history and examination are **key**. Other investigations to rule out reversible causes or if diagnosis uncertain.

PD FOCUSED EXAMINATION:

Hallmark features:
Bradykinesia – check finger thumb pinching
Rigidity – assess tone (lead pipe/cogwheel rigidity)
Resting tremor – ask to relax hands and count 20–0
Postural instability – shoulder-tug test
Gait – reduced arm swing, flexed posture, shuffling

UMN signs:
- hyperreflexia
- +ve Babinski
- clonus

Other:
- quiet speech (hypophonic)
- mask-like face (hypomimia)
- small writing (micrographia)

Prognostic determinants

- Age
- Genetics
- Comorbidities/frailty

Anti-PD medication complications

L-dopa
- **Dyskinesia:** uncontrollable wriggling/writhing
  ± confusion, depression, postural hypotension, insomnia

DA agonists
- Confusion/hallucinations
- **Impulsive control disorder:** gambling, hobbyism, hypersexuality

RFs: young, unmarried, smoking, FHx of impulsivity

MOAB inhibitors
- Postural hypotension

COMT inhibitors
- Sleepiness, hallucinations, impulsiveness

Often impact life more than motor symptoms
→ ensure to ask about these at follow-up

Management[11]

Liaise with Parkinson's specialist

MEDICAL

1. **L-dopa monotherapy** (dopamine precursor)
   - ► Combined with <u>carbidopa</u> to prevent peripheral metabolism to dopamine
   - ► Complications may arise after 4–6y & efficacy reduces (narrowed therapeutic window)
   - ► **Time and dose = critical for controlling 'on–off' fluctuations DYSKINESIA = BIGGEST SIDE-EFFECT**

2. **Dopamine agonist patch** (e.g. rotigotine patch)
   - ► if nil by mouth / early stages of disease
   - ► can also be used as L-dopa adjunct later in disease

3. **L-dopa dual therapy**
   + MOAB inhibitors (selegiline/rasagiline)
   - ► can increase duration of response to L-dopa
   + COMT inhibitors (entacapone)
   - ► block L-dopa metabolism
   + Amantadine
   - ► useful if prominent dyskinesias as SE of L-dopa therapy

4. **Treatment of non-motor symptoms**
   - ► Daytime sleepiness – **INFORM DVLA**, consider modafinil
   - ► REM sleep disorder – clonazepam/melatonin
   - ► Psychosis – beware of antipsychotics due to neuroleptic sensitivity
   - ► Dementia – cholinesterase inhibitor
   - ► Postural hypotension – medication review, consider midodrine
   - ► Depression – antidepressants
   - ► Drooling – consider glycopyrronium bromide
   - ► Constipation – laxatives

PSYCHOLOGICAL

- Patient education, e.g. advice to minimise 'freezing', e.g. using laser pointer
- Therapy for depression / mood symptoms

SOCIAL

- Social support
- Physio/OT
- SALT
- Nutrition review / dietitian input

PD medications need regular review. At follow-up clinic always ask about:
- non-motor symptoms
- fluctuations in motor capabilities
- hallucinations
- dyskinesias
- → **enquire how any symptoms relate to timing of dopaminergic therapy – adjust time and dose accordingly**

Later life depression

Aetiology

'Monoamine hypothesis' → deficiency of DA, NA, 5-HT
= most common mental illness in the older person (affects 1 in 5, F>M)

Epidemiology / risk factors

Biological	Psychological	Social
Chronic pain	PMHx of depression/anxiety	Social isolation
Long-term conditions	Loss – spouse, job, independence	Not able to drive / lost mobility
Recent physical illness	Previously a highly independent person	Death of close friends/family
Medications, e.g. steroids, opioids		Elderly neighbours – can't offer support

Steroids also cause:
- psychosis
- anger/aggression

Diagnosis

1. ICD-10 diagnostic criteria: symptoms present for >2w

Core symptoms	Other symptoms ('GAAPPSS')
• **Low mood** ▸ worse in morning	**G**uilt/hopelessness
	Appetite reduced / weight loss
• **Anhedonia** ▸ loss of pleasure in activities	**A**gitation (more common in elderly)
	Psychosomatic (pain, GI complaints)*
• **Fatigue**	**P**sychosis (hallucinations/delusions)
	Suicidal thoughts / **S**elf-harm
	Sleep disturbance / poor memory

Criteria for diagnosis

MILD: 2 core + 2 other
MODERATE: 2/3 core + 3 other
SEVERE: 3 core + 5 other

*Depression in elderly often presents with **excessive concern over physical health**

Psychotic depression
= **most common presentation in elderly**
- Paranoid delusions
e.g. food being poisoned
- Nihilistic delusions
e.g. internal organs are blocked
- Guilt delusions
e.g. feel they need to be in prison

2. Geriatric Depression Scale (GDS)
= 15 YES/NO questions to help **screen for, assess severity of & monitor** clinical depression in an older person

Management[12]   *ASSESS SUICIDE RISK*

MEDICAL
- **Antidepressants:** SSRIs (1st line) e.g. sertraline
- ± antipsychotic or mood stabiliser if psychosis, e.g. olanzapine/lithium
- ± anxiolytics for anxiety: benzodiazepines → **SHORT-TERM ONLY**
- ± hypnotics for sleep: Z drugs → **SHORT-TERM ONLY**
- ECT – for severe depression that is life-threatening or Tx-resistant

PSYCHOLOGICAL
- CBT/IPT (interpersonal therapy)
- Supportive listening

SOCIAL
- Support networks/groups
- Social services referral
- Lifestyle: exercise/meaningful activity, limit alcohol, etc.

DDx of depressive symptoms

Endocrine/metabolic disease
- Hypothyroidism
- Anaemia
- Hypercalcaemia

Long-term physical illness
- Malignancy
- Dementia
- PD
- MS

Possible investigations

- General physical examination
- FBC, U&Es, LFTs
- Ca levels, glucose
- TFTs
- B12, folate

---

[12] NICE (2009) *Depression in adults* [CG90]

Incontinence

For normal bladder control we need

Intact nerve pathways (autonomic and voluntary)
Normal muscle tone in the detrusors, sphincters & pelvic floor
Absence of any obstruction to urine flow
Normal cognition

PNS: initiates micturition reflex
Contraction of detrusor muscle in bladder: **S2–S4**
SNS: inhibits micturition reflex
Contraction of smooth muscle sphincter: **T11–L2**
→ **target with medication for incontinence**

Medications causing urinary incontinence

CCBs, antidepressants, antipsychotics:
↓ detrusor activity (overflow)
α-blockers: relax urinary sphincter
ACEis: cough worsens stress incontinence
Opioids: worsen constipation which causes pressure on the bladder
Sedatives: reduce awareness of need to micturate
Diuretics: including alcohol and caffeine

Causes of faecal incontinence

Diarrhoea: infection, overflow from constipation
Faecal impaction: severe constipation
Nerve damage: spinal cord injury, MS, DM
Anal damage: post radiotherapy
Cognitive: dementia, stroke
Other: IBD, malignancy, poor diet / fluid intake

DO NOT DO URINE DIP IN >65y AS 50% WILL HAVE BACTERIURIA → only treat for UTI if symptomatic

Urinary incontinence: the complaint of any involuntary leakage of urine **sufficient to be a health or social problem**
→ VERY COMMON in elderly (30% at home, 50% in care homes)
→ more common in women ≈ 2 in 5 women & 1 in 10 men >65y

Causes of acute urinary incontinence (reversible)

Delirium
Infection (UTIs)
Atrophic urethritis and vaginitis (from lack of oestrogen)   **DIAPERS**
Pharmaceuticals / **P**sychiatric disorders (especially depression)
Excess urine output (polyuria – diabetes/excess intake)
Restricted mobility
Stool impaction: leads to **overflow** incontinence

Total bladder volume = approx. 600ml
Urge to void at approx. 250ml

Adverse consequences of urinary incontinence

- **Reduced quality of life:** depression, isolation, stigmatisation
- **Burden to caregivers**
- **Pressure ulcers** due to skin irritation
- **Increased risk of falls:** due to urgency & hurrying
- **UTIs:** risk if incomplete bladder emptying

Investigating urinary incontinence

INVESTIGATIONS
- **History & examination**
- **Urinalysis, urine culture (MSU)**
  - ► Glucose – diabetes
  - ► Protein – kidney pathology
  - ► Blood – stones/malignancy
  - ► DO NOT use leukocytes/nitrites to diagnose UTI (diagnose on symptoms & **only then send an MSU**)
- **Bloods**
  - ► U&Es, FBC, glucose, calcium
- **Frequency/volume charts**
  - ► over 3d
  - ► >2000ml/24h = polyuria
- **Pre- & post-void bladder scan**
  - ► determine residual volume
  - ► >100ml = abnormal
- **Uroflowmetry** (only use when diagnosis uncertain)
  - ► good to diagnose outlet obstruction

EXAMINATION
- **Neurological exam**
  - ► mental status
  - ► spinal cord: **lower limb weakness is a RED FLAG**
  - ► perineal sensation
- **Abdominal exam**
  - ► palpate kidneys and bladder
- **Pelvic exam**
  - ► organ prolapse
  - ► wall weakness
- **Rectal exam**
  - ► faecal impaction
  - ► rectal masses
- **Cardiorespiratory**
  - ► chronic lung disease
  - ► CCF

Types of urinary incontinence

Type	Risk factors	History	Specific management
Urge incontinence 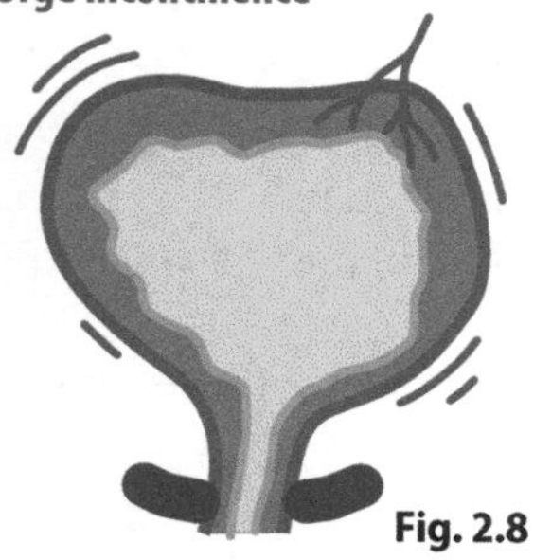 • Bladder oversensitivity • Abnormal neurological stimulation	**Most common type in elderly patients** • Idiopathic • Diuretics • UTIs • Caffeine/↑ fluid intake • Alcohol/smoking • Constipation • Neurogenic (MS, PD, stroke)	**Urgency** **Frequency** **Nocturia** ± stress incontinence Regular voiding of small volumes **Bladder retraining:** • at least 6w • resist urgency • void according to set timetable	**Lifestyle:** • ↓ fluids/caffeine • medication review • bladder retraining **Medical:** • anticholinergics, e.g. solifenacin/tolterodine avoid oxybutynin in elderly as increases risk of falls/confusion • botulinum toxin A block neuromusc transmission • intravaginal oestrogens
Stress incontinence 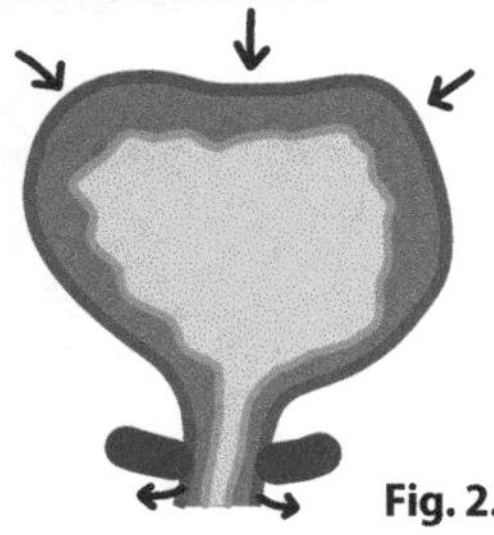 • Increased IAP • Weak pelvic floor	**Urethral sphincter weakness (cannot withstand ↑ IAP)** • pregnancy, obesity, age • previous vaginal delivery (long labour / forceps) • prolapse, hysterectomy • muscular diseases	**Leakage on exertion (e.g. cough/sneeze)** ↑ IAP causes bladder > urethral pressure	**Lifestyle:** • weight loss • pelvic floor training **Medical:** (only after pelvic floor training fails) • duloxetine ↑ sphincter activity • injectable bulking agents **Surgical:** • colposuspension
Overflow incontinence 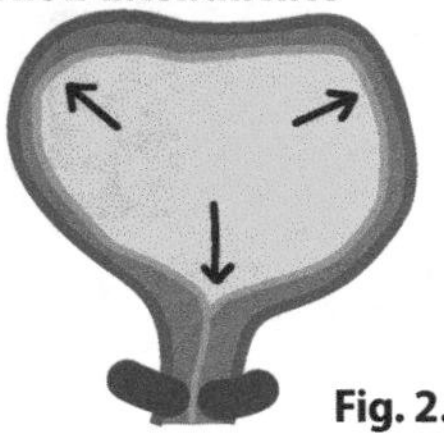 • Obstruction to outflow • Detrusor muscle failure	**Obstruction** • CONSTIPATION • pelvic surgery/strictures • BPH/prostate tumour • bladder calculi **Detrusor failure** • neurological/DM • medication	**Leakage on exertion OR continuous flow/dribble** Bladder overdistension → overflows (associated with chronic retention)	**Lifestyle:** • Intermittent self-catheterisation **Treat underlying cause** e.g. BPH, constipation

Fig. 2.8 / Fig. 2.9 / Fig. 2.10

Functional incontinence: cognitive failure to inhibit reflex, e.g. dementia/stroke
→ **Risk factors:** immobility, sedation, unfamiliar surroundings

Holistic management of urinary incontinence[13]

BIOLOGICAL
• Medication review – diuretics
• Treat any underlying cause, e.g. UTI, BPH
• Anticholinergics (tolterodine/solifenacin) for urge incontinence
• Oestrogen cream/pessary for vaginal/urethral atrophy

PHYSIO-/OCCUPATIONAL THERAPY
• Assess and improve mobility
• Equipment and changes to the home, e.g. downstairs toilet, commode
• Pelvic floor exercises

SOCIAL
• Smoking cessation, weight reduction
• Restrict fluids (especially in evenings)
• Reduce alcohol/caffeine
• Absorbent pads, commodes

> **Red flag symptoms**
> • Dysuria
> • Prolapse beyond vaginal opening
> • Suspicion of prostate cancer
> • Haematuria
> → **Need urology/gynaecology referral**

[13] NICE (2019) *Urinary incontinence and pelvic organ prolapse in women* [NG123]

Falls in the elderly

Fall: an event whereby an individual comes to rest on the ground or another lower level, with or without loss of consciousness

30% of >65s fall at least once per year
50% of >80s fall at least once per year
50% who fall will fall again within 1y
30% of falls result in injury

↳ *Should ask all elderly patients if they had a recent fall*

Consequences of falls

- Morbidity – complications of a long lie, fractures
- Mortality – 10% patients die within 1y following a hip fracture
- Financial cost – to NHS & patient/family if need further support/equipment/ institutionalisation
- Personal cost – fear of falling (reduced activity / social isolation, depression/ anxiety)

Risk factors for falls

Intrinsic	Extrinsic	Behavioural
Cardiovascular: • arrhythmias, syncope • postural hypotension	Poorly fitting footwear	Alcohol *Remember to ask about in the history!*
Balance & gait • neuropathy • muscle atrophy • foot deformities/arthritis • Parkinson's – shuffle, freeze	Inappropriate walking aid	Risky behaviour e.g. lifting, bending • no one to ask for help • want to maintain independence
Visual impairment • glaucoma, AMD, cataracts • presbyopia	Insufficient equipment	Rushing to answer phone, etc.
Cognitive impairment/confusion • dementia/delirium	Insufficient lighting	Poor diet/fluid intake
Incontinence – rushing to toilet	Unfamiliar environment	Non-compliance with advice
Malnourished – lack physical strength	Trip hazards, e.g. catheters, rugs, pets	Fear of falling
Medications • antihypertensives, anti-arrhythmics • diuretics, vasodilators • sedatives, opiates, hypnotics, antidepressants		Lack of exercise • lose muscle and balance

MUST ASK ABOUT HEAD INJURIES

Falls history

Before: dizziness, vision changes, palpitations, chest pain, position/movement pre-fall
During: LOC, time on floor, seizure activity, incontinence, injuries
After: post-ictal phase, confusion, injuries, ongoing pain

Investigations

KEY INVESTIGATIONS
- **History and examination** – gait (GALS), heart sounds, neurological, vision
- **ECG**
- **Lying and standing BP** – postural hypotension

} Must be done in all falls patients

OTHER INVESTIGATIONS

- FBC, U&Es, TFTs
- CRP – if suspicious of infection
- Creatine kinase – if a long lie (rhabdomyolysis)
- Bone biochemistry – for osteoporosis
- Tilt table test – if symptoms of syncope
- ECHO/24h tape – if ECG abnormal / cardiovascular symptoms
- CT – if head injury & on anticoagulants

Falls management[14]

PSYCHOLOGICAL

PATIENT EDUCATION, e.g. getting up slowly, using aids, don't use partner's glasses, etc.

PHYSIO-/OCCUPATIONAL THERAPY

- Strength and balance training
- Home hazards assessment
- Non-slip socks/mats/shoes

MEDICAL

- Analgesia
- Medication review
- Diagnose new medical conditions
- Optimise comorbidities – vision assessment and referral
- Cognitive screen
- Bone health assessment – FRAX score

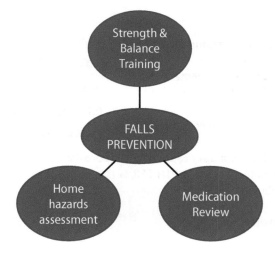

Fig. 2.11

MDT input is key in managing falls. Doctors, nurses, pharmacists, physios and occupational therapists all play an important role

---

ENCOURAGING MOBILITY IS KEY!
Encouraging sedentary behaviour to prevent falls can be counterproductive
→ **contributes to deconditioning and functional loss**
Try to ensure patient remains active and not sedentary post-discharge.

---

[14] NICE (2013) – *Falls in older people* [CG161]

Osteoporosis

Reduced bone mineral density with altered microarchitecture → weak & fragile

Common osteoporosis fractures

- Neck of femur*
- Colle's
- Vertebral crush

*Neck of femur fractures result in >4000 bed days per year, and cost the NHS £2 billion per year

Mnemonic for osteoporosis risk factors: 'SHATTERED'

Steroids/**S**moking
Hyperthyroid/parathyroidism/**H**ypocalcaemia
Alcohol/**A**norexia
Thin (low BMI)
Testosterone (low)
Early menopause
Renal/liver failure
Erosive bone disease (RA, malignancy)
Dietary (low vit D/Ca, malabsorption) / **D**isuse

*FRAX Risk Assessment Tool

Considers the following parameters to calculate % risk of a major hip fracture & major osteopenic fracture, over the next 10y:
Classified as LOW/INTERMEDIATE / HIGH fracture risk
- age, gender
- smoking/alcohol history
- rheumatoid arthritis
- BMI
- steroid use
- fracture history

**BMD measurement

T-score: number of SDs below average for **young adult male**
Z-score: number of SDs below average for **age-matched control**
Osteoporosis: T-score >**2.5** SDs **below** average
Osteopenia: T-score **1–2.5** SDs **below** average

***Counselling on bisphosphonates

- Tablets or injections once a week
- Swallow with water
- Sit upright for 30min after

Side-effects: GI upset, oesophageal ulcers, jaw necrosis (rare)

Aetiology

Bone resorption (osteoclasts) > bone formation (osteoblasts), resulting in:
- Gradual bone weakening – especially SPINE, HIP, WRIST
- Increased risk of fracture – e.g. from standing height / low trauma
- Back pain/kyphosis/loss of height

Risk factors

Primary: no other disease process present
- Age/female
- Genetics (determines peak bone mass)
- Low BMI
- Calcium/vit D deficiency
- Previous low trauma fracture

*Osteoporosis itself has no symptoms → Symptoms only **after** a bone has broken*

Secondary: osteoporosis contributed to by another disease process
- Chronic inflammation (RA, malignancy)
- Hyperthyroidism/hyperparathyroidism
- Malabsorption (coeliac disease, inflammatory bowel disease)
- Premature menopause (<45y)
- Steroid use (prednisolone >3m)
- Smoking
- Alcohol excess >3 units per day

Investigations

- **History and examination:** calculate FRAX score[15]*
- **X-ray** – if suspect fracture
- **DEXA scan (BMD measurement**)**
  - → Only if FRAX score in intermediate risk category
  - → High risk FRAX = immediately start treatment

Bone profile	Ca	PO$_4$	ALP
Osteoporosis	N	N	N
Osteomalacia	↓	↓	↑
Paget's disease	N	N	↑

- **Investigate for secondary cause of osteoporosis:**
  U&Es, bone profile, vit D, TFTs, PTH, ESR, LFTs, anti-TTG (coeliac), immunoglobulins (multiple myeloma)

Management[16]

SOCIAL/LIFESTYLE:
- Improve calcium intake
- Exercise (especially weight-bearing)
- Smoking cessation / reduced alcohol consumption

PHYSIOTHERAPY: reduce falls risk

MEDICAL: vit D & calcium supplements **PLUS**
1st line: bisphosphonates***
2nd line: denosumab (inhibits osteoclasts)
3rd line: teriparatide (PTH analogue which ↑ osteoblast activity) OR raloxifene (selective oestrogen reuptake inhibitor so ↑ oestrogen strengthens bones)

[15] FRAX Risk Assessment Tool – Centre for Metabolic Bone Diseases, University of Sheffield, UK
[16] NICE (2021) CKS – *Clinical scenario: Osteoporosis*

Nutrition in later life

Nutrition: intake of food, considered in relation to the body's dietary needs
Good nutrition: adequate, well-balanced diet combined with regular physical activity = cornerstone of good health
Malnutrition: a state of nutrition in which a **deficiency or excess of energy, protein and other nutrients** causes measurable **adverse effects on tissue/ body** form (shape, size, composition) and function to affect clinical outcome.
→ increased susceptibility to disease → impaired physical and mental development → reduced productivity

> **15%** of elderly people in the **community** = malnourished
> **50%** of elderly people in **hospital** = malnourished

Symptoms of malnutrition

- Loss of appetite
- Weight loss
- Tiredness / loss of energy
- Reduced physical performance
- Altered mood
- Poor concentration

> **DDx of weight loss in the elderly**
> - **Psychiatric disease** (depression/dementia)
> - **GI disease** (malabsorption/dysphagia)
> - **Systemic disease** (chronic conditions like COPD, malignancy)
> - **Iatrogenic** (medications)
> - **Age-related changes** (smell/taste, etc.)

Reasons for increased risk of malnutrition in the elderly

Cognitive	Physical	Social
• Unable to vocalise desires • Misinterpret sensation of hunger • Reduced appetite / early satiety • Depression/bereavement • Dementia/delirium	**Dental problems:** oral hygiene/gingivitis, dentures **GI complications:** delayed gastric emptying, malabsorption **Medications:** interactions and side-effects **Swallowing problems** **Poor mobility / reduced dexterity** **Reduced smell/taste**	**Access to food:** • inability to shop/prepare food • lack knowledge of food/cooking **Isolation/loneliness** • don't eat as a social activity **Finances**

Higher risk of malnutrition when hospitalised: unpleasant environment, can't access food (can't reach/open packets), limited provision for religious/dietary needs, nil by mouth, missed meals while having tests, increased nutritional needs

Screening for malnutrition in hospitals

Malnutrition Universal Screening Tool (MUST)[4] = 5-step tool to screen for malnourishment / risk of malnourishment
1. Calculate BMI
2. Note % unplanned weight loss
3. Establish acute disease effect and score
4. Add scores from 1–3
5. Develop appropriate care plan

> **MUST scores**
>
> **0 = low risk**
> - repeat screening weekly / if situation changes
>
> **1 = medium risk**
> - document intake for 3d then decide if further intervention is needed
>
> **≥2 = high risk**
> - dietetic support to improve intake & close monitoring
>
> *MUST score should be calculated within 24h of admission and repeated weekly (or sooner if patient's condition changes)*

Management of malnutrition[17]

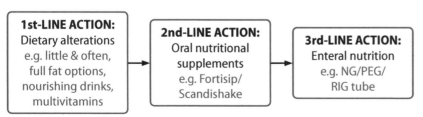

1st-LINE ACTION:
Dietary alterations
e.g. little & often,
full fat options,
nourishing drinks,
multivitamins

→

2nd-LINE ACTION:
Oral nutritional
supplements
e.g. Fortisip/
Scandishake

→

3rd-LINE ACTION:
Enteral nutrition
e.g. NG/PEG/
RIG tube

Must think about whether eating/swallow will ever improve, or if this is prolonging the inevitable → MDT discussion

---

[17] NICE (2006, updated 2017) *Nutrition support for adults* [CG32]

Pressure ulcers

Localised **injury** to the skin ± underlying tissue, usually **over a bony prominence**, due to **pressure/shearing/friction**

Common sites for pressure ulcers:
- sacrum
- ears
- heels
- elbows
- hips

Normally painful and pruritic unless co-existing neuropathic disease (e.g. DM)

Features of an ulcer

- **Base:** what you feel
  - ► if bone = risk of osteomyelitis
- **Floor:** what you see
  - ► necrosis/pus = suggests infection
- **Edge**
  - ► sloped = normal ulcer
  - ► undermined edges = TB
  - ► rolled up/everted = risk of malignancy

Risk factors

- Impaired mobility
- Impaired nutrition
- Impaired healing, e.g. DM, immunocompromised
- Neurologically compromised / reduced sensation
- Exposure to skin irritants, e.g. urine/faeces
- Poor posture
- Equipment without proper pressure relief

>65y = ↑ risk of all these so ↑ risk of ulcers

Screening and assessment

- **Skin inspection** – immediately on arrival to ward
- **Waterlow score**[18] – within 6h of admission to determine risk of pressure ulcer development
- **Nutritional assessment** – important for healing (FBC, iron profile, prealbumin, albumin)

Complications

- Skin and soft tissue infections, e.g. cellulitis
- Bone infections (osteomyelitis)
- Squamous cell carcinoma due to chronic inflammation
- Sinus tract formation due to chronic inflammation
- Sepsis

NB If non-healing ulcer, consider: INFECTION, MALNUTRITION or SQUAMOUS CELL CARCINOMA

Pressure ulcer DDx
- skin malignancy
- moisture lesion

Ix if suspect infection
- Wound swab & culture
- Blood culture
- Bloods: CRP, ESR, FBC, U&Es

Ix if suspect osteomyelitis
- X-ray, MRI

Ix if suspect squamous cell carcinoma
- Skin biopsy

---

[18]Waterlow J (1985) Pressure sores: a risk assessment card. *Nursing Times*, **81(48):** 49–55.

Diagnosis & staging

STAGE 1: Superficial	STAGE 2: Partial thickness	STAGE 3: Full thickness	STAGE 4: Full thickness	Moisture lesion: NOT a pressure ulcer
Non-blanching erythema, intact skin **(no ulcer)**	**Shallow ulcer** but subcutaneous tissue **not exposed**	**Deeper ulcer** and subcutaneous tissue (fat) **exposed** **Refer to tissue viability**	**Deep ulcer** & see **bone** Risk of osteomyelitis **Refer to tissue viability**	Redness ± partial skin loss Excessive skin moisture Due to **chronic exposure** to **urine/faeces/sweat**

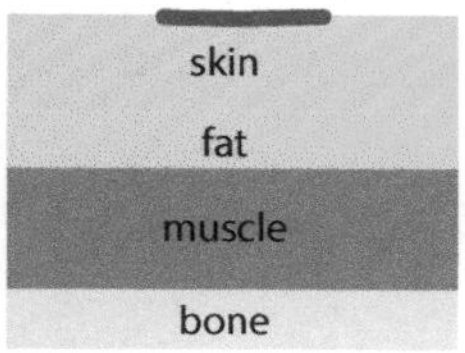

skin
fat
muscle
bone

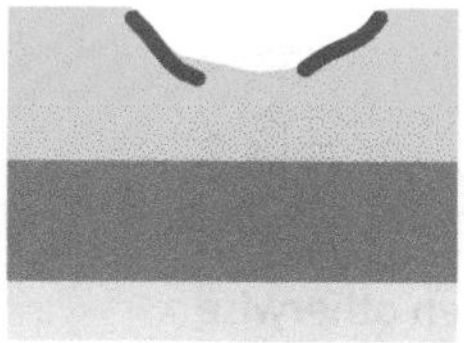

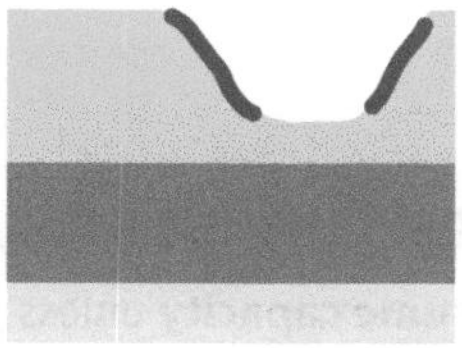

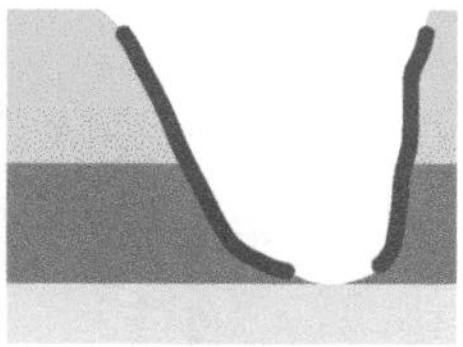

Fig. 2.12

Management[19]

PREVENTION
- **Offload pressure**
  - keep mobile/reposition (turn immobile patients every hour or 2)
  - use equipment (protective padding, support surfaces / special mattresses)
- **Other**
  - daily check for development of pressure ulcer
  - skin hygiene (keep dry, avoid irritants, avoid friction)
  - optimise nutrition (protein/calorie supplements, vitamin C, hydration)

TREATMENT
- **Wound care**
  - if it's dry, moisten to aid healing; if it's wet with exudate, dry it out to aid healing
  - cleaning – 0.9% NaCl
  - debridement – only if necrotic tissue present
- **Nutritional optimisation**
- **Antibiotics**
  - topical antibiotics if infection in the wound
  - systemic antibiotics **only** if cellulitis present / systemic symptoms
  - if osteomyelitis present, antibiotics needed for 6w
- **Surgery**
  - only in severe cases of ischaemia/necrosis

Pressure ulcers are a *clinical diagnosis* based on inspection

PREVENTION > CURE (ulcers hard to heal)
95% ulcers = avoidable

Prevention summary

Skin assessment
Keep moving
Incontinence/irritant avoidance
Nutrition assessment

[19]NICE (2014) *Pressure ulcers* [CG179]

Ethics and end-of-life decisions

Mental capacity

DEFINITION

Mental capacity is a person's ability to make their own decisions and choices
→ **It is DECISION- & TIME-SPECIFIC**
i.e. a person may have capacity to make simple decisions, but not more complicated ones
i.e. a person may not have capacity to make a decision when they are suffering from delirium, but do once they recover (interventions may be delayed until capacity is regained)

FIVE PRINCIPLES OF CAPACITY[20]

1. **Assume capacity** unless proven otherwise
2. Individuals should be **supported to make their own decisions** where possible **(facilitated)**
   ► All efforts must be made to help understanding of information / communication of decision, e.g. hearing aids, diagrams, demonstrations, interpreters
3. **Unwise decisions** must still be respected
4. If someone lacks capacity, must act in their **best interests**
   → Can have a '**best interests meeting**'
   ► Not based on age, appearance, etc.
   ► Consider person's wishes, feelings, beliefs, values
   ► Consider the views of close friends/family
   ► May consider the views of any IMCA*
   ► Consider whether they will **regain capacity**

NB If concerned that family are not acting in best interests, can refer to Court of Protection

5. If someone lacks capacity, must choose the **least restrictive option**

ASSESSING CAPACITY: 2-stage test

Stage 1:
Does person have an impairment of the mind or brain?
Temporary or permanent:
dementia, delirium, learning disability, stroke, alcohol/drugs, head injury

— No → No reason to question capacity

Yes ↓

Stage 2: Can the person:
- understand information?
- retain information (long enough to make decision)?
- weigh up consequences?
- communicate the decision?
If person cannot demonstrate 1 or more of the above, this indicates that they LACK CAPACITY related to a particular decision

*IMCA (Independent Mental Capacity Advocate)

An impartial, objective individual who helps decide what is in the patient's best interest.

Needed when someone lacks capacity but has no one else able to represent them.

When might we need to assess capacity?

- To gain consent for procedures
- Patient refusing interventions
- Patient wants to be discharged against medical advice
- Patient wants to be discharged without recommended support/POC
- Patient's behaviour puts self or others at risk
- Family members report concerns over patient's cognitive state

HOW TO APPROACH A CAPACITY ASSESSMENT

- **Explain to patient** what you are assessing capacity for / the decision that needs to be made.
- Explain the **risks and benefits/consequences** of both consenting and not consenting to this decision,
  i.e. why you want to do it & what could go wrong, as well as what could happen if they do not consent
- Ask if they understand → get them to **summarise/repeat back** what you've said to check understanding and ability to retain information.
- Ask them to **tell you their views / their decision**, based on the information you have given them.

Lasting power of attorney (LPA)

An LPA is a legal document that appoints an individual or individuals as attorney for the patient.
→ Attorneys are able to **make decisions on behalf of the patient**, should the patient lack capacity to do so themselves.
→ Attorneys must be appointed when the **patient has capacity**.
→ The LPA document is **legally binding**.

There are two types:
- **Financial** – decisions involving finances, e.g. buying/selling property, investing money
- **Health and wellbeing** – decisions on medical care, living situation, social contacts

Liberty protection safeguards (LPS)

Article 5 of Human Rights Act: no one should be deprived of their liberty unless in accordance with a procedure prescribed by law, e.g. if detained under the Mental Health Act / a deprivation of liberty safeguard is in place.

According to the Mental Capacity (Amendment) Act 2019[21]:
A doctor may deprive a patient of liberty if, by doing so, the doctor is enabling the care & treatment of the person who lacks capacity.

To apply for **deprivation of liberty** the following conditions must be met:

1. Lacks the capacity to consent to care and treatment **and**
2. The person subject to continuous supervision and control **and**
3. The person free to leave

RESTRAINTS AND CONSTRICTIONS
The Mental Capacity Act allows restraints/restrictions to be used if they are in the patient's **best interests**.

Restrictions and restraints must be **proportionate to the harm** we are trying to prevent.

→ Ensures the patient is managed in the least restrictive way possible

Examples of restraints/constrictions: locks/key pads, sedative medication, close supervision/isolation, restricting contact with friends/family, physically stopping patient doing something that will cause them harm

> **NOTE:** YOU CANNOT DEPRIVE SOMEONE OF LIBERTY IN THEIR OWN HOME

---

[21] Mental Capacity (Amendment) Act (2019), Chapter 18

Advance decision to refuse treatment (ADRT)

- **Made when patient has capacity** for if they lose capacity
- Has same weight in law as if patient still has capacity
- **Legally binding** – must be authorised
- Must be **very specific**
  - can set out the treatment they do not want and in which circumstances
  - **can refuse treatment, but not demand treatment,** *e.g. refusal of PEG if unable to self-feed, but cannot demand to be PEG fed*

Exception: *if patient is detained under **Mental Health Act**, they can still be treated for mental illness despite an ADRT*

→ *Cannot refuse **basic care***

CPR decision-making

CPR is a procedure we are performing on a patient and therefore, like all procedures, it is a **clinical decision.** Family and patient should be informed and the process explained, but the **final decision rests with the clinical team**[22].

By not providing CPR to a patient, we can instead **focus on their comfort and dignity** at the end of their life.

THINGS TO CONSIDER
- Survival chances[23]
- Quality of life after resuscitation – hypoxic brain damage/pain/broken ribs, etc.
- Will ITU be willing to support this patient post-arrest?

DNACPR
- **Only pertains to CPR** (once heart stops) and NOT other treatments that may aid recovery, *i.e. ABX, IV fluids*
- It is a **medical decision** but should be discussed with patient and family
  - need a **medical reason other than age,** e.g. not fit for ITU post-arrest/ frailty/terminal illness
  - team decision should be **signed by a consultant**

ReSPECT (Recommended Summary Plan for Emergency Care and Treatment)
- **Personalised recommendations** for clinical care in future, where the patient is unable to make or express decisions
- More **holistic summary** of end-of-life care; **covers details other than just CPR**, e.g. use of IV fluids/ABX
- Relevant for people with complex health needs / nearing the end of their lives / at risk of sudden deterioration
- **Is NOT legally binding.** Often used as part of an Advanced Care Plan (ACP) to help a patient and family discuss end-of-life wishes, which may help avoid unnecessary admissions to hospital.

Problems with ADRT
- Patients are often unaware of ADRTs / their legal validity
- Patients/doctors often uncomfortable discussing such topics
- Poor transfer of an ADRT from home/primary care to hospital
- May be **too vague**, e.g. refusal of 'life-sustaining treatment' may not help decisions about IV fluids
- **High level of competence is needed to complete an ADRT** – once patient has a diagnosis of dementia, they may not be able to complete one

Survival rates following CPR[23]
Most cardiac arrests occur in the community. Following out-of-hospital cardiac arrest, 30% of people achieved return of circulation, but only 9% survive to hospital discharge. Following in-hospital cardiac arrest, 53% achieved return of circulation with 23.6% surviving to discharge.

22 General Medical Council (2010) *Cardiopulmonary resuscitation guidance*
23 Resuscitation Council UK (2021) *Epidemiology of cardiac arrest guidelines*

Elder abuse

'A single or repeated act or lack of appropriate action, occurring within any relationship where there is an expectation of trust, which causes harm or distress to an older person.'[24]

Types of abuse

- **Financial**
  - ▶ misusing a patient's money in a way that controls or limits their life and/or actions

    sales scams, spending older person's money on themselves, pressuring older person to sign over their property / change their will
- **Emotional/psychological**
  - ▶ treating someone in a way that makes them feel threatened/belittled/ embarrassed

    shouting at person, insulting them, threatening them, ignoring them
- **Physical**
  - ▶ physically hurting someone

    slapping, hitting, rough handling, restraining
- **Sexual**
  - ▶ touching someone in a way that they don't want to be touched
  - ▶ also use of inappropriate sexual language / forcing someone to watch sexual material
- **Neglect/abandonment**
  - ▶ neglecting someone's needs: **NOT ALWAYS INTENTIONAL (passive neglect)**

    denied access to bathroom/food/phone
    left in soiled sheets / unsafe environment
    incorrect dose / timing of medication

May happen if there are frustrated relatives or poorly trained carers

Recognising abuse

Physical signs:
- Bruising (may be hidden – examine carefully)
- Unkempt appearance / soiled clothes
- Malnourished
- Low mood/self-esteem

Other signs:
- Behaviour/mood changes
- Strained relationships / spoken to harshly
- Appearing fearful/nervous around people
- Withdrawal from social activity
- Struggling financially

OUR RESPONSIBILITY

If you are concerned, you MUST TAKE ACTION
- Document concerns and escalate to someone more senior
- Consider an adults' safeguarding referral via *Multi Agency Safeguarding Hub*

Never agree to keep things secret
- Try to talk to the patient and reassure them that you are there to help

[24] WHO (2021) *Elder abuse factsheet*

GYNAECOLOGY

03

ABBREVIATIONS

AFP – Alpha fetoprotein
AIDS – Acquired immune deficiency syndrome
AMH – Anti-Müllerian hormone
ART – Anti-retroviral treatment
BMD – Bone mineral density
BPH – Benign prostatic hyperplasia
BSO – Bilateral salpingo-oophorectomy
BV – Bacterial vaginosis
CF – Cystic fibrosis
CIN – Cervical intraepithelial neoplasia
CL – Corpus luteum
COCP – Combined oral contraceptive pill
Cu – Copper
DEXA – Dual-energy X-ray absorptiometry
EC – Emergency contraception
ERPC – Extraction of retained products of conception
FCU – First catch urine
FISH – Fluorescence *in situ* hybridisation
FR – Failure rate
FSH – Follicle-stimulating hormone
FSU – First-stream urine
GBS – Group B Streptococcus
GDM – Gestational diabetes mellitus
GnRH – Gonadotrophin-releasing hormone
HIV – Human immunodeficiency virus
HMB – Heavy menstrual bleeding

HNPCC – Hereditary non-polyposis colorectal cancer
HPV – Human papillomavirus
HRT – Hormone replacement therapy
HSV – Herpes simplex virus
IAP – Intra-abdominal pressure
IBS – Irritable bowel syndrome
ICSI – Intracytoplasmic sperm injection
IMB – Intermenstrual bleeding
IUD – Intrauterine device
IUI – Intrauterine insemination
IUS – Intrauterine system
LBW – Low birth weight
LH – Luteinising hormone
LLETZ – Large loop excision of transformation zone
LMP – Last menstrual period
LN – Lymph node
LNG – Levonorgestrel
MS – Multiple sclerosis
MSU – Mid-stream urine
NAAT – Nucleic acid amplification test
(N)NRTI – (Non)-nucleoside reverse transcriptase inhibitor
OCP – Oral contraceptive pill
OHSS – Ovarian hyperstimulation syndrome
PCB – Post-coital bleeding
PCO – Polycystic ovaries

PCOS – Polycystic ovary syndrome
PCP – *Pneumocystis* pneumonia
PCR – Polymerase chain reaction
PGD – Pre-implantation genetic diagnosis
PI – Protease inhibitor
PID – Pelvic inflammatory disease
PMB – Post-menopausal bleeding
PMS – Premenstrual syndrome
POP – Progesterone-only pill
PROM – Premature rupture of membranes
PUFR – Perfect use failure rate
PV – Per vagina
RPOC – Retained products of conception
RUQ – Right upper quadrant
SNRI – Selective noradrenaline reuptake inhibitor
SSRI – Selective serotonin reuptake inhibitor
STI – Sexually transmitted infection
TOP – Termination of pregnancy
TSH – Thyroid-stimulating hormone
TUFR – Typical use failure rate
TV – Transvaginal
UPA – Ulipristal acetate
UPSI – Unprotected sexual intercourse
VDRL – Venereal disease research laboratory test
VE – Vaginal examination
VIN – Vulval intraepithelial neoplasia

Abnormalities of the uterus

Polyps

→ *small, benign tumours of the uterine cavity* – **endometrial origin**

↳ 0.2–1.5% become malignant

SYMPTOMS: may be asymptomatic
- HMB & IMB
- May prolapse through cervix

MANAGEMENT OPTIONS: (80% managed with outpatient hysteroscopy)
- Hysteroscopic resection with diathermy ⎫
- Hysteroscopy + morcellation* if large ⎬ *Complications of*
- Avulsion (twist & tear off polyp with forceps) ⎭ *bleeding & infection*
→ removed polyp sent for histology

INVESTIGATIONS:
- TV USS
- Hysteroscopy

Risk factors for polyps
- 40–50y
- high oestrogen (e.g. tamoxifen Tx)

*Morcellation = cutting uterine/fibroid tissue into smaller pieces to allow laparoscopic or hysteroscopic removal

Fibroids/leiomyomata

→ *benign tumours of the uterine cavity* – **myometrial origin**

↳ 25% women

PATHOLOGY
- **Location:** subserosal, intramural, submucosal — can form intracavity polyps
- **Size varies:** mm to cm
- **Growth** due to oestrogen/progesterone (stop & calcify after menopause)

SYMPTOMS
- **Asymptomatic:** 50%
- **HMB:** 30%
- **IMB** – if submucosal/polypoid
- **Pressure effects:** urinary freq./retention, hydronephrosis
- **Subfertility**

INVESTIGATIONS
- History & examination: **palpable, solid mass** in pelvis/abdo
- Bloods: Hb may be ↓ if HMB, or ↑ if fibroid secretes EPO
- TV USS: shows mass **continuous with uterus**
- MRI/laparoscopy: distinguish from ovarian mass & adenomyosis
- Hysteroscopy: assess uterine distortion

MANAGEMENT[1]
1. **No treatment:** if asymptomatic & slow growth
2. **Medical:** preserves fertility
   - GnRH: temporary shrinkage (max 6m use)
     → *often used for 2–3m pre-surgery*
3. **Surgical:** only myomectomy preserves fertility
   - Hysteroscopic transcervical resection of fibroid (TCRF) ± morcellation: if polypoid or submucosal <3cm
   - Myomectomy: failed medical Tx but **want to preserve fertility**
   - Hysterectomy: most effective
4. **Other:**
   - Uterine artery embolisation (UAE) → *cut off blood supply to fibroid*

HRT can cause continued growth after menopause

Risk factors for fibroids/leiomyomata
- Peri-menopausal
- Afro-Caribbean
- FHx polyps
- Nulliparous

COCP/progesterones = PROTECTIVE

Complications of fibroids
- **Torsion** of pedunculated fibroid
- **Degenerations**
  - ▶ *Red*: pain, haemorrhage, necrosis
  - ▶ *Hyaline/cystic*: liquefied & soft
  - ▶ *Calcification*: post-menopausal
- **Malignancy:** leiomyosarcoma (0.1%)

Trial tranexamic acid, NSAIDs, progesterones to control HMB: will be ineffective if HMB due to fibroid

Myomectomy complications: bleeding, infection, adhesions

---

[1] NICE (2018, updated 2021) *Heavy menstrual bleeding* [NG88]

Adenomyosis

→ *endometrial tissue growth within the myometrium*
  ↳ *exact cause unknown*

SYMPTOMS: may be asymptomatic
- HMB & IMB
- Dysmenorrhoea
- **Enlarged, tender uterus**

INVESTIGATIONS
- **MRI** gives definitive diagnosis

MANAGEMENT[2]
Medical:
- IUS/COCP ± NSAIDs (control HMB/dysmenorrhoea)

Surgical:
- **Hysterectomy** (usually required)

> **Risk factors for adenomyosis**
> - >40y
> - endometriosis
> - fibroids

Endometriosis

→ *endometrial tissue growth outside of uterus*
  ↳ *Affects 10% of women of fertile age*

PATHOLOGY
- **Growth:** oestrogen-dependent (regress after menopause)
- **Location:** anywhere in pelvis* (uterosacral ligaments & on/behind ovaries = common) *(rarely spreads outside pelvis)*
- **Disease process:** inflammation, progressive fibrosis & adhesions

SYMPTOMS: may be asymptomatic if mild
- **CHRONIC PELVIC PAIN = cyclical**
- Dysmenorrhoea before menstruation (peaks day 1)
- Deep dyspareunia
- Pain on passing stools
- **Subfertility** → endometriosis found in 25% subfertility Ix

SIGNS
- Retro-uterine/adnexal **tenderness &/or thickening**
- Uterus may be **retroverted & immobile**
- Nodule of endometrial tissue may be palpable on VE

INVESTIGATIONS
- TV USS
- Laparoscopy ± biopsy gives definitive diagnosis
- MRI: r/o adenomyosis
- Barium studies: assess ureteric, bladder, bowel involvement if necessary

MANAGEMENT[3]
No treatment: if asymptomatic
Medical: no improvement in fertility
- Analgesia: NSAIDs ± paracetamol or opiates
- Back-to-back COCP, POP, GnRH, IUS – suppress ovarian function & oestrogen levels

Surgical: may improve fertility
- Laparoscopic excision or laser/bipolar diathermy (ablation of lesions)
- Adhesiolysis
- Cystectomy of ovarian endometrioma
- Hysterectomy + bilateral salpingo-oophorectomy (BSO) if conservative Mx fails & fertility is not important

> **Risk factors for endometriosis**
> - 30–45y
> - nulliparous
> - genetics

Rarely spreads outside pelvis

> **Complications of endometriosis**
> - **Chocolate cyst (endometrioma):** accumulated, dark brown blood in ovaries
>   → **rupture causes acute pain**
> - **Frozen pelvis:** in very severe cases pelvic organs immobile due to adhesions

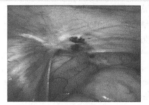

Fig. 3.1 Endometrioma.

active lesions = red vesicles/marks
less active lesions = white scars/brown spots ('powder burn')

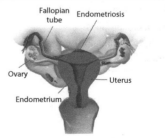

Fig. 3.2 Common locations of endometriosis.

> **Risks of surgery**
> Damage to bowel, bladder, vessels, ureters

---

[2] NICE (2018, updated 2021) *Heavy menstrual bleeding* [NG88]
[3] ESHRE (2013) *Management of women with endometriosis*

Disorders of the ovaries

Functional cyst: persistent corpus luteum
- very common & no Mx needed if <5cm

Mucinous cyst: can become enormous
- can cause pressure Sx (e.g. urinary freq.)
- 5% become malignant
- Mx: oophorectomy & histology

Dermoid cyst: contain hair/skin/teeth

Worrying cyst features:

>5cm / rapid growth, multi-loculated, post-menopausal development, ascites

Diagnostic criteria

PCO = ≥12 small follicles in an enlarged ovary

PCOS = ≥2 of:
- **PCO** on TV USS
- **irregular menstrual periods** (>35d apart)
- **hirsutism** (↑acne/hair or ↑serum testosterone)

Complications of PCOS
- T2DM (50% women)
- GDM (30% women)
- Endometrial cancer

Risk factors for PCOS
- Genetics
- ↑weight
- DM/FHx DM

FSH interpretation re anovulation

Raised: ovarian failure
Low: hypothalamic disease
Normal: PCOS

Ovarian cyst accidents

1. Rupture of cyst contents into peritoneal cavity → intense pain
2. Haemorrhage into peritoneal cavity → pain + hypovolaemic shock
3. Torsion of ovarian pedicle → severe pain + ovary/tube infarction
   ↳ urgent surgery needed

Polycystic ovary syndrome (PCOS)

PATHOLOGY
Raised LH (disordered production) & insulin levels (due to resistance) cause ↑**androgen production** in the ovaries
→ disrupts folliculogenesis = multiple small follicles
→ disrupts menstrual cycle = oligo-/amenorrhoea
→ physical manifestations = hirsutism

SYMPTOMS
- **Infertility** – cause of 80% anovulatory cases
- Obesity
- Acne / ↑hair (hirsutism)
- Oligo-/amenorrhoea (periods >35d apart)

INVESTIGATIONS: exclude other causes for symptoms
1. **Blood tests:** LH levels
   - **For anovulation:** FSH, prolactin, TSH, day 21 progesterone
   - **For hirsutism:** serum testosterone   albumin-bound
2. **TV USS:** for PCO
3. **Other:** fasting glucose & lipids (DM screen)

MANAGEMENT[4]
- Diet & lifestyle advice: ↓insulin resistance to improve symptoms
- Metformin ↑insulin sensitisation & improve hirsutism

If fertility not required:
- COCP (2nd line = anti-androgens) regulate menstruation & improve hirsutism

If fertility required:
- **Joint 1st-line:** clomifene (anti-oestrogen) triggers –ve feedback loop to ↑LH & FSH production & follicle development
- **Joint 1st-line:** letrozole (aromatase inhibitor) prevents conversion of androgens to oestrogens, ↑FSH & ovulation
- Laparoscopic ovarian diathermy
- Gonadotrophins (FSH ± LH) if clomifene has failed

[4]ESHRE (2018) *International evidence-based guideline for the assessment and management of polycystic ovary syndrome*

Disorders of the vulva & vagina

Vulval symptoms

- Pruritus – dermatological disease, neoplasia, infections
- Soreness/burning
- Superficial dyspareunia

Benign disorders

LICHEN SIMPLEX (CHRONIC VULVAL DERMATITIS)
→ chronic inflammatory skin condition
- **RFs:** sensitive skin/eczema, stress
- **Sx:** severe pruritus (worse at night), inflamed/thickened labia
- **Dx:** biopsy if unsure
- **Mx:** emollients, moderate potency steroid creams, antihistamines; avoid irritants

LICHEN PLANUS
→ dermatological disease commonly affecting mucosal surfaces
- **RFs:** ?autoimmune link
- **Sx:** flat papular purple lesions, pain
- **Mx:** high potency steroid creams

LICHEN SCLEROSUS → thinning of vulval epithelium due to collagen loss
- **RFs:** ?autoimmune link e.g. thyroid disease, vitiligo
- **Sx:** severe pruritus (worse at night), pain/dyspareunia, pink–white papules, parchment-like skin with fissures
- **Dx:** biopsy to exclude carcinoma
- **Mx:** ultra-potent topical steroids

VULVODYNIA (VULVAL PAIN)
→ can be provoked/spontaneous, local/generalised
- **RFs:** genital tract infections, use of OCP
- **Sx:** burning pain (generalised), superficial dyspareunia (localised)
- **Mx:** amitriptyline, gabapentin

BARTHOLIN'S GLAND CYST/ABSCESS
→ **CYST:** blocked duct causes mucus build-up
→ **ABSCESS:** infected cyst (E. coli / Staphylococcus)
- **Sx:** acutely painful red swelling
- **Mx:** incision & drainage

VAGINAL CYSTS → congenital
- **Sx:** smooth white lump ± superficial dyspareunia
- **Mx:** excision if symptomatic

VAGINAL ADENOSIS → columnar epithelium found in the normally squamous epithelium of vagina
- **RFs:** mother was given DES (diethylstilboestrol) during pregnancy (1940–70)
- **Mx:** usually resolves spontaneously BUT can **become malignant** (clear cell carcinoma)

VULVAL INTRAEPITHELIAL NEOPLASIA (VIN)
→ presence of atypical cells in vulval epithelium
- **RFs:** HPV 16, smoking, immunosuppression
- **Sx:** pruritus/pain, nodules/warts/papules/plaques
- **Mx:** emollients, mild topical steroids

Candida
HSV
Viral warts
Syphilis

Superficial dyspareunia = pain on initial penetration during intercourse
Deep dyspareunia = pain felt within the pelvis on deep penetration during intercourse

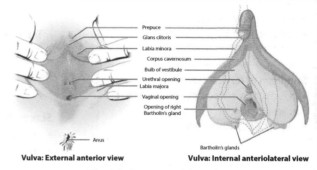

Prepuce
Glans clitoris
Labia minora
Corpus cavernosum
Bulb of vestibule
Urethral opening
Labia majora
Vaginal opening
Opening of right
Bartholin's gland

Anus

Bartholin's glands

Vulva: External anterior view

Vulva: Internal anteriolateral view

Fig. 3.3 Anatomy of the vulva.

Give ABX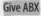

Drainage with Word catheter or marsupialisation (sutures to keep cyst open)

Conditions of the cervix

Frequency of screening

25–49y = every 3y
50–65y = every 5y
>65y = only if recent abnormal smear

Risk factors for cervical cancer
- **HPV 16 & 18** (↑ sexual contacts)
- Smoking
- Immunosuppressed/HIV
- Long-term OCP use (v. small risk)

Symptoms of cervical cancer
- bleeding between periods, after sex, after menopause
- change in vaginal discharge

Preventing cervical cancer:
HPV vaccine, barrier contraception, screening

CIN = cervical intraepithelial neoplasia
→ pre-cancerous changes to cells

Grade depends on **amount of dyskaryosis** (abnormal nuclei)

CIN I = atypical cells in ⅓ epithelium
CIN II = atypical cells in ⅔ epithelium
CIN III = atypical cells throughout
⅓ become malignant in 10y

Cervical screening

AIMS
1. Reduce incidence of cervical cancer by detecting pre-cancerous changes
2. Reduce mortality from invasive **cervical carcinoma**

METHOD: *cervical smear test*
- Insert **Cusco's speculum**
- Use brush to sweep around **transformation zone**
- **Liquid-based cytology** of cells collected (centrifuge + microscopy)
- HPV also tested for in this sample

Transformation zone = area of metaplasia between squamous and columnar epithelium
Oestrogen causes columnar epithelium to evert onto endocervix
→ exposure to acidic vagina causes metaplasia to squamous epithelium

HPV PRIMARY SCREENING[5]
Screen for high risk HPV (16 & 18) in smear before cytology for dyskaryosis
- high risk HPV present in 99.7% cervical cancers
- more sensitive test (fewer false negatives)

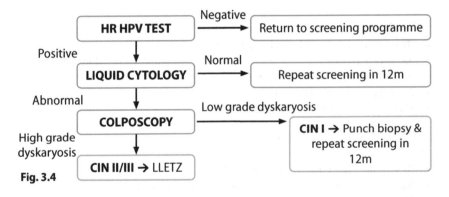

Fig. 3.4

Colposcopy

METHOD
- speculum to open vagina & colposcope to examine cervix
- **acetic acid** added to stain cells → abnormal cells turn white
- **biopsies taken** for histological examination & definitive diagnosis
  (CIN I, II, III or rarely cervical cancer)

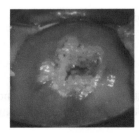

Fig. 3.5 Abnormal cells stained white with acetic acid.

---

[5] PHE (2021) *Cervical screening: programme and colposcopy management*

LLETZ = large loop excision of transformation zone

METHOD
- excision of abnormal cells under local anaesthetic
- diathermy (heat) can stop bleeding vessels

COUNSELLING POST-PROCEDURE
- avoid tampons & intercourse for 4w
- one treatment of LLETZ **doesn't reduce fertility**
- may have some bleeding / brown discharge (if offensive get ABX from GP)

Benign conditions of the cervix

Ectropion/erosion: area of eversion at transformation zone appears red
- **Sx:** may present with vaginal discharge or post-coital bleeding
- **Tx of bleeding:** cryotherapy*

Acute cervicitis: due to STIs (rare)

Chronic cervicitis: inflammation/infection usually of ectropion
- **Sx:** vaginal discharge
- **Tx:** cryotherapy ± ABX

Polyps: benign tumours of endocervical epithelium
- **Sx:** asymptomatic/IMB/PCB
- **Tx:** avulsion & histology

Cervical intraepithelial neoplasia (CIN)

→ *pre-malignant changes to cervical epithelium due to **HPV** (16 & 18)*
Epidemiology: peak 25–29y
RF: same as for cervical cancer
Pathology: exposure of cells at transformation zone to HPV results in incorporation of viral DNA into cells
Symptoms: asymptomatic but risk of cervical malignancy
Diagnosis: cervical smear screening programme
Management: if HPV positive refer to colposcopy

Complications/risks of LLETZ
- post-op haemorrhage (1–2%)
- cervical stenosis
- small increased risk preterm labour & PROM

Rule out carcinoma first with colposcopy

Reassure women with CIN that these are **pre-malignant** changes & colposcopic treatment is straightforward and very successful

Gynae-oncology

PALLIATIVE CARE: MDT of GP, cancer nurses, specialist gynae unit
1. PAIN CONTROL – analgesic ladder
2. N&V – antiemetics/antihistamines
3. HEAVY VAGINAL BLEEDING – high dose progesterones/radiotherapy (advanced cervical/endometrial cancers)
4. ASCITES/BOWEL OBSTRUCTION – paracentesis, antiemetics, stool softeners, antispasmodics (advanced ovarian cancers)

Indications for radiotherapy
1. **Primary therapy:** if unfit for surgery or gross metastases
2. **Adjunct therapy:** used pre- or post-op
3. **Recurrent disease**

Hysterectomy complications/risks
- Small bowel obstruction
- Bladder dysfunction
- Ureteral strictures
- Damage to other structures
- Blood loss
- Infection
- VTE/PE
- Fistulae

Definitions
PMB: post-menopausal bleeding

EUA: examination under anaesthetic

Trachelectomy: removal of 80% cervix + upper vagina

Type	Pathology	Epidemiology	RFs	Symptoms	Investigation	Staging	Treatment
Endometrial *Most common*	**90% adenocarcinoma** (columnar endometrial glands) (↓ prognosis); **10% adenosquamous carcinoma**; Uterine sarcomas = rare	Peak **60y**; 85% post-menopause; 75% 5y survival	**↑oestrogen > progesterone**: obesity, PCOS, nulliparous, late menopause, unopposed therapy (oestrogen/tamoxifen); DM, HTN, Lynch type 2; PROTECTIVE: COCP & pregnancy	**Post-menopausal**: Bleeding (10% risk), Discharge (50% risk); **Pre-menopausal**: IMB, recent onset HMB, atrophic vaginitis	TV USS; Endometrial biopsy a) Pipelle b) hysteroscopic = diagnostic; Hysteroscopy = staging; MRI/CXR = assess spread	**Pre-malignant**: atypical hyperplasia; **Stage 1**: uterus only; **Stage 2**: + cervix; **Stage 3**: through uterine wall/ LN involvement; **Stage 4**: bladder/bowel or distant mets; • Spreads via pelvic + para-aortic LNs	**Stage 1**: Hysterectomy + BSO + post-op radiotherapy if high risk LN involvement; **Stage >1**: Radiotherapy
Ovarian *Poorest prognosis*	**90% epithelial carcinomas**; **If <30y:** germ cell tumours most common	Peak **70–80y**; <35% 5y survival as presents late; Annual screening if BRCA1/2 mutations	**↑ovulations**: early menarche, late menopause, nulliparous, FHx BRCA1 or 2, FHx HNPCC (Lynch); PROTECTIVE: COCP, lactation, pregnancy	**Initially asymp.**; abdo distension, abdo/pelvic mass, early satiety, weight loss, pelvic/abdo pain, urine urge/freq., altered bowels, ascites; Similar to IBS Sx	**Women >50y**: CA125 levels, USS abdo/pelvis; **Women <40y**: + AFP & hCG (In case germ cell tumour); CT abdo/pelvis = assess spread	**Stage 1**: ovaries only; **Stage 2**: pelvis only; **Stage 3**: abdomen only; **Stage 4**: beyond abdo; • Mostly direct spread; • Also via para-aortic LNs	Total hysterectomy + BSO + partial omentectomy; **≥Stage 2**: + LN dissection + post-op chemo; **Advanced / unfit for surgery:** palliative

	Histology / prognosis	Peak / survival	Risk factors	Symptoms	Investigations	Staging	Management
Cervical	90% squamous cell carcinomas 10% columnar cell adenocarcinomas (↓ *prognosis*)	2 peaks: **30y & 80y** 65% 5y survival	**HPV 16 & 18** • ↑ sexual contacts • unvaccinated **Other** • smoking • immunosuppressed/ HIV • long-term OCP use (*very small risk*)	• PCB • IMB • PMB • offensive discharge **Later signs:** Pelvic pain, anaemia, uraemia, haematuria, rectal bleeding	Biopsy = *diagnostic* VE/DRE & EUA = *assess size* MRI = *size, spread, LN involvement*	**Pre-malignant:** CIN (1–3) **Stage 1:** cervix only **Stage 2:** + upper ²⁄₃ vagina **Stage 3:** + lower ¹⁄₃ vagina or pelvic wall or ureteric obstruction ± LNs **Stage 4:** bladder/rectum or further	**1a:** cone biopsy (*preserves fertility*) **1b–2a AND –ve LNs:** Radical hysterectomy OR Trachelectomy (*preserves fertility*) **≥2b OR +ve LNs:** Chemo–radiotherapy
Vulval	95% squamous cell carcinoma 5% melanoma, basal cell carcinoma, adenocarcinoma	Peak at **>60y** Stage 1: >90% 5y survival Stage 3–4: 40% 5y survival	• Lichen sclerosus • Paget's disease of vulva • Immunosuppression • Smoking	• Pruritus • Bleeding • Discharge • Ulcer/mass on labia/ clitoris • Lymphadenopathy	Biopsy	**Premalignant:** VIN **Stage 1:** vulva/perineum only **Stage 2:** adjacent spread (urethra/ vagina) but no LNs **Stage 3:** +ve LNs **Stage 4:** upper vagina, rectum/bladder, distant mets Superficial & deep inguinal LNs → femoral & external iliac	**Stage 1:** wide local excision **Stage >1:** wide local excision + groin lymphadenectomy + radiotherapy if LN +ve
Vaginal	Usually squamous cell carcinoma	50% 5y survival	Older women	• Bleeding • Discharge • Mass/ulcer	Biopsy	**Stage 1:** vagina only **Stage 2:** through vaginal wall **Stage 3:** reached pelvic wall **or** LNs **Stage 4:** bladder/rectum/ beyond pelvis	Intravaginal radiotherapy OR radical surgery

The menstrual cycle

Features of normal menstruation

Menarche <16y
Menopause >45y
Menstruation <8d
Blood loss <80ml

Cycle length 23–35d
No intermenstrual bleeding (IMB)

Stages of female puberty

>8y = ↑ GnRH = ↑ LH/FSH = ↑ oestrogen
9–11y: oestrogen causes development of 2° sexual characteristics
11–13y: menarche (onset of menstruation)

breasts → pubic hair → growth spurt → menarche

Oestrogen causes proliferative changes (thickening of endometrium, spiral artery growth)

Progesterone causes secretory changes (stromal cells ↑, glands swell, blood supply ↑)

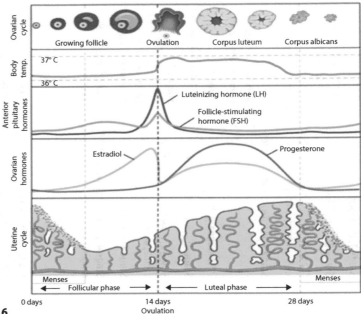

Fig. 3.6

1. FOLLICULAR PHASE (DAYS 1–14)

A) Menstruation (days 1–4): endometrium shedding + myometrial contractions

B) Proliferative phase (days 5–13):
- **GnRH pulses** from hypothalamus stimulate **LH & FSH release**
- FSH stimulates **follicle development** → follicles produce **oestrogen & inhibin**
- Low level oestrogen + inhibin = **–ve feedback** to inhibit >1 follicle developing
- **Graafian (dominant) follicle** continues to grow & produce oestrogen
- Oestrogen levels peak → **+ve feedback occurs** → **LH SURGE**

2. OVULATION (DAY 14/MID-CYCLE):
- 36h after LH surge = follicle rupture
- Graafian follicle becomes corpus luteum

3. LUTEAL/SECRETORY PHASE (DAYS 14–28)
- Corpus luteum produces progesterone > oestrogen = –ve feedback so ↓ FSH/LH
- **If no fertilisation:** corpus luteum degenerates after 14d = ↓ progesterone → endometrial degeneration & menstruation

Hormone	Gland	Effects
FSH	Anterior Pituitary	Acts on follicle granulosa cells in ovary: 1. Follicle development → oestrogen & inhibin production
LH	Anterior Pituitary	1. LH surge causes ovulation 2. Maintenance of corpus luteum
Oestrogen	Ovaries (follicle/CL)	1. Endometrial proliferation 2. Thinning of cervical mucus (better for sperm)
Progesterone	Ovaries (CL)	1. Stimulates secretory phase 2. Inhibits LH & FSH

Menorrhagia (HMB)

>80ml blood loss interfering with physical, social, emotional quality of life

CAUSES
- Idiopathic/dysfunctional uterine bleeding (majority)
- Uterine fibroids (30%)
- Polyps (10%)
- Adenomyosis
- Coagulopathies (rare)
- Consider IUD as cause

INVESTIGATIONS
- **History:** amount & timing of bleeding
- **Examination:** signs of anaemia, palpation of masses, pelvic tenderness
- **FBC:** Hb (TFTs & clotting if history suggests necessary)
- **TV USS:** exclude masses, detect polyps
- **Endometrial Pipelle biopsy:** exclude malignancy
- **Hysteroscopy:** allows biopsy & inspection of uterine cavity

MANAGEMENT[6]
1st-line: IUS – not suitable if want to conceive

+ may need iron supplements if anaemic

2nd-line:
- Tranexamic acid = antifibrinolytic
- NSAIDs – useful if + dysmenorrhoea
- COCP

3rd-line:
- Progesterones
- GnRH agonist – limited to 6m use

Surgical:
- Hysteroscopic polyp removal
- Endometrial ablation – destroy endometrium to ↓ bleeding
- Myomectomy – fibroid removal (GnRH first to ↓ size)
- Hysterectomy – last resort

> **Indications for endometrial biopsy (Pipelle/hysteroscopic)**
> - endometrial **thickness >10mm** (or >4mm post-menopausal)
> - **polyp** suspected
> - **>40y** with recent onset HMB/IMB/ treatment resistant
> - **RFs for cancer:** PCOS, FHx, HNPCC, obesity/DM

reduces fertility & pregnancy would be high risk → permanent contraception recommended

Inter-menstrual bleeding (IMB)*

→ *common in early or late reproductive years*

CAUSES
- Fibroids, polyps, ovarian cysts
- Adenomyosis
- Chronic pelvic infection
- Malignancy – recent onset/older

INVESTIGATIONS: **same as for HMB**
→ detect anaemia, exclude local pathology & malignancy

MANAGEMENT
Medical: if no anatomical cause detected
- IUS/COCP – lighter bleeding
- Progesterones – cause amenorrhoea
- HRT – if irregular bleeding during menopause

Surgical: same as for HMB
- Polyp removal, myomectomy, hysterectomy

*HMB often coexists

Ablation less effective in IMB

Dysmenorrhoea

→ *high prostaglandin levels cause painful uterine contraction & ischaemia*

PRIMARY[7]:**
- **Cause:** no organic cause
- **Tx:** NSAIDs/ COCP

50% women (esp. adolescents)

SECONDARY:***
- **Cause:** pelvic pathology – fibroids, adenomyosis, endometriosis, PID, malignancy
- **Sx:** ± deep dyspareunia, HMB
- **Ix:** pelvic USS, hysteroscopy
- **Tx:** depends on cause

**With start of menstruation

***Precedes & relieved by menstruation

---

[6] NICE (2018, updated 2021) *Heavy menstrual bleeding* [NG88]
[7] NICE (2018) CKS Clinical management scenario – *Dysmenorrhoea*

*Always abnormal (unless 1st intercourse)

Post-coital bleeding*

→ vaginal bleeding **after intercourse** that is **not menstrual loss**

CAUSES
- Endometrial instability – most common cause, especially with use of hormonal contraception
- Cervical carcinoma: <1% but MUST EXCLUDE
- Cervical ectropions/eversion – Tx with cryotherapy
- Benign cervical polyps – Tx with avulsion & biopsy
- Cervicitis, atrophic vaginitis

INVESTIGATIONS
- Cervical **inspection (speculum) & smear**
- Colposcopy if abnormal appearance of cervix

Amenorrhoea/oligomenorrhoea

→ absent/infrequent menstrual bleeding

PRIMARY: menstruation not started by 16y
1. **Delayed puberty:** secondary sexual characteristics not present by 14y
2. **Menstrual outflow problem:** imperforate hymen, transverse vaginal septum
3. **Congenital:** Turner syndrome (1 missing X chromosome), congenital adrenal hyperplasia

SECONDARY: menstruation ceases for ≥6m
1. **Hypothalamic hypogonadism** = ↓FSH/LH & therefore ↓oestrogen
   - **Causes:** psychological (stress), anorexia, excess exercise
   - **Tx:** oestrogen replacement (COCP/HRT)
2. **Hyperprolactinaemia** = inhibits GnRH
   - **Causes:** pituitary hyperplasia, benign adenoma (prolactinoma), medications (methyldopa, opiates, heroin)
   - **Tx:** bromocriptine, cabergoline + endocrine referral
3. **Hyper-/hypothyroidism**
4. **PCOS** – often oligomenorrhoea + subfertility   most common cause
5. **Premature menopause** 1 in 100 women

Causes cyclical lower abdo pain

Physiological causes of amenorrhoea
- Pregnancy/lactation
- Menopause
- Drugs

Investigations
- History & examination
- PREGNANCY TEST (urine hCG)
- FSH/LH, prolactin, testosterone
- TFTs
- Pelvic USS for PCOS
- MRI/CT if suspect tumours

Management: treat underlying cause & bone protection (HRT)

Stimulates ↑ dopamine release which inhibits prolactin

Premenstrual syndrome (PMS)
95% women
5% = severely debilitating

→ psychological, behavioural & physical **symptoms experienced regularly in luteal phase** of cycle

Cause:
Unknown – progesterone involved

Symptoms:
Psychological/behavioural: irritability, aggression, depression
Physical: bloated, GI upset, breast pain

Investigations:
Menstrual diaries: record mood & symptoms

Management[8]:
- **SSRIs** – continuous or intermittent
- **Oral contraception** – continuous
- **HRT** – oestrogen patches
- **GnRH agonists + add-back HRT** (if severe/Tx-resistant)

+ **Non-pharmacological:** diet, exercise, CBT

[8] RCOG (2016) *Management of premenstrual syndrome* [GTG48]

Subfertility

Where conception has not occurred **after 1y of UPSI** *15% couples*

Causes of subfertility

1. **Anovulation** (30%) = egg not produced
2. **Male factor problem** (25%) = inadequate sperm
3. **Disorders of fertilisation** (30%) = sperm doesn't reach egg
4. **Unexplained** (15%) = large proportion may result from defective implantation

Anovulation

DETECTING OVULATION

- **Serum progesterone** – day 21 (mid-luteal) increase
- **LH detecting kits (over the counter)** – detect LH surge
- **Temperature** – ↓0.2°C pre-ovulation & ↑0.5°C after
- **USS to detect follicle size/rupture** – not often used
- **Anti-Müllerian hormone (AMH)** – indicator of ovarian reserve

CAUSES OF ANOVULATION[9]

1. PCOS*
- **Causes:** disordered LH production (↑) & insulin resistance
- **RFs:** genetics, high BMI, T2DM
- **Symptoms:** infertility, oligomenorrhoea, hirsutism
- **Investigations**
  ▸ Bloods
  ▸ TV USS: for PCO
  ▸ DM screen: fasting glucose & lipids
- **Management**
  ▸ Clomifene citrate (anti-oestrogen) – triggers –ve feedback to ↑ LH & FSH for follicle development
  ▸ Metformin, diet & weight advice – insulin sensitisation
  ▸ Laparoscopic ovarian diathermy
  ▸ COCP/anti-androgens – regulate menstruation/hirsutism

2. Hyperprolactinaemia = ↑ prolactin = ↓ GnRH
- **Causes:** benign pituitary adenoma, pituitary hyperplasia, PCOS, hypothyroidism, psychotropic drugs
- **Symptoms:** oligo-/amenorrhoea, galactorrhoea, headaches, bitemporal hemianopia
- **Investigations:** bloods (↑ prolactin), CT scan
- **Management:** dopamine agonist (bromocriptine/cabergoline), surgery

3. Hypothalamic hypogonadism = ↓ GnRH release = ↓ LH/FSH & oestrogen
- **Causes:** anorexia nervosa / ↓ BMI, athletes, stress, Kallmann syndrome
- **Symptoms:** amenorrhoea
- **Investigations:** bloods (↓ GnRH, LH, FSH & oestrogen)
- **Management:** GnRH pump + bone protection (COCP/HRT), restore weight

4. Pituitary damage – causes include tumours & infarction
5. Premature ovarian failure
6. Gonadal dysgenesis
7. Hypo-/hyperthyroidism

> **Important to involve a trained counsellor / provide psychological support for the couple**

> **FSH interpretation re anovulation**
> **Raised:** ovarian failure
> **Low:** hypothalamic disease
> **Normal:** PCOS

*See notes on disorders of the ovaries

> **Pre-ovulation:** ↑ FSH, LH, oestrogen (& progesterone)
> **Post-ovulation:** fall in hormones if not fertilised

> **Blood test results in PCOS**
> - Raised LH
> - Raised testosterone
> - Raised AMH
> - Normal FSH/prolactin/TSH
> - Low 21-d progesterone

if fertility not required

> **Diagnostic criteria for PCOS**
> PCO = ≥12 small follicles in an enlarged ovary
> PCOS = ≥2 of:
> - **PCO** on TV USS
> - **irregular menstrual periods** (>35d apart)
> - **hirsutism** (↑ acne/hair or ↑ serum testosterone)

---

[9]NICE (2013, updated 2017) *Fertility problems* [CG156]

Ovarian hyperstimulation syndrome (OHSS)

- **Sx:** large, painful follicles (± oedema, ascites, SOB, hypovolaemia)
- **RF:** gonadotrophins, IVF, <35y, PCO
- **Ix:** FBC, U&Es/renal func, CXR, PV USS
- **Mx:** supportive – watch & wait (monitor closely) ± fluid tap
- **Prevent:** lowest dose gonadotrophins + USS monitoring

electrolyte imbalance

Drugs to induce ovulation

→ *First treat underlying cause*

1st-line: clomifene citrate (anti-oestrogens)

2nd-line:
- Gonadotrophins (FSH ± LH) – daily SC injections
- GnRH pump – in hypothalamic hypogonadism

Risks of ovulation induction:

>1 follicle develops = multiple pregnancy

Before offering ovulation stimulation:
1. Confirm anovulation with low 21-d progesterone
2. Ensure no tubal problems
3. Ensure no male factor problems

Male factor problem

SPERMATOGENESIS: **takes 70d**
- LH causes testosterone production in Leydig cells
- Testosterone & FSH control synthesis and transport of sperm in Sertoli cells

CAUSES OF INADEQUATE SPERM
- Idiopathic
- BMI
- Drugs – alcohol, smoking, anabolic steroids
- Industrial chemicals/solvents
- Varicocele – in 25% cases
- Anti-sperm antibodies – common after vasectomy reversal
- Infections – epididymitis, mumps, orchitis
- Congenital abnormalities / genetics, e.g. Klinefelter's (XXY), CF
- Hypothalamic problems / hypogonadotrophic hypogonadism

INVESTIGATIONS

Azoospermia + absent vas deferens = investigate for cystic fibrosis

1. **Semen analysis**
   - produced by masturbation after 2–7d abstinence
   - analysed within 1–2h
   - repeat for abnormal results in 12w
   - persistent abnormalities = scrotal exam & further investigations (see below)
2. **Blood tests:** FSH, LH, TSH, testosterone, prolactin
3. **Serum karyotype:** e.g. for Klinefelter's (XXY)

MANAGEMENT[10]

1. **Lifestyle advice**
   - reduce smoking/alcohol/drug exposure; weight loss
   - testicles below body temperature (*loose clothing / cooling methods*)
2. **Assisted conception**
   - **Mild oligospermia:** intrauterine insemination (IUI)
   - **Mod.–severe oligospermia:** IVF ± intracytoplasmic sperm injection (ICSI)
   - **Azoospermia:** sperm retrieval from testes + ICSI–IVF

> **Normal semen analysis**
> Volume: >1.5ml
> Sperm count: >15million/ml
> Progressive motility: >32%
>
> **Azoospermia:** no sperm
> **Severe oligospermia:** <5million/ml
> **Asthenospermia:** low motility

---

[10]NICE (2013, updated 2017) *Fertility problems* [CG156]

Disorders of fertilisation

1. TUBAL DAMAGE (25%)

- **Endometriosis:** → Tx = laparoscopic removal of deposits (IVF if unsuccessful)
- **Previous pelvic surgery:** cause adhesions around tubes
  → Tx = adhesiolysis/ salpingostomy (IVF if unsuccessful)
- **Infection:** PID/STIs cause adhesions around tubes → Tx = adhesiolysis/
  salpingostomy (IVF if unsuccessful)

2. CERVICAL PROBLEMS (<5%)

Causes: anti-sperm antibodies, infection ↓ mucus, cone biopsy
Mx: IUI to bypass cervix

3. SEXUAL PROBLEMS (5%)

Assisted conception[11]

offered after 2y of trying (& underlying causes treated)

INTRAUTERINE INSEMINATION (IUI): 15–20% success

- insert sperm into uterus – *often following gonadotrophin ovulation induction*
- cheaper than IVF but need patent fallopian tubes

IN VITRO FERTILISATION (IVF): 35% success per cycle (10% if >40y)

- sperm & oocyte mixed in Petri dish – *often following gonadotrophin ovulation induction*
- needs normal oocyte production → *not possible in ovarian failure*
- PGD if mother >37y / high risk genetic conditions

Steps:

1. **Follicular development:** 2w FSH ± LH then GnRH
2. **Ovulation induction:** identify mature follicles present with USS then single injection of LH/hCG
3. **Egg collection:** 35h later via transvaginal aspiration using USS guidance
4. **Fertilisation and transfer:** incubated with sperm and embryo transferred back to uterus at 3–6d

INTRACYTOPLASMIC SPERM INJECTION (ICSI): 90% success

- adjunct to IVF → sperm injected into oocyte

OTHER OPTIONS

- Oocyte donation from another woman, surrogacy, adoption

Increasing success rate

Summary of investigating subfertility

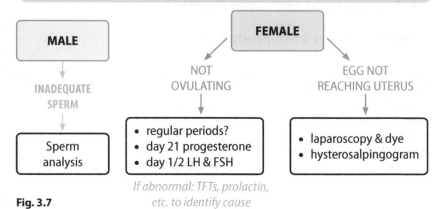

MALE

INADEQUATE
SPERM

Sperm
analysis

FEMALE

NOT
OVULATING

- regular periods?
- day 21 progesterone
- day 1/2 LH & FSH

If abnormal: TFTs, prolactin, etc. to identify cause

EGG NOT
REACHING UTERUS

- laparoscopy & dye
- hysterosalpingogram

Fig. 3.7

[11] NICE (2013, updated 2017) *Fertility problems* [CG156]

Incision in tube to clear blockage

12% are infertile after 1 episode of infection

Investigations

1. **Chlamydia serology**
2. **Laparoscopy & dye test** if chlamydia +ve or pain
   (assesses tube patency with flow of dye)
3. **Hysterosalpingogram:** if chlamydia –ve (use X-rays to visualise uterus & tubes)

Indications for assisted conception:

- all other methods have failed
- male factor subfertility
- unexplained subfertility (>2y)
- endometriosis / tubal blockage
- genetic disorders (allows PID)

Risks of IVF: infection, haemorrhage on egg collection, failure, multiple pregnancy, OHSS, ectopic

IVF criteria[11]

Women <40y offered 3 cycles if:

- 2y regular UPSI unsuccessful **OR**
- 12 cycles of IUI unsuccessful

Women 40–42y offered 1 cycle if:

- 2y UPSI **or** 12 cycles IUI unsuccessful **AND**
- never had IVF before **AND**
- no evidence of low ovarian reserve

If not eligible can pay for private Tx: £5000 per cycle

Pre-implantation genetic diagnosis (PGD)

- 2 cells removed before embryo retransferred to uterus
- PCR/FISH, etc. used to look for genetic abnormalities
- unaffected embryos selected and transferred to uterus

Indications: high risk of genetic conditions

Menopause

Average age of menopause = 51y

*continue HRT treatment until 51y

> **Osteoporosis:** T-score −2.5 or lower
> **Osteopenia:** T-score between −1 & −2.5
> T-score: number of standard deviations BMD differs from the mean

- **Menopause:** permanent cessation of menstruation due to loss of ovarian activity (**12m without a period**)
- **Perimenopause:** from first onset of symptoms to 12m after the last menstrual period
- **Post-menopause:** recognised after 12m since last menstrual period
- **Premature menopause:** menopause before 40y* → **1% women**

Symptoms

- **Vasomotor:** hot flushes & night sweats
- **Urinary problems** – frequency, urgency, nocturia, incontinence, infection
- **Vaginal atrophy** – dyspareunia, itching, burning, dryness
- **Loss of libido**
- **Psychological symptoms** – e.g. anxiety/depression, ↓ concentration
- **Risk of CVD**
- **Osteoporosis & fractures** – 1/3 women >50y
    - RFs: early menopause, long-term steroids, previous fracture, parental hip fracture

Investigations

1. To check ovarian reserve:
    - **FSH:** *raised* due to loss of −ve feedback from oestrogen
    - **Anti-Müllerian hormone:** *low* as normally produced by ovarian follicles
2. To rule out other causes of symptoms:
    - **TSH** – hyperthyroidism can cause hot flushes
    - **Catecholamines** – rule out phaeochromocytoma
    - **LH/oestradiol/progesterone**
3. To check for osteoporosis/fracture risk:
    - **DEXA scan & bone profile**
4. To check suitability for HRT:
    - **TV USS & endo biopsy** – for endometrial cancer
    - **Thrombophilia screen** – VTE risk

Management[12]

→ *aim of management = symptom relief*

HRT REGIMENS (oral, patch, gel, implant)
- **Oestrogen only:** post-hysterectomy
- **Oestrogen + progesterone:** if have uterus **or** endometriosis
    - ▸ **Perimenopausal:** *cyclical* combined HRT
        → daily oestrogen + 14d of progesterone
            ↳ a) every 4 w – monthly bleeds; b) every 13 w – 3-monthly bleeds
    - ▸ **Post-menopausal:** *continuous* combined HRT
        → daily oestrogen & progesterone = **amenorrhoea**
- **Topical oestrogens** (cream, pessary, ring): for vaginal & urinary symptoms
    → local action = ↓ risk of breast cancer

Duration of HRT: give for 5y at lowest effective dose, then review risks vs. benefits

Benefits of HRT	Risks of HRT
• Treats hot flushes within 4w	• Increases risk of VTE (especially oral preparations)
• Treats vaginal & urinary symptoms	• Increases risk of gallbladder disease (especially oral preparations)
• Reduces risk of osteoporosis and fractures	• **OESTROGEN ONLY:** endometrial cancer
• Reduces risk of colorectal cancer	• **COMBINATION:** breast cancer (risk reduces again after cessation)

Other SEs of HRT

- headaches, nausea
- mood swings
- abnormal PV bleeds
- fluid retention
- breast tenderness
- dyspepsia

---

[12] NICE (2015, updated 2019) *Menopause* [NG23]; NICE (2020, updated 2022) CKS *HRT*

NON-OESTROGEN THERAPIES: if oestrogen contraindicated
1. **Hot flushes / night sweats:** progestogens, SSRIs, clonidine
2. **Vaginal atrophy:** lubricants/creams/moisturisers
3. **Osteoporosis:** bisphosphonates, calcium/vit D, raloxifene, denosumab
4. **Reduced libido/energy:** consider testosterone

COMPLEMENTARY THERAPIES: little evidence

e.g. phyto-oestrogens, herbal remedies

Oestrogens: oestradiol, oestrone, oestriol

Progestogens: levonorgestrel, norethisterone

> **Tibolone:** synthetic steroid – metabolised to have oestrogenic, progestogenic & androgenic actions
> → enables amenorrhoea, preserves bone marrow density, treats vasomotor, psychological & libido problems

Post-menopausal bleeding (PMB)

→ *vaginal bleeding occurring* **at least 12m after the last menstrual period**

CAUSES

- **Endometrial or cervical carcinoma**
- **Endometrial hyperplasia ± atypia & polyps** } 20% of cases → MUST EXCLUDE
- Atrophic vaginitis
- Cervicitis
- Ovarian carcinoma
- Cervical polyps

INVESTIGATIONS

- Bimanual VE & speculum
- TV USS – measures endometrial thickness & visualise pathologies e.g. fibroids/cysts

Endometrial thickness **≥4mm** OR **>1 episode** of bleeding = **endometrial biopsy ± hysteroscopy**

SUMMARY OF INVESTIGATING PMB

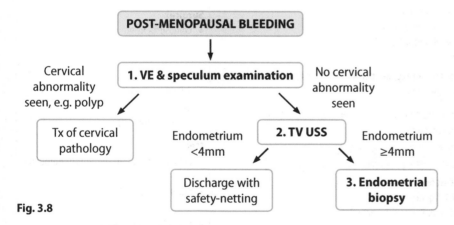

Fig. 3.8

> **Safety-netting:**
> Return to GP if gets worse/happens again

Premature ovarian failure (premature menopause/ amenorrhoea)

CAUSES

- Idiopathic
- **Iatrogenic:** surgery, chemo-/radiotherapy
- Autoimmune
- **Genetic:** Turner syndrome
- Viral infection
- Sickle cell disease

Urogynaecology

Investigations of the urinary tract

- **Urine dip**
  - ▸ **Blood:** carcinoma/calculi
  - ▸ **Protein/leukocytes/nitrites:** infection → send for MCS
  - ▸ **Glucose:** DM
- **Urinary diary*** – 1 week record of time & volume of fluid intake & micturition
- **Post-micturition USS** – exclude chronic retention
- **Renal tract USS** – excludes incomplete emptying & checks for congenital abnormalities/calculi/tumours
- **CT urogram** – determines integrity & route of ureter
- **Cystoscopy** – inspection of bladder cavity → identify fistulae, tumours, stones, cystitis
- **Cystometry (urodynamics)**
  - ▸ Leaking with coughing but no detrusor contraction = **urinary stress incontinence (USI)**
  - ▸ Involuntary detrusor contraction = **overactive bladder**

*especially for urge incontinence

measure bladder pressure via catheter + abdominal pressure via rectum

Urinary incontinence

Type	RF	History	Investigations	Management[13]
Stress (50%)	**Urethral sphincter weakness (cannot withstand ↑IAP)** • pregnancy, obesity, age • vaginal delivery (long labour / forceps) • prolapse, hysterectomy • muscular diseases	**Leakage on exertion (e.g. cough/sneeze)** ↑IAP causes bladder > urethral pressure **Pelvic floor muscle training (PFMT):** • at least 3m • taught by physio • 8 contractions 3× /d	1. Urine dip (r/o infection) 2. Cystometry (exclude OAB)	**Lifestyle:** • weight loss • pelvic floor training **Medical:** • Duloxetine SNRI to ↑ sphincter activity • Injectable bulking agents **Surgical:** • Colposuspension
OAB / urge (35%)	• idiopathic • detrusor overactivity (spinal cord injury/MS) • previous pelvic surgery	**Urgency, frequency, nocturia** ± stress incontinence Detrusor contraction causes bladder > urethral pressure **Bladder retraining:** • at least 6w • resist urgency • void according to set timetable	1. Urine dip (r/o infection) 2. Urine diary (high frequency, small volume) 3. Cystometry	**Lifestyle:** • ↓ fluids/caffeine • medication review • bladder retraining **Medical:** • anticholinergics (oxybutynin/tolterodine) ↓ detrusor activity • botulinum toxin A block neuromusc transmission • intravaginal oestrogens
Overflow (1%)	**Obstruction** • pelvic surgery/strictures • bladder calculi **Detrusor failure** • neurological • medication • DM	**Leakage on exertion OR continuous flow/dribble** Bladder overdistension → overflows (associated with chronic retention)	1. Urine dip (r/o infection) 2. Post-micturition USS	Intermittent self-catheterisation **Refer to relevant specialty to treat underlying cause** e.g. urology for BPH

[13] NICE (2019) *Urinary incontinence and pelvic organ prolapse in women* [NG123]

Acute urinary retention

Definition: unable to pass urine for ≥12h = very painful
Causes: childbirth, surgery, anticholinergics, pelvic masses, neurological disease
Management: catheterisation

Pelvic organ prolapse (POP)

→ *protrusion of pelvic organs into vaginal canal*

TYPES

1. **Apical:** uterus, cervix & upper vagina

2. **Anterior vaginal wall:**
   - cystocoele (bladder) – upper anterior wall
   - urethrocoele (urethra) – lower anterior wall
   - cysto-urethrocoele (bladder + urethra)

3. **Posterior vaginal wall:**
   - rectocoele (rectum) – lower posterior wall
   - enterocoele (pouch of Douglas) – upper posterior wall

CAUSES: weakness of supporting structures
- Vaginal delivery / pregnancy – large baby, long labour, instrumental
- Congenital – abnormal collagen (e.g. Ehlers–Danlos)
- Menopause – deterioration of collagen with ↓ oestrogen
- Chronic ↑ IAP – smoking, obesity, chronic cough/constipation, heavy lifting, pelvic mass
- Iatrogenic – pelvic surgery (e.g. hysterectomy/continence surgery)

SYMPTOMS
- Dragging sensation / feeling of a lump – worse at end of day / when standing
- Urinary/bowel symptoms – stress incontinence, frequency, double-voiding, etc.
- Severe cases: problems with intercourse, bleeding, discharge

INVESTIGATIONS
- Abdo/bimanual examination – visualise externally if severe, exclude pelvic mass
- DRE – differentiate entero- & rectocoele
- Sim's speculum – inspect vaginal walls (can see bulge)
- Pelvic USS – r/o pelvic mass if suspected **or post-menopausal bleeding**

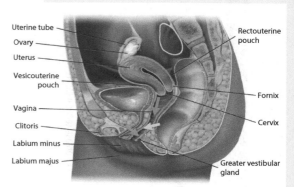

Fig. 3.9 Arrows show direction of prolapse: blue = apical, green = anterior wall, yellow = posterior wall.

MANAGEMENT[14]

1. **Conservative:**
   - **lifestyle:** weight loss, stop smoking
   - **topical oestrogen:** if vaginal atrophy
   - **pelvic floor muscle training:** ≥16w

2. **Pessaries:** 'artificial pelvic floor'
   - ring or shelf
   - changed every 6–9m

3. **Surgical:**
Uterine prolapse:
- vaginal hysterectomy – uterus & cervix removed via vaginal incision
- hysteropexy – uterus & cervix attached to sacrum with mesh

Vaginal vault prolapse (often follows hysterectomy):
- sacrocolpopexy – vagina attached to sacrum with mesh
- sacrospinal fixation – vagina stitched to sacrospinous ligament

Vaginal wall prolapse:
- anterior & posterior wall repair – may use mesh

---

[14]NICE (2019) *Urinary incontinence and pelvic organ prolapse in women* [NG123]

Contraception

yellow highlight = important point to remember

1. Combined hormonal contraceptives (oestrogen-containing)

Method	Frequency	Method of action	Cautions/CIs	Advantages	Disadvantages	Safety-netting
COCP (e.g. Microgynon) PuFR = 0.2% TuFR = 8%	3w on, 1w off (withdrawal bleed) **OR** back-to-back	• **Inhibits ovulation** • Thins endometrium • Thickens mucus	• VTE, CVA, IHD • migraine with aura • severe HTN • breast/endometrial cancer • BMI >40 • breastfeeding <6w • pregnancy • smokers >35y • >40y	• periods lighter, less painful • improve acne • protective against endometrial, ovarian, bowel cancer • protective against fibroids, ovarian cysts, endometriosis	**SEs:** nausea, headaches, dizziness, ↓ libido, breast tenderness → can become ineffective with ABX **Major complications** • VTE, MI/CVD • CVA, migraine • HTN, jaundice • breast/cervical cancer	1. **Condoms first 7d** 2. Diarrhoea/vomiting within 2h = take another 3. >2 missed pills = 7d condom use 4. Leg/chest pain, haemoptysis, headaches = SEE GP 5. Stop 4w before major surgery
Transdermal patch (Evra) PuFR = 0.2% TuFR = 8%	New patch weekly for 3w then 1w off					
Vaginal ring (Nuvaring) PuFR = 0.2% TuFR = 8%	Worn for 3w then removed for 1w, followed by new ring					

2. Progesterone-only contraceptives

Method	Frequency	Method of action	Cautions/CIs	Advantages	Disadvantages	Safety-netting
POP 'minipill' (e.g. Micronor, Cerazette) PuFR = 1% TuFR = 7%	Take **every day at same time** with no break	• **Inhibits ovulation** • Thickens mucus • Thins endometrium *(older pills like Micronor may not inhibit ovulation in all women, but work mainly to thicken mucus & thin the endometrium)*	Breast cancer in past 5y *Safest method!*	• Can be used where COCP is contraindicated • Periods may be less painful • Not affected by broad-spectrum ABX	**SEs** • breakthrough bleeds/spotting • breast tenderness • acne • mood changes, ↓ libido • ovarian cysts	1. Good timekeeping (within 3h) NB desogestrel = 12-h window 2. Missed pill/diarrhoea/vomiting within 2h = take another & **condom for 2d**
Depo-Provera (IM injection) PuFR = <1% TuFR = 4%	Every 3m Noristerat = injection every 8w as short-term cover		• Current breast cancer • Osteoporosis risk (adolescents/elderly) • Obesity	• May have less painful, lighter periods • Unaffected by V&D	• irregular bleeding (at start) • weight gain • headaches, nausea, mood • breast tenderness • delayed return to fertility (warn if considering pregnancy) • initial bone density decrease (restored on cessation)	1. **Condoms for first 7d** 2. Infection at site – fever, red, swollen, hot, pain = SEE GP
Implant (Nexplanon) PuFR = <0.1%	Every 3y		• Current breast cancer • Liver enzyme inducers	• immediate return to fertility • compliance not an issue • easy to remove	• irregular bleeding (esp. start) • headaches, nausea, mood • breast tenderness	1. **Condoms for first 7d** 2. Infection at site – fever, red, swollen, hot, pain = SEE GP 3. Changed position, skin, shape, pain = SEE GP

LARC: long-acting reversible contraceptive

3. Intrauterine devices

Method	Frequency	Method of action	Cautions/CIs	Advantages	Disadvantages	Safety-netting
IUS (hormonal coil) PUFR = <0.5%	Jaydess = 3y Levosert, Mirena, Kyleena = 5y	**Prevents implantation:** • Thickens mucus • Thins endometrium	**Both** • endometrial cancer • cervical cancer • active/recent pelvic infection • pregnancy • previous ectopic **IUS** • breast cancer	**IUS** • Lighter, less painful periods (Mirena = only one licensed for menorrhagia) • Hormonal SEs ↓ as localised action	**Complications** • expulsion • perforation of uterus • infection • ectopic • bleeding	**IUS: use condoms first 7d** **IUD: immediate protection** 1. Check threads after each period – SEE GP if not felt 2. Pelvic pain/discharge/signs of pregnancy = SEE GP 3. Intermenstrual bleeding = SEE GP
IUD (copper coil) PUFR = <0.5%	5–10y	**Blocks fertilisation:** Toxic to sperm	**IUD** • menorrhagia	**Both** • Unaffected by D&V • Rapid return to fertility	**IUD:** can cause menorrhagia	

4. Barrier methods

Male & female condoms, caps + spermicides
- PUFR = 2%   TUFR = 15%
- Physically prevent sperm entering cervix
- Provide STI protection

5. Sterilisation

Female: FR = 0.5%
1. **Filshie clips** – occlude lumen
→ COMPLICATIONS: failure, post-op pain

Male: FR = 0.05%
1. **Vasectomy** – ligation and removal of section of vas deferens
→ COMPLICATIONS: failure, haematoma, infection, chronic pain

Counselling before sterilisation:
- Must be certain
- Have discussed alternative forms of contraception
- Warn of risk of failure (0.5% or 0.05%)
- Risk of ectopic pregnancies
- Risks of surgery

Key:
FR = Failure rate
PUFR = Perfect use failure rate
TUFR = Typical use failure rate

Emergency contraceptives (ECs)

→ *measures used after UPSI to help prevent pregnancy*

ORAL

- Levonelle (levonorgestrel, LNG) = progesterone that **delays ovulation**
- ellaOne (ulipristal acetate, UPA) = selective progesterone receptor modulator that **delays ovulation for ≥5d**

Should offer oral EC while waiting for fitting of IUD

INTRAUTERINE

- Copper IUD* = copper is **toxic to sperm** and **prevents implantation**

LNG can do no harm even if implanted pregnancy — if in doubt, give it!

Method	When to take	Cautions/CIs	Efficacy	Side-effects	Safety-netting
'Morning after pill'	Levonelle (LNG): within **72h**	• previous ectopic • severe malabsorption • hepatic impairment • CYP450-inducing drugs **LNG:** • BMI >26 ↓s efficacy **UPA:** • progesterone ↓s efficacy	90%	• N&V • headaches • skin reactions • menstrual cycle irregularities Next period may be earlier or later than expected	Go on to ovulate so **need other contraceptive method in place** • if vomit within 3h, take another • take **pregnancy test in 3w** to ensure worked • wait 7d before restarting COC/POP
	ellaOne (UPA): within **120h**		95%		
Cu-IUD	**Within 5d** of UPSI OR within 5d of expected ovulation	• pregnancy • previous ectopic • endometrial/cervical cancer • menorrhagia • gonorrhoea/chlamydia (treat before fitting)	99%	Heavier, longer, painful bleeds <u>Complications</u> • expulsion • infection • ectopic • uterine perforation	Can be used as **contraceptive method going forward** Immediate protection

Expected ovulation = length of cycle – 14d
e.g. 28-d cycle, ovulation at day 14, so Cu-IUD by day 19 (14+5)

QUICK START: starting long-term contraception immediately after EC given.

→ cannot quick-start hormonal contraceptives after UPA as progesterone will ↓ efficacy of UPA **(wait 5d)**

OTHER FACTORS TO CONSIDER WITH EC:

- Ensure not already pregnant before offering EC
- Consensual intercourse / domestic violence
- STI risk – assessment and screening
- Starting long-term contraceptive as well

Summary of choosing an emergency contraceptive

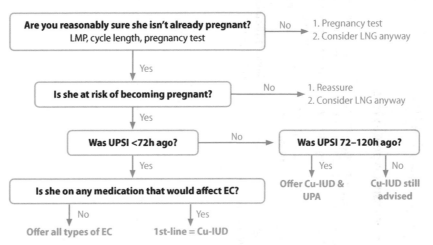

Fig. 3.10

Unintended pregnancy & abortion

Symptoms of early pregnancy

- Missed/light period
- Nausea (esp. in morning)
- Breast tenderness
- Tiredness
- Urinary frequency
- Constipation

- Period-like pains/cramps
- ↑ vaginal discharge (w/out soreness)
- Strange metallic taste
- Going off things, e.g. coffee, tobacco, fatty food

Methods of abortion[15,16]

→ *depends on gestation & patient's choice*

1. First do blood tests: Hb, G&S, rhesus status → if Rh−ve, give Anti-D
2. Discuss contraception going forward
3. Ensure emotional support
4. Advise pregnancy test after 3w to ensure TOP successful

MEDICAL: suitable up to 14w   **24–48h after**
- **MIFEPRISTONE** (antiprogesterone) + **MISOPROSTOL** (prostaglandin)
- **If >22w:** inject fetal heart/umbilical cord with **KCl** → prevents live birth
  ↳ COMPLICATIONS: haemorrhage, infection (10%), failure (1%)

SURGICAL: give preop ABX cover
- **<14w:** vacuum aspiration (under general or local anaesthetic)
- **≥14w:** dilation & evacuation (or vacuum aspiration with large-bore cannula)
  ↳ COMPLICATIONS: haemorrhage, infection (10%), uterine perforation, cervical trauma, risk of preterm delivery (stretched cervix), failure (0.2%)

Ethical issues surrounding TOP: Abortion Act 1967[17]

1) **2 doctors must agree** that TOP is in best interests of woman by considering the following
<24w AND:
- continuation would involve **risk to the physical or mental health of the mother**
- continuation would involve **risk to the physical or mental health of existing children**

Any time if:
- continuation would involve risk of **serious permanent physical or mental injury or death** to the mother
- there is a high risk that the born **child would be seriously handicapped** by physical or mental abnormalities

2) Conscientious objection
- Must clarify exactly what they will & will not do in relation to abortion & ensure the team are aware
  ▸ **MUST NOT:** Restrict/delay access to abortion care OR coerce woman not to have an abortion

3) Pregnancy in under 16s   *<13s unable to consent to sex so MUST refer to social care*
- Explain limits of confidentiality
  ▸ Assess Gillick competence / use Fraser guidelines
  ▸ Safeguarding assessment
- Explore support available – parents/school/nurses, etc.

Actions to take if unwanted pregnancy

1. **Confirm pregnancy**
2. **Estimate gestation** – from 1st day of LMP
3. **Consider complications:** ectopic, pre-existing conditions
4. **Provide information** on available options
5. Assist patient in making the right choice for them
6. Determine **rhesus status** & give prophylaxis if needed
7. Refer to necessary services
8. Provide **contraceptive advice:** at time of abortion
9. **Assess STI risk** & test as appropriate

Contraindications for medical TOP

- HTN/CVD
- smoker >35y
- oral steroid use
- bleeding disorder/anticoagulant
- renal disease
- breastfeeding
- fibroid/uterine anomaly
- poorly controlled diabetes

NB Abortion is illegal in Northern Ireland

Fraser guidelines

1. They **understand** advice
2. They cannot be persuaded to **inform parents**
3. Likely to continue **sexual intercourse**
4. Without contraception **health likely to suffer**
5. In their **best interests**

---

[15] NICE (2019) *Abortion care* [NG140]
[16] RCOG (2015) *Best practice in comprehensive abortion care.* Paper No. 2
[17] Abortion Act 1967, Section 1

Genital tract infections

grey highlight = key feature

Non-sexually transmitted

Organism	Aetiology/RFs	Signs & symptoms	Complications	Diagnosis	Management
Bacterial vaginosis (*Gardnerella*)	Overgrowth of normal lactobacilli RF: douching, smoking	• Grey-white discharge • Fishy odour	• Preterm labour • 2° infection in PID	• High vaginal swab • Raised pH • 'Clue cells' on microscopy	Metronidazole gel/PO or clindamycin cream
Candidiasis/thrush (*Candida albicans*) = common (20% women)	• Immunocompromised • Diabetes • Pregnancy • ABX use	**Often asymptomatic** • 'Cottage-cheese' discharge • Vulval itching • Dyspareunia & dysuria	Recurrence in diabetes or immunocompromised	• High vaginal swab → culture	Antifungal pessary/cream (clotrimazole) **Or oral fluconazole** (NOT IF PREGNANT)

Sexually transmitted: *screen for concurrent STIs, partner notification & screening, education on barrier contraception*

Organism	Signs & symptoms	Complications	Diagnosis	Management
Trichomoniasis (*Trichomonas vaginalis*)	**May be asymptomatic** • Offensive grey-green discharge	• Preterm/LBW child • Postpartum sepsis • HIV transmission	• Wet film microscopy • High vaginal swab	Metronidazole PO one-off
Chlamydia (*Chlamydia trachomatis*) = 5–10% women aged 20–30	**Usually asymptomatic** • Watery/milky vaginal discharge • (± PCB) • Urethritis	**PID:** subfertility, chronic pelvic pain **Reiter's syndrome:** urethritis, conjunctivitis, arthritis **Neonatal conjunctivitis**	**Men:** first catch urine (FCU) for NAAT analysis **Women:** endocervical/vaginal swab for microscopy	Azithromycin PO one-off Doxycycline PO 7d OD *Opportunistic screening programme*
Gonorrhoea (*Neisseria gonorrhoeae*)	**Often asymptomatic** • White/yellow discharge (M&F) • Urethritis • Bartholinitis • Cervicitis	• Bacteraemia • Acute septic arthritis • PID **Neonatal conjunctivitis**	• FCU for NAAT analysis • Endocervical swab for microscopy **→ Gram –ve diplococcus** • Culture to check ABX sensitivities	IM ceftriaxone **Ciprofloxacin** = alternative but resistance common
Syphilis (*Treponema pallidum*)	**1° syphilis:** • Chance (painless genital ulcer) **2° syphilis:** • Rash (soles/palms), flu symptoms • Warty genital & peri-oral growths • Multi-organ problems	• Congenital syphilis *if pregnant* **3° syphilis:** • aortic regurgitation • skin/bony swellings (gummata) • dementia • tabes dorsalis (neural tract degen.)	**Serological tests (blood test)** • Enzyme immunoassay • VDRL	IM/IV penicillin one-off (10–14d PO doxycycline if penicillin allergy)
Genital warts: HPV 6 & 11 (Condylomata acuminata)	**Multiple warts: varied appearance** • Flat patches • Papilliform swellings (cauliflower-like)	HPV 16 & 18 associated with **cervical intraepithelial neoplasia (CIN)** • high recurrence rate	• On inspection	• Topical podophyllin/imiquimod cream • Cryotherapy • HPV vaccination

Condition	Symptoms	Diagnosis	Treatment
Genital herpes: HSV 1 & 2	• **Multiple, small, painful vesicles** • Dysuria & itchy genitals • Malaise, fever, headache • Local lymphadenopathy **Reactivation:** dormant in dorsal root = less severe symptoms **Neonatal herpes:** high mortality	• On inspection • PCR of viral swabs	• Aciclovir
HIV/AIDS = retrovirus infecting CD4 helper T cells	**Seroconversion:** rash + flu-like Sx **Often asymptomatic = latent period** until CD4 count low enough **Opportunistic infections** • TB, PCP, meningitis • Genital infections **Malignancy:** • CIN – *recommend annual smears* • Kaposi sarcoma (skin) • Non-Hodgkin lymphoma	Antibody/antigen test on blood/saliva **CD4+ <200 cells/mm³ = AIDS**	**2NRTIs +** • **1 NNRTI** OR • **Boosted PI** OR • **Integrase inhibitor**

Diagnosing genital tract infections

Triple swab:

1. High vaginal (charcoal): BV, trichomoniasis, candida, GBS
2. Endocervical (charcoal): gonorrhoea
3. Endocervical (pink): chlamydia

National Chlamydia Screening Programme (NCSP)

= opportunistic screening of those at risk (sexually active <25s)

- Offered at GP & sexual health clinics ↳ *Assess Gillick competence if <16y*
- Must have fully-informed consent from patient (patient info leaflet)

Management of positive results:

- Treat infection: prevent possible complications
- Partner tracing & treatment: reduce transmission & reinfection
- Exclude other STIs
- Educate on transmission method & barrier contraception

> **WINDOW PERIOD:** time from infection until detectable by test
>
> **Gonorrhoea & chlamydia =** 2w
> **Blood-borne viruses, e.g. HIV =** 6w

AIDS = now a *treatable, chronic condition* with normal life expectancy

Side-effects of ART

- hyperlipidaemia
- lipodystrophy
- T2DM
- hypersensitivity
- peripheral neuropathy
- renal impairment
- hepatic toxicity
- pancreatitis

PREP (pre-exposure prophylaxis): combination of 2 reverse transcriptase inhibitors to prevent acquiring HIV even if have sex with HIV-positive partner

PEP (post-exposure prophylaxis): if had sex with HIV-positive partner can give *within 72h* to prevent infection

HIV/AIDS

RISK FACTORS FOR TRANSMISSION

- Anal intercourse / males having sex with males = 46%
- Multiple sexual partners / paid sex worker
- Overseas partners (especially Africa)
- Percutaneous injury (needle-stick)
- Blood products from abroad
- IVDU = 2%
- Vertical transmission = 2%

MANAGEMENT[18]

HOLISTIC Mx: medical, psychological, social

1. **Antiretroviral treatment (ART)**
   - 2 NRTIs + NNRTI / protease Inhibitor / integrase inhibitor
2. **Treatment & prophylaxis for opportunistic infections** (Hep A/B, flu vaccines)
3. **Monitor:**
   - CD4 count & viral load
   - Routine bloods: FBC, U&E, LFT, glucose, lipids
   - STI screening
4. **Healthy lifestyle advice** – have higher risk of CVD & metabolic abnormalities
5. **Psychological support**
6. **Contact tracing**

Summary of STI symptom differentials

Symptom	Differentials	Investigations
Urethritis	<ul><li>Chlamydia</li><li>Gonorrhoea</li><li>Non-specific urethritis</li></ul>	<ul><li>Microscopy & culture</li><li>Urine NAAT</li><li>Bloods</li></ul>
Ulcers	<ul><li>Genital herpes (HSV 2) = *multiple, painful*</li><li>Syphilis = *single, painless*</li><li>Chancroid = *bacterial infection*</li><li>Behçet's disease = *vessel inflammation (rare)*</li></ul>	<ul><li>Microscopy</li><li>PCR</li><li>Bloods</li></ul>
Vaginal discharge	<ul><li>Trichomoniasis</li><li>Chlamydia</li><li>Gonorrhoea</li><li>Candidiasis</li><li>BV</li></ul>	<ul><li>Triple swabs</li><li>Bloods</li><li>Pregnancy test</li></ul>
Systemic symptoms	<ul><li>HIV</li><li>Hep A/B/C</li><li>PID</li></ul>	<ul><li>Swabs</li><li>Blood antibody/antigen</li></ul>
Lumps/bumps	<ul><li>Genital warts (HPV 6 & 11)</li><li>Molluscum</li><li>Scabies</li><li>Pubic lice</li></ul>	<ul><li>Triple swabs</li><li>Bloods</li><li>Biopsy</li></ul>

---

[18] NICE (2021) CKS Clinical management – *HIV infection and AIDS*

Infections of the uterus & pelvis

Endometritis

→ *infection confined to the uterine cavity*

CAUSES
- Instrumentation to uterus: coil insertion, C-section, laparoscopy
- Miscarriage/termination if RPOC

SYMPTOMS
- **Heavy, persistent bleeding**
- Pain
- ± fever

SIGNS
- Uterine tenderness
- Cervical **os open**

COMPLICATIONS
- Septicaemia
- Spread to pelvis

INVESTIGATIONS
- Vaginal & cervical swabs
- FBC
- Pelvic USS (identify RPOC)

MANAGEMENT
- **Broad-spectrum ABX**
- **ERPC** if RPOC seen on USS or symptoms persist

Acute pelvic infection (PID)

→ *sexually transmitted pelvic infection*

↳ Salpingitis = infection of fallopian tubes (form of PID)

Chlamydia & gonococcus = 60%

↳ *If discharge = more likely gonococcus than chlamydia*

CAUSES
- Ascending bacteria from vaginal/cervical infection (endometritis often coexists)
- Uterine instrumentation & RPOC – may introduce non-sexually transmitted bacteria

SYMPTOMS
- **Often asymptomatic** until complications present
- **Deep dyspareunia**
- Abnormal vaginal bleeding/**discharge**

Risk factors for / causes of PID
- Multiple partners
- Unprotected intercourse
- Younger
- Nulliparous

SIGNS
- **Bilateral lower abdo pain**/RUQ pain/peritonism
- Bilateral adnexal tenderness
- Cervical excitation*   *pain on moving cervix
- ± pelvic mass (abscess)

DDx
- Appendicitis ⎫ Usually
- Ovarian cyst rupture ⎬ *unilateral*
- Ectopic pregnancy ⎭ pain

INVESTIGATIONS
- **PREGNANCY TEST** – r/o ectopic
- Endocervical swabs – for gonococcus & chlamydia
- Blood cultures – if fever
- WBC, CRP
- Pelvic USS – exclude abscess/ovarian cyst
- **Laparoscopy + fimbrial biopsy & culture = GOLD STANDARD**

Complications of PID
- Abscess/pyosalpinx
- Tubal obstruction/subfertility
- Chronic pelvic infection/pain
- 6× ↑ risk ectopic pregnancy

MANAGEMENT[19]
- Analgesia (+ IV fluids if febrile)
- IM ceftriaxone + PO doxycycline + PO metronidazole – **start empirically**
- R/V at 24h – no improvement = laparoscopic lx
- Pelvic abscess may need drainage – rupture = life-threatening
- **If septic = hospital admission, sepsis 6, bloods, senior review**

PLUS contact tracing of all sexual partners in past 6m & contraceptive advice

---

[19]NICE (2019) CKS: Scenario – *Management of pelvic inflammatory disease*

Chronic pelvic infection (PID)

→ *persisting infection from untreated PID*

SYMPTOMS

- **Chronic pelvic pain**
- Dysmenorrhoea, deep dyspareunia
- Heavy, irregular menstruation
- Chronic PV discharge

INVESTIGATIONS

- Laparoscopy

SIGNS

- Dense pelvic adhesions
- Fluid/pus obstructs & dilates fallopian tubes
- Abdominal & adnexal tenderness
- **Fixed, retroverted uterus**

MANAGEMENT

- Analgesia + antibiotics
- Adhesiolysis (cutting adhesions)
- Salpingectomy

> **General investigations for infective symptoms**
>
> - FBC, CRP, LFTs
> - MSU for culture and microscopy – for UTIs
> - FSU or high vaginal swabs – for STIs

Chronic pelvic pain (CPP)

→ *intermittent or constant for >6m & not exclusive to menstruation or intercourse*

DDX:

- Endometriosis } *cyclical*
- Adenomyosis
- Chronic PID
- Adhesions (trap tissue)
- IBS
- Neurological (fibromyalgia)
- Psychological (sleep disorders / depression)
- Idiopathic (never find cause)

INVESTIGATIONS:

- Full & careful history
- Triple swabs
- TV USS
- MRI
- Laparoscopy

MANAGEMENT: depends on suspected cause

- **Cyclical pain:** COCP or GnRH analogue + HRT
- **IBS:** diet + antispasmodics
- **Psychological:** counselling + psychotherapy
- **Pain management:** gabapentin, amitriptyline

Vaginal discharge

1. **Physiological** – increases at ovulation & if using COCP
2. **Infection** – bacterial vaginosis, candidiasis, chlamydia, gonorrhoea, trichomonas
3. **Atrophic vaginitis** – oestrogen deficiency (pre-menarche, in lactation, post-menopause)
4. **Foreign body** – very offensive discharge
5. **Malignancy** – bloody & offensive discharge = RED FLAG

Summary of vaginal discharge features

Cause	Discharge	Odour	pH	Itching	Redness	Treatment
Ectropion/eversion	Clear	Normal	Normal	No	No	Cryotherapy
Candidiasis	White	Normal	Normal	Yes	Yes	Imidazoles
Bacterial vaginosis	Grey-white	Fishy	Raised	No	No	ABX
Trichomoniasis	Grey-green	Malodorous	Raised	Yes	Yes	ABX
Atrophic	Clear	Normal	Raised	No	Yes	Oestrogen/HRT
Malignancy	Red-brown	Malodorous	Variable	No	No	Biopsy

OBSTETRICS

04

ABBREVIATIONS

ACEi – Angiotensin-converting enzyme inhibitor
ADHD – Attention deficit hyperactivity disorder
AFP – Alpha fetoprotein
AP – Anterior-posterior
APH – Antepartum haemorrhage
AROM – Artificial rupture of membranes
BB – Beta-blocker
B-hCG – Beta human chorionic gonadotrophin
BW – Birth weight
CF – Cystic fibrosis
CMV – Cytomegalovirus
CO – Cardiac output
COCP – Combined oral contraceptive pill
CRL – Crown–rump length
C-section – Caesarean section
CTG – Cardiotocography
CVP – Central venous pressure
DC twins – Dichorionic twins
DCDA – Dichorionic diamniotic
DIC – Disseminated intravascular coagulation
DM – Diabetes mellitus
ECV – External cephalic version
ERPC – Evacuation of retained products of conception
EUA – Examination under anaesthetic

FBS – Fetal blood sampling
FFP – Fresh frozen plasma
FHR – Fetal heart rate
GBS – Group B strep
GDM – Gestational diabetes mellitus
HG – Hyperemesis gravidarum
HIE – Hypoxic ischaemic encephalopathy
HPL – Human placental lactogen
ILGF – Insulin-like growth factor
IOL – Induction of labour
IUD – Intrauterine device
IUFD – Intrauterine fetal death
IUGR – Intrauterine growth restriction
IVF – *In vitro* fertilisation
LGA – Large for gestational age
LLETZ – Large loop excision of the transformation zone
LSCS – Lower section caesarean section
MC twins – Monochorionic twins
MCDA – Monochorionic, diamniotic
MCMA – Monochorionic monoamniotic
NICU – Neonatal intensive care unit
NT – Nuchal translucency
NTD – Neural tube defect
NVD – Normal vaginal delivery
NVP – Nausea & vomiting in pregnancy
OA – Occipito-anterior
OGTT – Oral glucose tolerance test
OP – Occipito-posterior

OT – Occipito-transverse
PAPP-A – Pregnancy-associated plasma protein A
PCOS – Polycystic ovary syndrome
PGS – Pre-implantation genetic screening
PID – Pelvic inflammatory disease
POP – Progesterone-only pill
PPH – Postpartum haemorrhage
PPROM – Premature prelabour rupture of membranes
PROM – Prelabour rupture of membranes
PV – Per vagina
Rh – Rhesus
ROM – Rupture of membranes
RPOC – Retained products of conception
RUQ – Right upper quadrant
SCA – Sickle cell anaemia
SFH – Symphysial fundal height
SGA – Small for gestational age
STI – Sexually transmitted infection
SV – Stroke volume
TENS – Transcutaneous electrical nerve stimulation
TOP – Termination of pregnancy
TV – Transvaginal
VBAC – Vaginal birth after caesarean section
VE – Vaginal examination

Antenatal care

Antenatal care involves the MDT including midwives, obstetricians & GPs

Aims

- Detect & manage pre-existing maternal disorders which could affect pregnancy
- Prevent/detect & manage maternal/fetal complications of pregnancy
- Detect congenital fetal problems – if requested
- Plan delivery to ensure maximal safety and satisfaction
- Provide education & lifestyle advice

Visits

1. BOOKING VISIT: as early as possible in pregnancy (before 10w)

Components of the booking visit

1. Assess risk – determines frequency of visits
2. Check gestation / arrange dating scan
3. Prenatal screening discussed
4. Give information

Booking visit history for risk

Age <17 or >35

Past obstetric disorders (may recur)
- preterm/small-for-date/growth-restricted
- stillbirth/miscarriages
- haemorrhage
- pre-eclampsia, gestational diabetes
- rhesus disease

Gynaecological Hx: subfertility increases risk
NB assisted conception ↑ chance multiple pregnancy

Medical conditions increasing risk of problems
- HTN, diabetes, autoimmune, thromboembolic
- Cardiac, renal
- Psychiatric illness, especially depression

NB should also check FHx

Drugs: stop if contraindicated in pregnancy, ensure on vitamins/folate
Social: smoking, alcohol, illicit drugs, housing/support*

Vaccines offered:
Flu & whooping cough

Booking visit routine examinations

General health
- Nutrition
- BMI: >30 or <18 = ↑ risk GDM, pre-eclampsia, NTDs
- BP: HTN increases pre-eclampsia risk
- Urine dip: glucose, protein, leucocytes, nitrites

Abdo, vaginal and pelvic examination
- Auscultate fetal heart, check pelvic capacity

*Ask if feel safe at home

Booking visit routine investigations

Blood screen
- FBC: anaemia
- Blood group & anti-D antibodies
- Glucose tolerance: if woman is at risk of GDM
- Syphilis
- Rubella immunity: postnatal vaccination if needed
- HIV & Hep B: counselling & screening offered
- Hb electrophoresis: SCA, thalassaemias (test dad if positive)

Other tests
- Infection screening, e.g. chlamydia
- Urinalysis: glucose, nitrites, protein
- Urine MCS if asymptomatic bacteriuria → 20% get pyelonephritis

USS (dating scan): between 11–13 + 6w
- Check gestation (measure crown–rump length: CRL)
- Detect multiple pregnancies
- Screen for trisomies (13, 18, 21): combined/triple test

Lifestyle advice

Diet: well balanced, approx. 2500kcal
- avoid unpasteurised milk, soft cheese, pâté
- avoid alcohol (esp. first 12w) & caffeine (2 cups/day)
- avoid smoking (offer nicotine replacement therapy)

Exercise: avoid contact but swimming and other gentle exercise is advised

Sleep: left lateral position

risk of listeria, salmonella, toxoplasmosis

2. REGULAR VISITS:
History
- Brief review
- Physical & mental health check-up
- Fetal movements

Medication advice

- Avoid medications in first trimester if possible
- Folic acid supplementation = 400mcg/d until week 12
- Vit D supplementation = 10mcg/d if BMI >30 / low sun
- Iron supplementation = if anaemic (Hb <10.5)
- Vaccines: flu & whooping cough

Frequency of visits

16–28w = monthly
28–36w = fortnightly
36w onwards = weekly

Examination
- BP & urinalysis (glucose, protein, leucocytes/nitrites)
- Abdo exam: fetal heartbeat, lie & presentation

Management
- **Reassess pregnancy risk**
- Offer advice/info: lifestyle, gestation, breastfeeding

Summary of antenatal appointment schedule[1]

*nulliparous women also have appointments at 25w & 31w

8–12w	**Booking appointment:** • History, examination, investigations • USS: dating scan (combined test)
16w	• Screening & blood results from booking • BP & proteinuria • OGTT if high risk (prev. GDM/current DM)
20w	• USS: anomaly scan
25w*	• SFH & BP + urine dip
28w	• BP & proteinuria • Symphysial-fundal height measured • FBC & antibodies checked • OGTT if indicated (FHx DM, glycosuria, etc.) • **Anti-D given if rhesus negative**
31w*	• SFH & BP + urine dip
34, 36, 38, 40 weeks	• BP & proteinuria • SFH measured • Fetal lie & presentation checked • Info given on birth plan & labour • Info given on caring for newborn, etc. • USS: presentation & placental location
41w	• Offer membrane sweep • Discuss IOL (offered at 42w)

Substance use in pregnancy

Risks of illicit drugs in pregnancy:
- Low birth weight / fetal growth restriction
- Preterm delivery
- Cardiac defects – with Ecstasy
- Sudden infant death syndrome
- Neonatal withdrawal syndrome – especially opiates and benzodiazepines

Risks of smoking/nicotine in pregnancy:
- Low birth weight / fetal growth restriction
- Preterm delivery
- Miscarriage/stillbirth

Risks of alcohol in pregnancy:
- Miscarriage
- Reduced birth weight / IUGR
- Intellectual impairment
- Fetal alcohol syndrome
  ↳ small head & eyes, saddle nose, thin lips, cerebral palsy, learning difficulties, behaviour/attention problems, hearing/vision problems, cardiac defects

[1] NICE (2021) CKS Scenario: *Antenatal care in uncomplicated pregnancy*

Routine USS

12w (dating): gestation & nuchal translucency

20w: fetal anomaly scan, e.g. cardiac, spina bifida

+ 36/38w: if low-lying placenta at 20w scan

+ serial growth scans if high risk:
4-weekly from 28w
2-weekly if monochorionic twins

Isoimmunisation: Rh-negative mother & Rh-positive fetus → mother develops IgG antibodies against fetal RBCs
Result = fetal haemolysis → jaundice, anaemia and hydrops fetalis

Management: identify fetal anaemia with Doppler & give blood transfusion / deliver if >36w

Prevention: Sensitisation can occur at previous birth, amniocentesis, APH/vaginal bleeds, miscarriage, TOP, ectopics
Give Anti-D at 28w ± within 72h of event: neutralises fetal antigens before mother's immune system can create IgGs

Side-effects
- local pain/tenderness, fever, malaise, headaches
- **rarely hypersensitivity reaction** (monitor for 20min)

Refer for external cephalic version (ECV) if breech

Indications for consultant-led care
- Maternal disorders: epilepsy, diabetes, HTN
- Previous pre-eclampsia/GDM
- BMI >30 or <18
- Age <16 or >40
- Any previous preterms
- High risk SGA
- Any previous C-sections
- Multiples
- IVF
- Grand multiparity (>6)

Indications for high dose (5mg) folate in pregnancy
- Epilepsy
- Diabetes
- BMI >30
- Hx of baby with spina bifida

Congenital abnormalities

2% pregnancies

Increased AFP	Decreased AFP
• NTDs • Multiple pregnancies	• Down's • Edward's • Maternal diabetes mellitus

Larger NT = higher risk of trisomies & structural abnormalities
Normal NT: 2.5–3.5mm

Possible risks of tests

• miscarriage	• rhesus sensitisation
• infection	• fetal trauma

Amniocentesis allows diagnosis of:
• chromosomal abnormalities
• infection (CMV, toxoplasmosis)
• inherited disease (CF, SCA, thalassaemia)
→ results = 98–99% definitive

Chorionic villus sampling allows diagnosis of:
• chromosomal abnormalities
• inherited disease abnormalities

Anencephaly = incomplete development of brain & skull → fetal death

Fetal hydrops = excess fluid in 2 or more areas
→ can result from rhesus antibodies, chromosomal or structural abnormalities, anaemia
1 in 500, high mortality

Screening tests

If these suggest high risk, offer diagnostic tests

BLOOD TESTS
• **NTDs:** increased AFP
• **Chromosomal (trisomy 21, 18, 13):**
  altered B-hCG, pregnancy-associated plasma protein A (PAPP-A), AFP, oestriol

ULTRASOUND SCAN
• **Combined test:** nuchal translucency + blood hCG + PAPP-A
• **Triple test (if >14w):** AFP + B-hCG + oestriol
  ↳ *PAPP-A, AFP & oestriol = low in Down's*
  B-hCG = high in Down's
• **Anomaly scan:** at 20w

Diagnostic tests

If screening suggests high risk (>1:150)

NON-INVASIVE DIAGNOSTIC TESTS
• **Fetal MRI:** diagnose intracranial lesions
• **3D/4D USS:** better visualisation of abnormality
• **Preimplantation genetic diagnosis:** if had IVF

INVASIVE DIAGNOSTIC TESTS
• **Amniocentesis:** 1% risk miscarriage
  ▸ removal of **amniotic fluid** via fine-gauge needle & USS
  ▸ safest **after 15 weeks'** gestation

• **Chorionic villus sampling:** 1–2% risk miscarriage*
  ▸ take sample of **placental cells** via fine-gauge needle
  ▸ under local anaesthetic
  ▸ done **at 11–13 weeks'** gestation – early enough for TOP

but earlier on in pregnancy so figure may be skewed by higher rate of spontaneous miscarriage anyway

Chromosomal abnormalities

• Down syndrome (trisomy 21)
• Edwards syndrome (trisomy 18)
• Patau syndrome (trisomy 13)
• Klinefelter syndrome
• Turner syndrome

Structural abnormalities

• **NTDs:** spina bifida, anencephaly → preconceptual **folic acid for 3m** reduces risk
• **Cardiac:** in 1% pregnancies → often associated with chromosomal disorders
• **Abdo wall:** exomphalos → bowel extrudes in peritoneal sac
• **Chest:** diaphragmatic hernia
• **GI:** oesophageal/duodenal fistulas/atresia

Hypertensive disorders in pregnancy

Pre-existing/chronic hypertension

= BP >140/90mmHg **before pregnancy or 20 weeks'** gestation or taking an antihypertensive
→ Increases risk of pre-eclampsia **so give prophylactic ASPIRIN & MANAGE BP**

Pregnancy-induced hypertension (5–7%)

= BP >140/90mmHg **after 20 weeks'** gestation
→ Due to pre-eclampsia or transient HTN

Pre-eclampsia (5%)

= BP >140/90mmHg **AND proteinuria >0.3g/24h** after 20 weeks' gestation
- **Mild/moderate pre-eclampsia** = BP 140/90–159/109 → asymptomatic
- **Severe pre-eclampsia** = BP >160/110 and/or symptoms → headache, N&V, oedema, visual disturbance, RUQ/epigastric pain, reduced urine output, hyper-reflexia, seizures

PATHOPHYSIOLOGY

Multisystem disease caused by complex interaction between immunological & vascular adaption
↳ **Stage 1 (<20w):** incomplete invasion of trophoblast into spiral arteries
   → poor placental perfusion
↳ **Stage 2 (>20w):** ischaemic placenta induces endothelial damage
   → vasoconstriction, ↑permeability, clotting dysfunction   ↑ BP & proteinuria

COMPLICATIONS FOR FETUS
- **IUGR** (<34w needs pre-term delivery) ⎫
- Increased risk placental abruption ⎬ ↑ morbidity & mortality

COMPLICATIONS FOR MOTHER
- **Eclampsia** – grand mal seizures due to cerebral vasospasm – Tx: Mg sulphate
- Cerebrovascular haemorrhage
- Renal failure – Tx: may need dialysis
- Pulmonary oedema – Tx: O_2 + furosemide
- **HELLP syndrome** (liver failure)
  - **H:** Haemolysis – dark urine, ↑LDH, anaemia
  - **EL:** Elevated Liver enzymes – RUQ/epigastric pain, liver failure, clotting dysfunction
  - **LP:** Low Platelets – DIC may occur

INVESTIGATIONS
- BP & urinalysis
- Bloods: FBC, LFTs, clotting, U&Es/uric acid level
- USS (umbilical artery Doppler) & CTG

Management (of pre-eclampsia and existing HTN)[2]

MILD/MODERATE: as outpatient → **deliver at 37–39w**
- BP & urine twice a week (clinic or midwife)
- USS every 2–4w (fetal growth)

SEVERE: admit for careful monitoring → **deliver at 34–36w**
- **Magnesium sulphate IV** – seizure control
- **Antihypertensives** – if >150/100 (labetalol, nifedipine)
- **Steroids** – promote fetal pulmonary maturation
- **Restrict fluids** – reduce risk pulmonary oedema

[2] NICE (2019) *Hypertension in pregnancy* [NG133]

Avoid ACEis in pregnancy
→ give labetalol
→ + aspirin 75mg

BP in normal pregnancy: aim for 135/85
- BP drops to <90/60mmHg in 2nd trimester
- Rises again to pre-pregnancy levels by term

Prognosis: resolves after 24h post-delivery

Risk factors
- Nulliparity
- Previous pre-eclampsia
- FHx pre-eclampsia
- Older age (>35y)
- Chronic HTN/DM
- Obesity
- Twin pregnancies
- Renal disease
- Autoimmune disease

Ix for complications

ALT/LDH (↑), plts (↓), Cr (↑), Hb (↑), USS, umbilical artery Doppler, CTG

Risk reduction

1. Booking Ix identifies risk
   - Hx, BP, proteinuria
2. Aspirin 150mg OD (12w–birth)
   - if deemed high risk

Postpartum care

GP review
- **Close fetal monitoring**
- **Maternal monitoring:** BP, FBC, LFTs, U&Es, fluids
- **Maintain BP:** at 140/90mmHg

IF FETAL DISTRESS / MOTHER AT RISK
→ **consider delivery**
(mechanism depends on individual situation)

1. 4-hourly BPs
2. Fluid balance
3. 24h urine
4. Reflexes **(for Mg)**

Glycaemic disorders in pregnancy

Glycaemic changes in pregnancy:
- Transplacental glucose transport (reflects mum's levels)
- ↑ HPL, progesterone, cortisol cause **insulin resistance**
  - → results in ↑ maternal glucose levels

in 2nd trimester

Diagnostic criteria for GDM
1. Fasting glucose >5.6mmol/L
2. OGTT >7.8mmol/L (2h after 75g oral glucose)

Further Ix
- HbA1c (check not T2DM)
- Abdo palpation (SFH, lie, pain)
- USS & fetal artery Dopplers

Risk factors for GDM
- PHx/FHx GDM
- 1st-degree relative with DM
- BMI >30kg/m²
- Black Caribbean, South Asian
- Previous large fetus (>4.5kg)
- Previous unexplained stillborn

OGTT done ASAP if previous GDM/DM

Polyhydramnios / persistent glucosuria

*>50% diagnosed with DM in 10y postpartum
→ fasting glucose test at 3m postpartum*

Glucose = teratogenic

Pre-existing diabetes mellitus (1%)

MANAGEMENT:
MDT team → consultant-led care
- **Pre-pregnancy:**
  - optimise glycaemic control (education)
  - folic acid 5mg daily
- **During pregnancy:**
  - increase insulin dose to maintain normoglycaemia
- **aspirin 150mg daily** to reduce pre-eclampsia risk
- regular BG, HbA1c, BP & renal monitoring (& screen for retinopathy)
- regular fetal monitoring (20w USS + regular growth scans, fetal echocardiography)
- → **Delivery by 39w**

Gestational diabetes mellitus (GDM) (13.5%)

DEFINITION: glucose intolerance **first diagnosed in pregnancy**
→ may or may not resolve after

AETIOLOGY: Beta islet cells unable to compensate for raised maternal glucose levels in pregnancy → hyperglycaemia

SCREENING:
- **Booking appointment:** screen for high-risk group
- **28 weeks*:** OGTT if identified as high-risk
- **Any time in pregnancy:** OGTT if RFs develop

MANAGEMENT[3]:
stepwise approach for optimising glucose control + regular review
1. **Lifestyle advice:** diet & exercise
2. **Oral agents:** if not controlled with lifestyle (e.g. metformin)
3. **Insulin:** if still not controlled (discontinued after pregnancy)
4. **75mg aspirin:** prophylaxis for pre-eclampsia
5. **Folic acid:** 5mg
6. **Regular fetal growth/USS scans** – every 4w

POSTPARTUM CARE
- Educate on increased lifetime risk* of DM: diet/exercise advice
  - ↳ very important
- Educate on increased recurrence of GDM
- Carefully monitor fetus: prefeed blood glucose for 24h

Complications of hyperglycaemia in pregnancy

MATERNAL COMPLICATIONS
- **Hypoglycaemia/ketoacidosis** (rare)
- **Infection:** UTI, endometritis, wound infection
- **Pre-eclampsia:** more common if pre-existing DM
- **Deterioration of pre-existing disease:** retinopathy, nephropathy

NEONATAL COMPLICATIONS
- **Hypoglycaemia** As developed compensatory hyperinsulinaemia in womb
- **Respiratory distress syndrome** Due to reduced pulmonary maturity

FETAL COMPLICATIONS
- **Congenital abnormalities** (↑×3) – NTDs, cardiac
- **IUGR/IUFD**
- **Macrosomia** (↑ birth weight) – hyperglycaemia causes ↑ fetal insulin & fat deposition → C-section if >4.5kg
- **Polyhydramnios** – due to ↑ fetal weight causing ↑ fetal urine
- **Preterm labour** (10%)
- **Birth complications:** trauma, dystocia, fetal distress/death
  - ↳ C-section/instrumental delivery more likely

[3] NICE (2015, updated 2020) *Diabetes in pregnancy* [NG3]

Other maternal disease in pregnancy

Thromboembolic disease

EPIDEMIOLOGY
- **Risk of VTE is increased ×6**
- Greatest risk is postpartum
- PE = important cause of maternal death

SIGNS/SYMPTOMS
- Calf tenderness
- Cough
- Chest/abdo/groin pain

PROPHYLAXIS: with LMWH*
Antenatally: only if high risk
Postnatally: if >1 moderate risk factor

INVESTIGATIONS
PE: CXR, ABG, CT or V/Q scan
DVT: Doppler USS
D-dimer not useful in pregnancy

Pregnancy = prothrombotic state

***warfarin contraindicated in pregnancy**

Risk factors for thromboembolic disease: assess at booking & postpartum

High risk:
- previous VTE
- prolonged immobility/hospitalisation

Moderate risk:
- BMI >30
- age >35
- IVDU/smoker
- immobility
- thrombophilia
- varicose veins
- C-section
- pre-eclampsia

Anaemia

→ *Hb drops to 11g/dl (symptoms if <9g/dl)*

PROPHYLAXIS:
- Dietary advice
- Folic acid 5mg OD
- Iron supplements

DIETARY ADVICE:
Iron-rich: kidney, liver, eggs, green vegetables
Folate-rich: fish, raw green vegetables

Thrombophilias

→ *antiphospholipid syndrome, protein S/C deficiency, factor V Leiden*

ACA antibody

COMPLICATIONS
- VTE
- Miscarriage
- Placental abruption
- IUGR
- Pre-eclampsia
- Fetal death

MANAGEMENT: as high-risk pregnancy
- Aspirin & LMWH
- LMWH continued postnatally

Cardiac disease

PATHOPHYSIOLOGY: During pregnancy ↑ HR & SV to ↑ CO by 40%

↑ *blood flow causes systolic ejection murmur in 90%*

IMPACT
- Major cause of maternal mortality: pre-existing cardiac condition may mean heart cannot cope with increased demand during pregnancy
- Problems usually occur >28w or during labour
- Fetal cardiac abnormalities occur in 3%

MANAGEMENT
1. Treat conditions before pregnancy if possible e.g. valve disease
2. Stop contraindicated drugs: warfarin, ACEi
3. Regular checks: of BP, anaemia, fetal abnormalities

> Reassure that 9 out of 10 women with epilepsy have a healthy baby

vomit up anti-epileptic medication

> **Safest drugs:** carbamazepine, lamotrigine
> **Contraindicated drugs:** sodium valproate

Epilepsy

IMPACT
- Significant cause of maternal mortality:
  - ► **seizure control reduced:** in labour, if sleep-deprived, during morning sickness
- Increased risk of **congenital defects (NTDs)** – mainly due to drug therapy
- 3% risk of fetus developing epilepsy

MANAGEMENT[4]: *consultant-led care*
1. **Seizure control:** with as few drugs as possible at lowest dose
2. **Folic acid supplementation** 5mg OD pre-conception
3. **Vitamin K for baby at birth:** 1mg IM
4. Offer **high resolution USS** abnormality scan at 18–20w + **serial growth scans**

→ *involve neurology team* → *DO NOT CHANGE MEDS without their advice*

Obesity

20% pregnant women have BMI >30

MATERNAL RISKS	**FETAL RISKS**
• Thromboembolism	• Congenital abnormalities
• Pre-eclampsia	• Mortality ↑ ×2.5
• GDM	• Miscarriage/stillbirth
• C-section	• NTDs
• Postpartum haemorrhage	• Macrosomia (shoulder dystocia)
• Wound infection	

ANTENATAL MANAGEMENT[5]
1. **Preconceptual advice:** weight, diet, exercise
2. **Supplementation:** 5mg folic acid & vit D
3. **Thromboprophylaxis**
4. **Prophylactic aspirin:** 75–150mg OD to prevent HTN
5. **Monitor:** blood glucose, BP
   - OGTT at 28w
   - Serial growth scans from 24w

LABOUR/POSTNATAL MANAGEMENT
1. **IOL** if large baby (elective C-section may be discussed)
2. **Continuous CTG in labour**
3. **Thromboprophylaxis:** clexane, stockings, up & moving
4. ↓ **risk of haemorrhage:** IV syntocin for 4h
5. ↓ **risk of infection:** regular checks, expose to air if possible

---

[4] RCOG (2016) *Epilepsy in pregnancy* [GTG 68]
[5] RCOG (2018) *Care of women with obesity in pregnancy* [GTG 72]

Early pregnancy problems

→ 15% pregnancies

Miscarriage

→ *fetus dies or delivers dead **before 24 completed weeks** of pregnancy*

↳ majority before 12 weeks

CAUSE: Significant chromosomal abnormality in 60% cases

SYMPTOMS: Lower abdo **pain** (crampy/ 'period-like') & vaginal **bleeding**

↳ Bleeding before pain

INVESTIGATIONS: in order

1. **Speculum** – open os is suggestive of miscarriage
2. **TV USS** – shows if fetus is intra-uterine & viable / any RPOC
3. **48h serum hCG** – rise >66% in viable pregnancies, remains low in miscarriage
4. **Check FBC, CRP, Rhesus status, G&S**

↳ CRP often raised

TYPES OF MISCARRIAGE

*RPOC: retained products of conception

Type	Symptoms	On examination	Mx
Threatened	Pain, bleeding – fetus still alive (only 25% miscarry)	Os closed, uterus normal for date	Home
Inevitable	Pain, **heavy** bleeding – fetus may/may not be alive	Os open	1, 2 or 3
Incomplete	Pain, bleeding – **some** fetal parts passed	Os open, **some RPOC***	1, 2 or 3
Complete	Slowed bleeding – **all** fetal parts passed	Os closed, uterus not enlarged, **no RPOC***	Home
Missed	May be **asymptomatic** – fetus dead/not developed	Os closed, uterus small for date (often picked up on 1st dating scan)	1, 2 or 3
Septic	Pain, **offensive vaginal loss** ± fever	Uterine tenderness, endometritis	ABX & 3

MANAGEMENT[6]

1. **Conservative/expectant:** wait to see if miscarriage occurs naturally → **80% successful**
   - R/V at 14d
     ‣ no bleeding/pain = pregnancy test at 3w to confirm miscarriage
     ‣ still bleeding/pain = re-scan & consider medical/surgical management

2. **Medical:** give medication to cause completion of miscarriage → **80% successful**
   - **PO/PV misoprostol** (prostaglandin) ± **mifepristone** (anti-progesterone)
   - + Analgesia & anti-emetics PRN
   - Pregnancy test at 3w to confirm miscarriage
   - **Risks:** bleeding*, infection, failure

3. **Surgical:** remove tissue surgically under local or general anaesthetic
   - **Vacuum aspiration** + histological examination to exclude molar pregnancy
   - **Complications:** partial removal of endometrium, perforation/scarring of uterus

Asherman's syndrome ↵

Recurrent miscarriage

→ ***3 or more** miscarriages in succession*

1% couples

CAUSES

- **Antiphospholipid antibodies** – cause thrombosis → Tx: aspirin & LMWH
- **Chromosomal defects** – refer to geneticist & consider IVF/PGS (rare)
- **Uterine abnormalities, e.g. LLETZ, fibroid** – USS to identify → Tx depends on cause
- **Hormonal:** thyroid problems
- **Other:** obesity, smoking, higher maternal age, PCOS

Interpreting USS results

CRL <7.2mm on 1st scan
= very early pregnancy OR miscarriage
→ rescan in 7–10d to be sure

CRL >7.2mm + no cardiac activity
= miscarriage diagnosed
→ at this size heartbeat should be present

Additional management considerations[6]

1. Give anti-D prophylaxis if Rh −ve & >12w gestation AND are having SURGICAL MANAGEMENT
2. Give PV progesterone BD for pregnant women with vaginal bleeding & history of miscarriage

SEs of misoprostol = diarrhoea & fever

*Risk of excess bleeding

All have approx. 3% risk of infection

Emotional support/counselling = very important in these cases

---

[6]NICE (2019, updated 2021) *Ectopic pregnancy and miscarriage* [NG126]

→ 1% pregnancies

Ectopic pregnancy

→ *embryo implants outside of the uterine cavity*

RISK FACTORS: particularly things that **scar tubes**

- Advanced maternal age
- Previous ectopic pregnancy
- IVF pregnancy
- PMHx chlamydia/pelvic infection/PID
- Previous abdo/tubal surgery
- Use of progesterone-only pill or IUD (the coil)

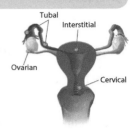

Fig. 4.1 Locations of ectopic pregnancy.

→ *Pain before bleeding*

SIGNS & SYMPTOMS: can be variable & vague!

- **Lower abdominal pain**
  - ▶ initially colicky then constant
  - ▶ rebound tenderness
  - ▶ uterine & adnexal tenderness
- **Abnormal vaginal bleeding** – scanty, dark
- **Signs of intraperitoneal blood loss**
  - ▶ dizziness & *shoulder-tip pain (referred)
  - ▶ *syncope/collapse in extremes
- **Amenorrhoea 4–10w**
  - ▶ may be unaware of pregnancy & interpret bleed as period
- **Uterus small for date & closed cervical os**

INVESTIGATIONS:

1. **Urine hCG pregnancy test:** will show +ve in ectopics
2. **TV USS** to exclude intrauterine pregnancy
   - BUT won't show very early uterine pregnancies
   - May show clot / free fluid in tubes
3. **Serum βhCG** to distinguish early & ectopic pregnancies
   - Early pregnancy: ↑ by >60% in 48h
   - Ectopic = slower ↑ or decrease
   - **If already >1000IU/ml would see pregnancy in uterus unless it is ectopic**
4. **Laparoscopy:** most sensitive but invasive*

MANAGEMENT[7]:

1. **Admit to hospital:** ABCDE, IV access, X-match, **Anti-D if Rh –ve**
2. **Medical:** *If unruptured AND no cardiac activity AND hCG <1500 IU/L*
   - Single dose IM methotrexate → 15% need 2nd dose, 10% need surgical escalation
   - Followed by serial hCG level monitoring
3. **Surgical:**
   - Laparoscopic salpingectomy (tube removal)
     - → consider **salpingostomy** (remove ectopic & leave tube) if other tube is damaged – allows future conception
     - → **Risks:** bleeding, infection, damage to other structures, hernia from incisions, DVT/PE, anaesthetic risks

Counselling points

1. **If medical management or salpingostomy:** explain possibility ectopic remains
   - → need for serial hCG levels
   - → know warning signs of rupture: severe abdo pain, pale/clammy, tachycardic, LOC/collapse
2. **Information about increased risk of ectopic in future** BUT reassure 70% go on to have future successful pregnancy
3. **Emotional support/counselling**

> In a woman of child-bearing age, abdominal pain + abnormal PV bleed = ectopic until proven otherwise.
> → Must do a URINE PREGNANCY TEST!

*RED FLAGS

*Used if clinical picture strongly suggests ectopic, i.e. USS showing empty uterus + serum hCG >1500IU/ml

Side-effects of methotrexate
- Mouth ulcers
- Liver dysfunction

---

[7]NICE (2019, updated 2021) *Ectopic pregnancy and miscarriage* [NG126]

Hyperemesis gravidarum

↳ 1 in 750 women

= Severe N&V in early pregnancy causing **dehydration, electrolyte disturbances, 5% weight loss, ketosis**

- starts at 4–7w, resolves by 16w

Severity	Prevalence	Symptoms	Treatment
Mild NVP*	50%	Nausea, occasional vomiting	No treatment needed
Moderate NVP	5%	More persistent vomiting	Often need admission
Severe NVP (hyperemesis gravidarum)	0.15%	Vomiting causing systemic Sx	Hospital admission

INVESTIGATIONS: Physical exam for signs of dehydration

- BP & pulse – for **hypovolaemia**
- Urine dip/urinalysis – for **ketonuria** & exclude UTI
- FBC – raised haematocrit if dehydrated
- U&Es – raised urea & Cr if dehydration causes AKI, hyponatraemia, hypokalaemia
- Calcium – exclude hypercalcaemia as cause of vomiting
- Pelvic USS – check viability of pregnancy & RFs for hyperemesis gravidarum

COMPLICATIONS

- DVT/PE – TED stockings ± LMWH prophylaxis
- Wernicke's encephalopathy – due to thiamine deficiency
- Hypokalaemia – IV/PO potassium replacement
- Mallory–Weiss tear – due to excessive vomiting
- Oesophageal rupture/pneumothorax – very rare!

MANAGEMENT[8]

Dehydration: IV fluids (Hartmann's/saline) → may need added K⁺ if hypokalaemia
N&V: antiemetics (IV/IM/SL if oral intake not tolerated)
Close monitoring: BP, pulse, renal function
Complications: TED stockings/LMWH, thiamine/Pabrinex, Gaviscon, folic acid

Gestational trophoblastic disease

→ *trophoblastic tissue* proliferates more *aggressively* than normal   excess hCG

TYPES: from blastocyst

1. **Hydatidiform mole:** localised & non-invasive proliferation
   - **Complete:** sperm fertilises empty oocyte = mitosis of 46XX tissue → no fetal tissue
   - **Partial:** two sperms fertilise oocyte = forms triploid zygote (69XXX/XXY/XYY) → variable evidence of fetus
2. **Invasive mole:** invasion localised to within the uterus ⎫ **Malignant:** need
3. **Choriocarcinoma:** invasion followed by metastases ⎭ further Ix/Tx
   outside of the uterus

SYMPTOMS

- Vaginal bleeding – may be heavy
- Severe vomiting
- Uterus large for date
- Early pre-eclampsia & hyperthyroidism

INVESTIGATIONS

- **USS** – swollen villi = 'snowstorm appearance'
- **Serum hCG** – very high
- **Histology** = diagnostic

MANAGEMENT

- **Suction curettage** – removes trophoblastic tissue
- **Serial hCG levels** – persistent/rising suggests malignancy*

---

[8]RCOG (2016) *The management of nausea and vomiting of pregnancy and hyperemesis gravidarum* [GTG 69]

*NVP = nausea & vomiting in pregnancy
Feel dizzy/faint
Oliguria

Risk factors

- Multiparous
- Multiple pregnancy
- Molar pregnancy

Differential diagnosis

- UTI
- Gastroenteritis
- Trophoblastic disease

Possible antiemetics

- Promethazine
- Cyclizine
- Metoclopramide
- Ondansetron

RARE: 1 in 700 pregnancies

Gestational trophoblastic neoplasia: persistently elevated hCG resulting from persistence of any form of trophoblastic tissue

---

*Malignancy
Diagnosed if: persistent/rising hCG **OR** persistent vaginal bleeding **OR** blood-borne metastases

Mx: chemotherapy

Late pregnancy problems

Give anti-D if Rh −ve
Kleihauer test: estimates fetal Hb & therefore amount of anti-D to give

Classification of placenta praevia

Minor: placenta not covering os
Major: partially/fully covering os

90% low-lying placentas will move upwards after 20w with growth of the uterus in the 3rd trimester

Delivery of placenta praevia

Elective C-section at 36–37w
- Earlier if severe bleeding

If placenta accreta/percreta
- Rusch balloon compression/total hysterectomy after C-section to ↓ bleeding

↳ *Intra-operative/postpartum haemorrhage = common*

CTG to monitor wellbeing

*Blood ≠ severity. Pain without bleed = 'concealed' abruption

Delivery in placental abruption

- **No fetal distress >37w:** IOL with amniotomy
- **No fetal distress <37w:** monitor on antenatal ward, steroids if <34w
- **Fetal distress = urgent C-section**
- **Fetus is dead:** IOL with amniotomy + blood & FFP transfusion

↳ *Intra-operative/postpartum haemorrhage = common*

Antepartum haemorrhage (APH)
→ *bleeding from the genital tract after 24 weeks' gestation*

Common causes
- Undetermined
- Placental abruption
- Placenta praevia

Rarer causes
- Genital tract pathology
- Uterine rupture
- Vasa praevia

PLACENTA PRAEVIA – *placenta implants in lower section of uterus*
→ *Complicates 0.4% pregnancies*

Risk factors
- Twins
- High parity
- Increased maternal age (>40)
- Scarred uterus, e.g. previous C-section/surgery, previous placenta praevia
  - ↳ **Placenta accreta:** implantation so deep into scar that **placental separation is prevented**
  - ↳ **Placenta percreta:** implantation so deep into scar that it **penetrates uterine wall** into surrounding structures e.g. bladder

Symptoms
- Intermittent, **painless** bleeds → increase in frequency & intensity
- Breech presentation, transverse lie, fetal head not engaged

Investigations: avoid vaginal examination → can provoke massive bleed
- **Ultrasound scan**
  - detects low-lying placenta at 20w → **safety-net:** straight to hospital if bleed occurs
  - repeat at 32w to exclude praevia

Management[9]
- **Presentation without bleeding: delay admission until delivery**
- **Presentation with bleeding: admit & keep until delivery**
  - FBC, clotting studies, cross-match
  - monitor fetal and maternal wellbeing: CTG, IV access
  - IV steroids if <34 weeks' gestation
  - anti-D if woman is Rhesus −ve

PLACENTAL ABRUPTION – *part or all of placenta separates before delivery of the fetus*
→ *Complicates 1% pregnancies*

Risk factors
- Hx of placental abruption (6%)
- Pre-eclampsia / pre-existing HTN
- IUGR
- Multiple pregnancy
- High parity
- Autoimmune
- **Smoking / cocaine use**

Investigations
USS: exclude placenta praevia
→ *may not show abruption*

Symptoms
- **Painful**, dark bleeds*
- Tender, contracting uterus → labour often ensues
- **If severe** = 'woody-hard' uterus, hypotension, ↑HR
- Decreased fetal movements

Management: admit
- FBC, clotting studies, cross-match
- Monitor fetal and maternal wellbeing: CTG, CVP, IV access
- IV steroids if <34w gestation
- Anti-D if woman is Rhesus −ve

[9]RCOG (2011) *Antepartum haemorrhage* [GTG 63]

VASA PRAEVIA – *fetal blood vessels run in the membranes in front of the presenting part*
→ when membranes rupture, fetal vessels do too = MASSIVE FETAL BLEED

Symptoms	**Management**
• Moderate, **painless** vaginal bleed when membranes rupture	URGENT C-SECTION
• Severe fetal distress	

UTERINE RUPTURE
→ occasionally occurs before labour in women with scarred / congenitally abnormal uterus **but very rare**

BLEEDING OF GYNAECOLOGICAL ORIGIN
Causes
- **Cervical carcinoma** → suspect if small recurrent or post-coital bleeding
- Cervical polyps   ↳ check with speculum & colonoscopy
- Ectropions   if smear overdue
- Vaginal lacerations

BLEEDING OF UNKNOWN ORIGIN
→ Small, painless bleeds in absence of placenta praevia → **likely minor placental abruptions**

Prolonged pregnancy

DEFINITION: >42w

RISKS

To fetus/neonate
- Meconium aspiration
- Macrosomia: prolonged labour, shoulder dystocia
- Neonatal seizures/encephalopathy
- IUGR (due to placental insufficiency)
- Stillbirth / neonatal death

To mother
- Prolonged labour
- Instrumental delivery/C-section
- Perineal damage
- PPH
- Infection

MANAGEMENT
Offer IOL after 41w
If IOL declined, increased monitoring: CTG 2× per week

usually too slow to save fetus if not in hospital

Risk factors for prolonged pregnancy
- Hx post-term pregnancy
- Primigravidity
- High BMI
- Higher maternal age
- Genetics

Chorioamnionitis
        ↳ 5% pregnancies
DEFINITION: acute **inflammation of the amniotic fluid/membranes** 2° to ascending bacterial infection

RISK FACTOR: Prelabour ROM

INVESTIGATIONS
- FBC, CRP
- High vaginal swab – culture & sensitivities
- CTG

SYMPTOMS
- Uterine tenderness
- Maternal signs of infection: fever, tachycardia, leucocytosis

MANAGEMENT: Medical emergency
- Prompt delivery under IV ABX
     → may need C-section

Preterm delivery

↳ *5–8% of deliveries*

DEFINITION: delivery between 24w & 37w (if <24w = miscarriage)

↳ *<34w = highest risk to neonate*

CAUSES
- Spontaneous preterm labour (50%)
- Iatrogenic – IOL by doctor due to fetal/maternal risk or PPROM

COMPLICATIONS
For neonate:
- Prematurity = **80% NICU occupancy**
- Chronic morbidity
- Death

Lung disease, blindness/hearing loss, cerebral palsy, neurological impairment

For mother:
- Infection (endometritis = common)
- Increased need for C-section

SYMPTOMS
- Painful contractions → 50% resolve & no preterm delivery
- Dull suprapubic ache & increased discharge **if cervical incompetence**
- Antepartum haemorrhage
- Fluid loss → suggests ROM

Prevention: *only high-risk women,* e.g. previous preterm labour[10]
- **Offer cervical cerclage:** sutures to strengthen cervix & keep it closed
  - ▸ elective at 12–14w if recurrent early loss
  - ▸ cervical length scans at 16w, 18w, 20w & offer sutures if <25mm
  - ▸ 'rescue suture' of dilated cervix can be performed if first presentation
- **Progesterone supplementation:** suppositories from early pregnancy
- **Treatment of maternal medical disease**
- **Avoid unnecessary ABX:** treat UTIs, STIs, bacterial vaginosis but caution for other infections
- **Multi-fetal reduction:** of higher order multiples
- **Treatment of polyhydramnios:** needle aspiration (amnioreduction) or NSAIDs (reduce fetal urine output)

MANAGEMENT[11]: <27w transfer to NICU

Do not continue tocolytics >24h or if infection present

1. **Steroids & tocolysis:**
   - Steroids if <34w to promote pulmonary maturity
   - Take 24h to work so delay delivery with tocolysis → e.g. nifedipine
2. **IV ABX:** only given antenatally if PPROM
3. **MgSO$_4$ if <32w:** reduces risk of intraventricular haemorrhage and cerebral palsy
4. **Delivery:** VAGINAL WHERE POSSIBLE – ensure in optimal environment (neonatal unit)
   - C-section if breech or other obstetric indications → increases risk of fetal respiratory distress
   - No artificial rupture of membranes if <34w
   - Forceps only if necessary
   - **Antibiotics*** – given intrapartum as GBS prophylaxis (regardless of mum's GBS status)

Risk factors for preterm delivery

General
- Hx of preterm labour
- Younger/older mothers
- Lower socioeconomic status
- Short inter-pregnancy interval

Biggest risk factor

Fetal survival response
- Maternal disease, e.g. renal, thyroid, DM
- Pregnancy complications – IUGR, pre-eclampsia
- Antepartum haemorrhage

Damage to uterus/cervix
- STIs/UTIs/vaginal infections
- Hx cervical surgeries
- Uterine abnormalities/fibroids

Infection indicated in 60%

Not enough space
- Multiple pregnancy
- Polyhydramnios

Predicting preterm labour

1. **Hx & VE**
2. **Transvaginal USS:**
   Serial cervical length
3. **Fetal fibronectin**
   Levels rise shortly before labour
4. **QUiPP app[10]** to calculate risk

---

*ABX only started in baby if red flags for sepsis

---

[10] QUiPP version 2.0, released Oct 2017, © King's College London
[11] NICE (2015, updated 2019) *Preterm labour and birth* [NG25]

Preterm pre-labour rupture of membranes (PPROM)

DEFINITION: membranes rupture before labour at <37w

CAUSES
- Often unknown
- Any of the causes of preterm labour

COMPLICATIONS
- **Preterm delivery** – occurs within 48h in 50%
- **Infection of fetus, placenta, or cord** (chorioamnionitis/funisitis)
- Prolapse of umbilical cord
- Pulmonary hypoplasia / postural deformities (due to lack of liquor)

SYMPTOMS
- Gush of clear fluid + further leaking
- **Chorioamnionitis Sx:**
  - ▶ contractions
  - ▶ abdominal pain / uterine tenderness
  - ▶ fever, tachycardia
  - ▶ offensive liquor

INVESTIGATIONS
- **Speculum:** pool of fluid in posterior fornix
- **USS:** may show reduced liquor **BUT normal liquor volume doesn't exclude PPROM**
- **Point of care tests*:** ILGF binding protein / placental alpha microglobulin
- **Infection screen:** high vaginal swab, FBC, CRP ± amniocentesis & culture
- **Assess fetal wellbeing:** CTG

Management[12]: balance risks of infection vs. risks of preterm delivery
No signs of infection
- Admit & monitor for signs of infection
- Corticosteroids if <34w (promote lung maturity of fetus)
- Prophylactic erythromycin (for maximum of 10d)
- IOL if reach 37w

Signs of infection
- Immediate IV ABX & delivery
- IV ABX & septic screen in baby when born

*not entirely reliable

remember ↑ WCC in pregnancy anyway

---

[12] RCOG (2019) *Care of women presenting with suspected preterm prelabour rupture of membranes* [GTG 73]

Multiple pregnancies

↳ **Twins:** 1/80 pregnancies
↳ **Triplets:** 1/1000 pregnancies

Risk factors
- Assisted conception
- Increasing maternal age
- Higher parity
- Genetics

All obstetric risks increased!

Definitions

Dizygotic twins (2/3) – fertilisation of **2 different oocytes** by **2 different sperm**
Monozygotic twins (1/3) (identical) – meiotic division of a **single oocyte**

↳ **Division before day 3** = dichorionic diamniotic (DCDA) — 2 placentas, 2 amnions **(30%)**
↳ **Division in days 4–8** = monochorionic diamniotic (MCDA) — 1 placenta, 2 amnions **(70%)**
↳ **Division in days 9–13** = monochorionic monoamniotic (MCMA) — 1 placenta, 1 amnion **(rare)**
↳ **Incomplete division** = conjoined twins

Complications*

MATERNAL
- Gestational diabetes, pre-eclampsia, anaemia = more common
- Spontaneous miscarriage – one fetus dies in 50% cases
- Preterm labour – 40% twins, 80% triplets
- Malpresentation of 1st twins at labour – 20%
- Postpartum haemorrhage – atonic uterus is common

FETAL
- ↑ ×6 mortality/stillbirth → prematurity = big cause of mortality
- ↑ ×5 handicap (e.g. cerebral palsy)
- Congenital abnormalities more common in MC twins
- IUGR – ⅔ cases: especially in MC twins but can occur in any twin pregnancy due to **placental insufficiency**
  ↳ Usually one twin is smaller

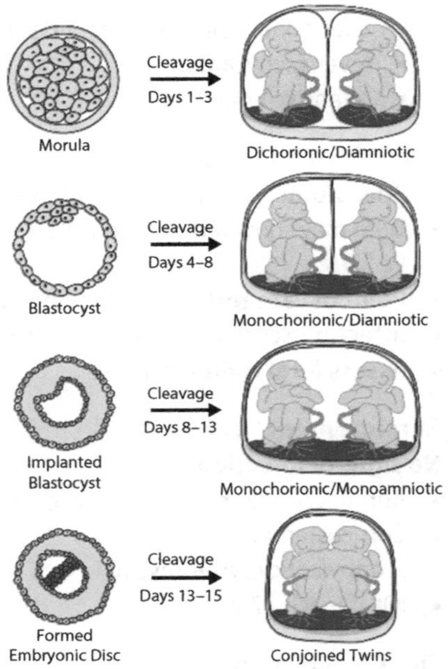

Morula — Cleavage Days 1–3 → Dichorionic/Diamniotic

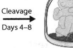

Blastocyst — Cleavage Days 4–8 → Monochorionic/Diamniotic

Implanted Blastocyst — Cleavage Days 8–13 → Monochorionic/Monoamniotic

Formed Embryonic Disc — Cleavage Days 13–15 → Conjoined Twins

Fig. 4.2

Biggest risk of complications is in MC twins due to shared blood supply

Specific complications of monochorionicity

TWIN–TWIN TRANSFUSION SYNDROME (TTTS) – in MCDA only (15%)
- **Unequal blood distribution** through anastomoses in placenta
- **Donor twin:** volume depletion, anaemia, IUGR, oligohydramnios
- **Recipient twin:** volume overload, polycythaemia, cardiac failure, polyhydramnios

Management
→ complete laser photocoagulation of placental interface via USS & fetoscopy (seal blood supply between twins)
→ USS amnioreduction (draw out some amniotic fluid)

Outcomes of TTTS
- Severe preterm delivery
- IUFD

Prognosis of TTTS
- Both survive: 50%
- One survives: 80%

TWIN REVERSED ARTERIAL PERFUSION (TRAP) – rare (1%)
- Fetal blood systems connected
- One twin (pump) = normal & other twin (acardiac) = **abnormal/missing heart & upper limbs**

SELECTIVE FETAL GROWTH RESTRICTION – 10–15%
- Due to superficial artery–artery anastomoses causing **intermittently absent or reversed blood flow** to 1 twin
- Sudden IUFD in 20%

CO-TWIN DEATH
- Death of one twin causes **acute transfusion of blood to surviving twin**
- Results in hypovolaemia → **death/neurological damage in surviving twin**

MONOAMNIOTIC TWINS – rare
- **Cords are always entangled** → blood shunting between twins via cord anastomoses → IUFD = common

Management[13]

ANTENATAL MANAGEMENT: consultant-led as high risk
- **Early USS to determine chorionicity**
  - **DC twins:** thicker dividing membrane as meets placenta (λ sign)
  - **MC twins:** thinner dividing membrane, perpendicular to placenta (T sign)
- **Regular USS checks for IUGR**
  - **DC twins:** every 4w from 28/40
  - **MC twins:** every 2w from 12/40
- **Selective reduction:** discussed at 12w if triplets or more
  - reduces chance of preterm delivery & associated fetal death/handicap
- **Birth plan / method of delivery discussed** by 28w

DELIVERY:
- **Timing:** DC twins = 37w, MC twins = 36w
- **Location:** in hospital
- **Staff:** consultant, 2× midwives (1 senior), paediatricians
- **Continuous CTG**
- **Analgesia:** epidural recommended
- **Mode:** LSCS commonly used for multiple pregnancies, but evidence does not suggest different outcomes to NVD
  - **NVD:** only viable if 1st twin = cephalic
  - **fetal distress:** speed delivery with **ventouse or breech extraction**
  - **after 1st twin is born:** check lie of 2nd twin → ECV if needed & amniotomy → 2nd baby may need C-section
- **Active 3rd stage (oxytocin):** high risk of PPH due to uterine atony

Additional considerations
- Iron & folate supplements
- Postnatal home help discussed
- Educate patient on signs of preterm labour & complications (e.g. PPROM)

Absolute indications for C-section
- Malpresentation of 1st twin
- Hx of antepartum complications
- Triplets or more

↑ risk death in 2nd twin delivered: hypoxia, cord prolapse, placental abruption

[13] NICE (2019) *Twin and triplet pregnancy* [NG137]

Mechanism of labour

Normal labour: lasts 10–12h
- Spontaneous onset at 37–42w
- Low risk at start & throughout
- Baby born in vertex position

*At brim transverse = widest,
At outlet AP = widest*

Reasons for admission

- Established labour (regular contractions)
- ROM
- Bleeding
- Green discharge
- Mother feels unwell
- Fetal movements stop
- Strong urge to push

Counsel to stay home as long as possible to reduce iatrogenic risk / unnecessary interventions. Advice to give whilst at home:
- Warm bath / heat packs
- Hip rocking / birthing ball
- Paracetamol
- Light, plain food

Mechanical factors of labour

1. POWERS – uterine contractions
- **Start at fundus** and pass inwards and downwards
- Muscle fibres contract to pull cervix up (effacement) & cause dilatation
- Assist with descent & expulsion of fetus

2. PASSAGE – pelvis, cervix, vagina, pelvic floor
- **Pelvic dimensions** change between brim & outlet*
- **Ischial spines are used as reference** point to describe the level of descent (also known as 'station')

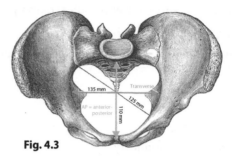

135 mm   Transverse
AP = anterior-posterior 125 mm
110 mm

Fig. 4.3

3. PASSENGER – fetus, placenta, membranes
- **Size:** fetal head greatest in diameter AP → sutures & fontanelles enable compression of head = 'moulding'
- **Attitude:** degree of flexion of fetal head (ideal = well flexed 'vertex position') → *chin tucked into neck*
- **Position:** degree of rotation of the head → *ideally starts transverse & rotates 90° in pelvis to become OA*

Signs of onset of labour

- **Regular, painful uterine contractions:** every 2–3min, lasting 45–60s
  ► triggered by an increase in oxytocin production
- **'Show' (operculum):** expulsion of mucous plug
  ► gloopy/Vaseline-like mucus discharge from vagina → may be blood-streaked
- **Spontaneous rupture of membranes (SROM):** labour doesn't always follow immediately
  ► offer IOL within 24–48h as **risk of infection**

Stages of labour

Stage 1: onset of **regular, painful contractions** to **full dilation of cervix (10cm)**
- **Latent:** slow dilation to 3cm over several hours
- **Active:** faster dilation of 1–2cm/h

Stage 2: From full dilation of cervix to **delivery of baby**
- **Passive:** until head reaches pelvic floor
- **Active:** mother is pushing (usually for 20–40min before delivery)

Stage 3: From delivery of baby to **separation & delivery of placenta & membranes**
- Normally lasts 15min
- **Controlled cord traction:** inject **IM Syntometrine** (oxytocin analogue) to induce placental separation

Management of labour[14]

Maternal monitoring

1. **Basic observations**
   - BP, RR, temperature, urine output every 4h
   - FHR every 15min
   - Pulse every hour
   - Liquor colour – check for **meconium**
2. **Abdominal palpation:** lie, presentation, position, SFH
3. **Monitoring progress:**
   - **Cervical dilation:** record every 4h (up to 7cm) & plot on **partogram** (check more regularly after 7cm)
   - **Contractions** – frequency and length

   Also record of maternal vital signs (BP, temp., pulse, urine) & fetal HR

Encourage
- **Hydration:** isotonic drinks and water
- Frequent micturition
- Movement

Meconium: bowel contents of fetus which stain amniotic fluid ('pea soup') → can be aspirated by fetus = pneumonitis

Fetal monitioring

Detecting & managing fetal distress/hypoxia:

Auscultate FHR every 15 mins (& after contractions)

Start CTG if abnormal FHR, labour >5h, high risk labour, meconium, PV bleeding

→

CTG / fetal scalp electrodes

If ominous abnormalities not resolved by simple measures: **FBS**

If bradycardia >3min = **prepare for emergency LSCS**

→

FBS* (fetal blood sample)

pH <7.20 or BE <−10 = immediate section

= More reliable measure of FHR
Use if start to lose CTG trace/CTG is worrying

amnioscope inserted into vagina and makes small cut on fetal scalp → collect blood in tube & analyse pH & base excess

Pain relief

- **Entonox (gas & air):** NO + O_2
  - mild analgesia, rapid onset
  - SEs: nausea, light-headedness, tearful
- **TENS (transcutaneous electrical nerve stimulation):** stimulation of nerves through 4 patches stuck on back
  - distracts from pain
  - must be put on **at start of labour** & no pool births
- **Systemic opioids:** morphine, pethidine → IM by midwife/doctor
  - mild analgesia, fairly rapid onset
  - SEs: N&V, sedation, **cross placenta** (respiratory depression in baby)
- **Epidural:** fentanyl (opioid) + bupivacaine (anaesthetic)
  - injected by anaesthetist into **epidural space between L3–L4**
  - very effective
  - complete sensory (except pressure) & partial motor blockade from injection site downwards

Indications for epidural
- Long labour
- Pre-eclampsia (reduces BP)
- For instrumental delivery / C-section
- Twins

Contraindications for epidural
- Sepsis
- Coagulopathy/anticoagulant therapy
- Spinal abnormalities/neurological disease

Problems with epidural
- Hypotension
- Itching/toxicity
- Urinary retention (reduced sensation)
- Poor mobility
- CSF tap (if insert too far) → big headache
- Complete spinal analgesia (rare)
- **Reduced ability to push** = higher instrumental delivery rate

Poor progress in labour

CAUSES

Power	Passenger	Passage
• Dehydration/ketosis	• Multiples	• Size & shape of pelvis (genes)
• Maternal exhaustion	• Abnormal presentation (breech/brow)	• Pelvic deformities / cysts
• Epidural / other medication	• Abnormal position (OP/OT)*	• Cervical abnormalities
• Overactive uterus (placental abruption & fetal hypoxia)	• Macrosomia	• Low-lying placenta / fibroid

Insufficient uterine activity: #1 cause of slow progress
→ needs augmentation

*Rotate with ventouse/forceps

[14]NICE (2014, updated 2017) *Intrapartum care for healthy women and babies* [CG190]

AUGMENTATION OF LABOUR

1. If dilation <1cm/h in active phase (post 3cm)

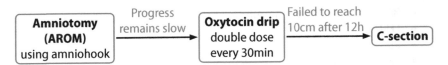

2. If been pushing for 1h (multips) or 2h (nullips) and delivery not imminent

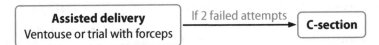

Induction of labour (IOL)

→ Determine **BISHOP'S SCORE:** based on degree of effacement & dilatation of cervix, station & position of fetus   Likelihood of IOL success
→ Mother and fetal monitoring: **CTG & Obs**

METHODS

- **Membrane sweep:** use fingers to separate membranes from uterus/cervix
- **Prostaglandin E$_2$ gel (Propess):** into posterior vaginal fornix
- **Mechanical:** Dilapam sticks and AROM
- **Amniotomy** (+ oxytocin if no induction after 2h)
- **Oxytocin:** following amniotomy OR if membranes already ruptured

COMPLICATIONS OF IOL

→ Slow labour (insufficient uterine activity) = increases risk instrumental delivery
→ Cord prolapse
→ Infection
→ Postpartum haemorrhage

Assisted delivery

INSTRUMENTAL DELIVERY: 20% nullips, 2% multips
Indication: if delayed second stage of labour or concern over baby's wellbeing

C-SECTION DELIVERY: 20–30% deliveries in the world
- **Emergency:** failure to progress in labour, fetal distress
- **Elective:** breech, placenta praevia, severe IUGR, multiples, diabetes, severe pre-eclampsia

Procedure: 40–50min in theatre → epidural or spinal anaesthetic

Complications of C-section

- Haemorrhage – G&S, X-match, transfusion ready
- Infection – prophylactic ABX
- VTE – prophylactic thrombolysis + TED stockings
- Postoperative pain and immobility
- Damage to visceral organs/fetus
- **Cannot drive for 4–6w**

→**Future problems** due to adhesions & scarring → risk of placenta praevia / uterine rupture

---

Indications for IOL
- Term + 10
- Multiples
- Pre-eclampsia
- Diabetes/GDM
- IUGR
- PROM*

*PROM: prelabour (term) ROM
= gush clear fluid then trickle

→ risk of infection & cord prolapse
NB most start labour spontaneously

Contraindications for IOL
- Abnormal lie
- Placenta praevia
- Pelvic obstruction
- >1 previous C-section

C-section causes future risk of placenta praevia (accreta & percreta) due to scar tissue

Labour complications

Vaginal birth after C-section (VBAC)[15]

→ *75% success rate (higher if previous vaginal delivery)*

BENEFITS OVER REPEAT C-SECTION
- Quicker recovery
- No anaesthetic risk
- Reduced risk of bleeding, infection, VTE
- Increased chance of normal vaginal delivery in future pregnancies

RISKS
- Rupture of previous uterine scar (0.5% = 1 in 200) → need emergency C-section
- Risk of perianal trauma

PROBLEMS WITH REPEAT C-SECTION
- Increased complications from adhesions
- Increased risk of placenta praevia in future pregnancies

MANAGEMENT OF VBAC
- Consultant-led care – final delivery plans discussed at 36w
- Hospital delivery with:
  - **continuous CTG monitoring**
  - **maternal obs:** BP, HR, RR, temperature, regular VEs
  - **IV access & FBC:** G&S in case of emergency C-section
  - **pool birth not recommended** – discuss with consultant
- Emergency C-section if failure to progress / fetal distress / uterine rupture*

Elective C-section

done around 39w → confirm decision/plan at 36w

BENEFITS
- Lowers risk of scar rupture if previous C-section
- Avoids risk of perianal trauma
- Lower risk of HIE
- Can plan delivery date

RISKS/DISADVANTAGES
- Longer recovery
- Increased risk of bleeding and infection
- Increased chance will need C-section in future

> **If IOL for a woman with previous C-section, must be done MECHANICALLY**
> i.e. with Dilapam sticks + AROM

> **Contraindications to VBAC**
>
> - ≥2 previous C-sections
> - Vertical uterine scar
> - Current indications for C-section
>   - placenta praevia
>   - abnormal lie
>   - severe IUGR

*scar pain, PV bleeding, maternal collapse
→ if cannot stop bleed may need hysterectomy

---

[15] RCOG (2015) *Birth after previous caesarean birth* [GTG 45]

PRESENTATION: part of fetus occupying lower section of uterus
LIE: relationship of fetus to long axis of uterus

Unstable lie: continually changing position
→ *commonly caused by too much room to turn*

Breech presentation affects
→ 3% term pregnancies
→ 25% preterm labours

Contraindications to ECV

- Multiple pregnancy
- Fetal distress
- Recent APH / active PV bleed
- Ruptured membranes
- Uterine abnormality

Risks: bleed, fetal distress

External cephalic version (ECV): low risk

- No analgesia but ± uterine relaxant (tocolytic)
- Manipulation of fetus with hands on abdomen
- Ultrasound-guided
- CTG monitoring & anti-D given immediately after

Risks: uterine rupture, placental abruption, fetal distress
CIs: ROM, twins, recent APH, fetal distress, placenta praevia

Abnormal lie & breech presentation

CAUSES OF ABNORMAL LIE

- **Preterm labour**
- **↑ room to turn:** polyhydramnios, high parity (stretched uterus)
- **↓ room to turn:** uterine/fetal abnormalities, multiple pregnancy
- **Prevention of engagement:** placenta praevia, pelvic tumour
- **Fetal abnormalities:** IUGR/macrosomia, short cord, hydrocephaly

COMPLICATIONS OF ABNORMAL LIE

- Cannot deliver fetus!
  - ▶ arm or umbilical cord prolapse
  - ▶ uterine rupture

MANAGEMENT OF TRANSVERSE/UNSTABLE LIE:

<37w: no action needed
>37w: admission & USS to exclude polyhydramnios/placenta praevia
  → **if spontaneous version:** discharge
  → **continued abnormal lie to 41w or labour:** C-section
    (ECV & amniotomy are options if expert available)

BREECH PRESENTATION

Risk factors
- Previous breech presentation (8%)
- Preterm labour/prematurity
- RFs for abnormal lie

Complications
- Fetal abnormalities
- Long-term neurological handicap
- Cord prolapse
- Late detection of trapped head
  → fetal hypoxia/death

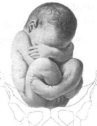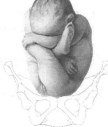

Flexed Breech   **Extended Breech**

Fig. 4.4 Types of breech presentation.

Diagnosis: only important >37w or if in labour

1. **Symptoms:** upper abdo discomfort & palpable fetal head
2. **USS:** confirms diagnosis & helps identify abnormalities

Management[16]

1. **External cephalic version (ECV):** attempt after 37w → 50% successful for primips, 70% for multips
2. **Elective C-section:** advised if ECV failed or contraindicated
3. **Vaginal breech birth:** if patient chooses over C-section
→ ↑ risk of fetal compromise & cord prolapse
  ↳ pushing not advised until buttocks are visible
  ↳ CTG & epidural advised
  ↳ prepare for emergency C-section:
    FBC, G&S, paediatrician, theatre ready

---

[16]RCOG (2017) *Management of breech presentation* [GTG20b]

Obstetric emergencies

Shoulder dystocia

→ *normal downwards traction fails to deliver the shoulders after the head*

COMPLICATIONS

- Brain damage (hypoxia) ⎤
- Damaged brachial plexus → Erb's palsy ⎦ *baby*
- Perineal injury / uterine rupture ⎤
- PPH ⎦ *mum*

MANAGEMENT[17]: RAPID SKILLED INTERVENTION → CALL FOR HELP ('SOAPS')

1. **McRobert's manoeuvre:** hyperextend legs + suprapubic pressure
2. **Wood's screw manoeuvre:** manual internal rotation of shoulders (need episiotomy)
3. **Grasp posterior arm:** gently pull down and rotate body as it follows
4. **Last resort:** symphysiotomy, Zavanelli manoeuvre, C-section → often too late by this point

Cord prolapse

→ *following ROM, the cord descends **below the presenting part***

PRESENTATION

- Cord felt on VE
- Pathological CTG signs

COMPLICATIONS

- Cord compression/spasm → fetal hypoxia (15–20% mortality in hospital)

MANAGEMENT[18]: GET HELP ('SOAPS' + prepare theatre for C-section)

1. **Stop cord compression:**
   - Use finger to push presenting part upwards **and keep in** / get woman on all 4s
   - Fill bladder with 500–750ml – push baby's head off cord
   - Tocolytics given, e.g. terbutaline
2. **If cord is out of introitus:** keep warm & moist but do not force back inside
3. **Delivery:** keep patient on all 4s while prepare for safest delivery*

Uterine rupture

→ *de novo tear OR opening of previous scar* **Risk = 1 in 200 if previous C-section**

COMPLICATIONS

- Extrusion & hypoxia of fetus
- Massive internal maternal haemorrhage

MANAGEMENT

1. **Maternal resuscitation:** IV fluids & blood + clotting, X-match, FBC
2. **If blood loss too fast:** urgent laparotomy to deliver fetus & repair/remove uterus

PREVENTION: caution with oxytocin if previous section

Amniotic fluid embolism

→ *liquor enters maternal circulation, causing anaphylaxis*

COMPLICATIONS (FOR MOTHER)

- Dyspnoea, hypoxia, hypotension ⎤
- Seizures, cardiac arrest, acute heart failure ⎬ *can result in death*
- DIC, pulmonary oedema, respiratory distress ⎦

MANAGEMENT

1. **Maternal resuscitation:** IV fluids, O_2, blood & FFP for transfusion + clotting, X-match, FBC

Prevalence

Shoulder dystocia: 1 in 200
Cord prolapse: 1 in 500

⎧ **S**enior midwife
⎪ **O**bstetrician
⎨ **A**naesthetist
⎪ **P**aediatrician
⎩ **S**cribe

Risk factors for shoulder dystocia
- **Large baby** (>4kg)
- Previous shoulder dystocia
- High maternal BMI
- Maternal diabetes
- IOL / instrumental delivery

Risk factors for cord prolapse
- Preterm labour / low birth weight
- Breech/OP/abnormal lie
- Multiples (2nd twin)
- Polyhydramnios
- Multiparous (↑ risk unstable lie)

>50% following artificial amniotomy when presenting part still high

usually C-section but instrumental may be possible if fully dilated

Risk factors for uterine rupture
- Scarred uterus (e.g. previous C-section, myomectomy)
- Neglected obstructed labour
- Congenital uterine abnormalities

Risk factors for amniotic fluid embolism
- Polyhydramnios
- Very strong contractions

Typically occurs at ROM, C-section or TOP

---

[17] RCOG (2012) *Shoulder dystocia* [GTG42]
[18] RCOG (2014) *Umbilical cord prolapse* [GTG50]

Fetal monitoring

Low BW: <2.5kg
Very low BW: <1.5kg
Extremely low BW: <1kg

Small for gestational age (SGA): smaller than 10th percentile for gestation
Large for gestational age (LGA): weight/length/head circumference above 90th percentile for gestation
IUGR: small for date AND evidence of compromised growth *i.e. drop in linear growth on chart / abnormal umbilical artery Doppler*

IUGR affects 5 in 1000 births (0.5%)

Complications of IUGR

- Meconium aspiration
- Hypotension, hypoglycaemia, hypothermia
- Jaundice, sepsis
- Increased risk stillbirth / neonatal death
- Increased risk neuro-behavioural abnormalities (ADHD, dyspraxia, dyslexia)
- Increased risk of development of adult diseases (obesity, T2DM, CVD)

Methods of fetal growth surveillance

- **Symphysis-fundal height (SFH)**
- **Serial USS:** measure abdominal & head circumference, identify abnormalities
- **Doppler scan umbilical artery:** increased resistance to flow can indicate placental insufficiency
- **Doppler scan fetal circulation:** mainly middle cerebral artery to detect brain sparing in IUGR or suspected anaemia
- **USS of biophysical profile & fluid volume:** measures limb movements, tone, breathing movements, liquor volume
- **Cardiotocography (CTG):** records fetal heart rate for up to 1h

Small for gestational age

CAUSES:
- **Physiological**
- **Pathological** (IUGR)
  - maternal disease (e.g. pre-eclampsia, DM, SLE) → often causes **placental insufficiency**
  - drugs, smoking, alcohol
  - diet / low BMI
  - infection
  - chromosome abnormalities, e.g. Down syndrome → often no other obvious reasons
  - dichorionic twins → often no other obvious reasons

INVESTIGATIONS:
1. Serial SFH measurements
   - Small but linear growth suggests small fetus
   - Drop in growth suggests IUGR
2. Uterine artery Doppler USS
3. Fetal abnormality screen
4. Infection testing
5. Karyotyping in severe cases

MANAGEMENT:
- Monitor closely in **consultant-led care**
- Delivery by 39w if SGA → may be earlier if static growth / fetus at risk
- May need NICU for baby

Cardiotocography (CTG)

→ *records fetal heart rate & uterine contractions*

FEATURES:

1. **BASELINE FHR** – average fetal HR within 10min
   - **Normal:** 110–160bpm
   - **Tachycardia:** chorioamnionitis, anaemia, hypoxia, prematurity
   - **Bradycardia:** fetal heart block, maternal hypotension, fetal distress

2. **VARIABILITY** – short-term variation in HR* representing fetal autonomic system
   = *difference between highest peak & lowest trough of a 1-min segment*
   - **Normal:** 5–25bpm
   - **Non-reassuring:** <5bpm for 30–90min
   - **Abnormal:** <5bpm >90min OR sinusoidal

3. **ACCELERATIONS** – increase in baseline FHR of ≥15bpm for ≥15s
   = *represent autonomic activity*
   - **Presence:** reassuring – occur with movements & contractions

4. **DECELERATIONS** – decrease in baseline FHR of ≥15bpm for ≥15s
   - **Early decelerations:** synchronise with contractions in response to head compression → quickly recover = benign
   - **Variable decelerations:** fall in HR with variable recovery phase → often reflect cord compression → hypoxia
   - **Late decelerations:** persist after contraction, suggesting placental insufficiency → hypoxia

Describing decelerations

- individual depth & duration
- timing in relation to contractions
- how long they have been present
- whether they occur in >50% contractions

Overall impression of CTG

Category	Features
Normal	All reassuring
Suspicious	1 non-reassuring AND 2 reassuring
Pathological	1 abnormal OR 2 non-reassuring
Urgent intervention	Bradycardia OR single deceleration >3min

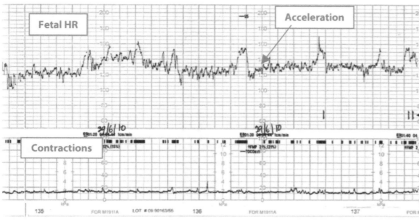

Fig. 4.5 Example CTG.

CTG indications during pregnancy
- Pre-eclampsia & GDM
- Recurrent APH
- IUGR
- Oligohydramnios

CTG indications during labour
- IOL or use of oxytocin
- Suspected chorioamnionitis/sepsis
- New onset fresh vaginal bleeding
- Breech presentation
- Preterm labour
- Twins/multiples
- VBAC

*Reasons for reduced variability
- Fetal sleep
- Premature <32w
- Fetal acidosis/hypoxia
- Medications: opioids, BBs, Mg^{2+}

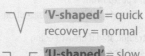
'V-shaped' = quick recovery = normal
'U-shaped' = slow recovery = worrying

Periods of variable decelerations **lasting >30–60min** OR single deceleration **lasting >3min** = ABNORMAL

Interpreting CTGs:
Dr C BRaVADO

DR: Define Risk
- maternal illness
- pregnancy complications e.g. IUGR

C: Contractions
- number in 10min
- regular/irregular?
- **amplitude ≠ strength**

BRa: Baseline Rate
V: Variability
A: Accelerations
D: Decelerations
O: Overall impression

NB NICE criteria for CTG assessment are more complex, but this remains a useful and applicable approach

The puerperium

The puerperium = 6w period following delivery → body returns to prepregnant state

Physiological changes

- **Genital tract**
  - ► uterus contracts & shrinks
  - ► internal os closes (by day 3 unless RPOC)
  - ► lochia (uterine discharge) = blood-stained to week 4 then yellow/white
  - ► menstruation restarts at 6w if **not lactating** (lactation delays restart)
- **Cardiovascular, renal & electrolyte values renormalise**
- **Haematological:** platelets & clotting factors rise → **VTE risk**

Postnatal care

- Monitor BP, temperature, pulse, FBC, lochia
- Fluid balance & perineal wounds checked regularly
- Analgesics if necessary
- **Offer vit K for baby** (single IM or course of oral drops)
- Pelvic floor exercises
- **Contraceptive advice**
- Risk assess & plan for psychiatric illness

Hormone changes

- ↓ oestrogen & progesterone
- ↑ prolactin & oxytocin

Contraceptive advice

- At risk of pregnancy from 21d postpartum
- Start contraception ASAP if possible or at least by week 3/4 postpartum
- Lactation alone = inadequate contraception

COCP = contraindicated if breastfeeding
POP/IUD = safe if breastfeeding

Breastfeeding

- **Prolactin** stimulates milk secretion (yellow 'colostrum' secreted for first 3d)
- Rapid **fall in oestrogen & progesterone** post-delivery enables lactation (normally inhibits prolactin)
- **Oxytocin** stimulates milk release on nipple-sucking
- **Give vitamin K supplementation**

Advantages of breastfeeding: immune protection, bonding, cheaper
↓ risk sudden infant death, asthma/atopies, childhood obesity/DM

Possible problems with breastfeeding: engorgement, mastitis, nipple trauma

Postpartum problems

Postpartum haemorrhage (PPH)[19]

PRIMARY PPH: loss of >500ml blood within 24h of delivery (or >1000ml after C-section)
↳ 10% women

Causes: 4Ts
- **Tone:** uterine atony (80%)
- **Trauma:** vaginal & cervical tears, episiotomy (20%)
- **Tissue (retained placenta):** partial separation causes accumulation of blood in uterus – may not see external loss
- **Thrombin (coagulopathies):** congenital disorders, anticoagulant therapy, DIC

Prevention
- Routine **oxytocin** in 3rd stage (placental delivery)
  - → avoid ergometrine/Syntometrine in hypertensive women

Management: GET SENIOR HELP
1. **Resuscitation:** nurse flat, O$_2$, IV fluids ± blood transfusion (X-match, FBC, clotting)
2. **Identify cause:** abdo palpation, VE/EUA, examine placenta, TV USS
3. **Treat cause:** *for RPOC*
   - **Retained placenta:** remove manually if bleeding or not delivered in 60min
   - **Uterine atony:** IV oxytocin/ergometrine (contracts uterus) → prostaglandin if persists
   - **Persistent haemorrhage:** SURGERY (Rusch balloon, brace suture, hysterectomy)

SECONDARY PPH: excessive blood loss between 24h and 6w after delivery

Causes
- **Endometritis** ± retained placental fragments

Management[19]
- Evacuation of retained products (ERPC)
- Antibiotics

Postpartum pyrexia

→ *maternal fever >38°C in first 14d*

CAUSES
Infection
1. **Genito-urinary**
   - → Offensive lochia
   - → Frequency, urgency, dysuria
   - → Enlarged, tender uterus
2. **Wounds/post-op**
   - → Inflamed, tender wound/incision sites
3. **Mastitis**
   - → Painful, hard, red breast
   - → Cellulitis
   - → Flu-like symptoms
4. **Other infections**
   - → Chest: SOB, cough, etc.

DVT / PE
Swollen, painful calves, SOB

RFs = prolonged labour, grand multiparity, fibroids, overdistension (multiples/polyhydramnios)

Risk factors for PPH
- Previous PPH
- Previous C-section
- Antepartum haemorrhage
- Instrumental/C-section delivery
- Prolonged labour
- Coagulopathies
- Multiparity, multiples
- Polyhydramnios
- Uterine abnormalities

Common causative organisms:
Group A strep, staphylococcus, *E. coli*

C-section = major risk

Management: must exclude sepsis
- **Inspection:** of abdomen, breasts, calves, IV access points, wounds
- **Obs:** temperature, BP
- **Cultures:** high vaginal, blood, urine
- **Broad-spectrum ABX**
- Paracetamol for pain relief: mastitis, wound infection, etc. (safe in breastfeeding)

---

[19]RCOG (2016) *Prevention and management of postpartum haemorrhage* [GTG52]

Thromboembolic disease = leading cause of maternal mortality

Suicide = major cause of death postpartum

Risk factors for postnatal depression
- Previous postnatal depression
- PHx of moderate–severe depression

Risk factors for puerperal psychosis
- FHx of puerperal psychosis
- Primigravid

Thromboembolic disease

Prevention
- Early mobilisation & hydration
- Prophylactic LMWH if ≥1 moderate RF

Detection
PE: CXR, ABG, CT
DVT: Doppler USS

Management: subcutaneous LMWH

Psychiatric problems

Baby blues: temporary emotional lability 3–4d post-delivery = 50% women

Postnatal depression: depressive Sx (often feelings of guilt/incapability) ± thoughts of harming baby = 10% women

Management
- SSRIs
- Social support
- Psychotherapy

Puerperal psychosis: sudden onset psychotic Sx around day 4 = 0.2% women

Management
- Psychiatric admission
- Tranquilisers

More detail on postpartum mental health in Chapter 6: Psychiatry

PAEDIATRICS

05

ABBREVIATIONS

5-ASA – 5-aminosalicylic acid
AABR – Automated auditory brainstem response
ACTH – Adrenocorticotrophic hormone
ADHD – Attention deficit hyperactivity disorder
AEDs – Anti-epileptic drugs
ALL – Acute lymphoblastic leukaemia
AML – Acute myeloid leukaemia
AOM – Acute otitis media
APH – Antepartum haemorrhage
APTT – Activated partial thromboplastin time
BCG – Bacillus Calmette–Guérin (anti-tuberculosis vaccine)
BMD – Becker muscular dystrophy
BR – Bilirubin
BW – Birth weight
CAH – Congenital adrenal hyperplasia
CMV – Cytomegalovirus
CVC – Central venous catheter
DDH – Developmental dysplasia of the hip
DMD – Duchenne muscular dystrophy
EBV – Epstein–Barr virus
EDD – Estimated delivery date
ELBW – Extremely low birth weight
EPO – Erythropoietin
ET tube – Endotracheal tube
FOOSH – Fall on outstretched hand
FTT – Failure to thrive
G6PD – Glucose 6 phosphate dehydrogenase
GBS – Group B streptococcus
GDD – Global developmental delay
GH – Growth hormone

GORD – Gastro-oesophageal reflux disease
Hep – Hepatitis
HLHS – Hypoplastic left heart syndrome
HPLC – High performance liquid chromatography
HPV – Human papillomavirus
HSP – Henoch–Schönlein purpura
HSV – Herpes simplex virus
HUS – Haemolytic uraemic syndrome
ID – Intellectual disability
ILGF – Insulin-like growth factor
ITP – Immune thrombocytopenic purpura
IUGR – Intrauterine growth restriction
IVH – Intraventricular haemorrhage
JIA – Juvenile idiopathic arthritis
LA – Left atrium
LBW – Low birth weight
LLSE – Lower left sternal edge
LMN – Lower motor neurone
LP – Lumbar puncture
MCH – Mean corpuscular haemoglobin
NAI – Non-accidental injury
NEC – Necrotising enterocolitis
NIPE – Newborn & infant physical examination
NIPPV – Non-invasive positive pressure ventilation
NTD – Neural tube defect
OAE – Otoacoustic emissions
OME – Otitis media externa
ORT – Oral rehydration therapy
PCP – *Pneumocystis* pneumonia
PCV – Pneumococcal conjugate vaccine
PDA – Patent ductus arteriosus
PET – Positron emission tomography

PICU – Paediatric intensive care unit
PKD – Polycystic kidney disease
PKU – Phenylketonuria
(P)PROM – (Premature) Prelabour rupture of membranes
PT – Prothrombin time
PTA – Pure tone audiometry
PTH – Parathyroid hormone
RDS – Respiratory distress syndrome
RIF – Right iliac fossa
ROM – Rupture of membranes
RSV – Respiratory syncytial virus
SBO – Small bowel obstruction
SCA/D – Sickle cell anaemia/disease
SCID – Severe combined immunodeficiency
SLE – Systemic lupus erythematosus
STI – Sexually transmitted infection
SVC – Superior vena cava
TGA – Transposition of the great arteries
TIBC – Total iron-binding capacity
TM – Tympanic membrane
TMJ – Temporomandibular joint
TOF – Tetralogy of Fallot
TPO – Thyroid peroxidase
TTP – Thrombotic thrombocytopenic purpura
UC – Ulcerative colitis
U(L/R)SE – Upper (left/right) sternal edge
URTI – Upper respiratory tract infection
VLBW – Very low birth weight
VO crises – Vaso-occlusive crises
VUR – Vesicoureteric reflux
VZV – Varicella zoster virus
WOB – Work of breathing

Neonatology

Neonate = up to 4w

Apgar score[1]

	0	1	2
Appearance	Blue/pale	Pink body, Blue extremities	Pink
Pulse	Absent	<100	≥100
Grimace (reflex response)	Absent	Small (grimace)	Large (cries/coughs)
Activity	Absent/flaccid	Some limb flexion	Moving/active
Respiration	Absent	Gasping/irregular	Strong cry/regular

Measure at 1, 5, 10min after birth

The normal neonate

Passing urine & meconium: within 24h
Regaining birth weight: 5–10% loss of BW in first 5d → regained by day 10
Weight gain: ×2 in 18w (in 6w if preterm)
Fontanelle closure: posterior = 2nd month, anterior = 12–18m

Neonatal screening & surveillance

Newborn: NIPE + hearing screening (OAE/AABR)
5–9d: biochemical screening (heel-prick)
First 2w: midwife visits
6–8w: GP examination
Pre-school: orthoptist vision screening

Childhood immunisation schedule[2]

Age	Vaccination
2m	• **6 in 1** (diphtheria, tetanus, polio, whooping cough, Hib, hep B) • Oral rotavirus • Men B
3m	• **6 in 1** (diphtheria, tetanus, polio, whooping cough, Hib, hep B) • Oral rotavirus • PCV
4m	• **6 in 1** (diphtheria, tetanus, polio, whooping cough, Hib, hep B) • Men B
12–13m	• Hib • PCV • Men B & Men C • **MMR** (measles, mumps, rubella)
2–8y	• Annual flu vaccine
3–4y	• **4 in 1** (diphtheria, tetanus, polio, whooping cough) • **MMR** (measles, mumps, rubella)
12–13y	• HPV
13–18y	• **3 in 1** (diphtheria, tetanus, polio) • Men ACWY

Interpreting Apgar scores

0–3 = low
4–6 = moderate
7–10 = good

LBW <2.5kg
VLBW <1.5kg
ELBW <1kg

Biochemical screening: Guthrie/heel-prick test:

6 inherited metabolic diseases
• PKU
• Homocystinuria
• Isovaleric acidaemia
• Glutaric aciduria type 1
• MSUD (maple syrup urine)
• MCAD (medium-chain acyl-CoA DH deficiency)
Mitochondrial condition resulting in hypoglycaemia

+ 3 other congenital diseases:
• Hypothyroidism
• SCA & thalassaemia
• CF

Preterm babies should still get first vaccines at 2m & follow the normal schedule (regardless of gestation & BW)

BUT be aware of increased risk of adverse side-effects

Live vaccines

Not if immunocompromised
• Oral polio
• Nasal flu
• MMR
• BCG

Contraindications to vaccines

• Previous anaphylaxis
• Immunocompromised
• Pregnancy (some vaccines)
• Hx of intussusception (rotavirus vaccine only)

[1] Apgar V. (2015) A proposal for a new method of evaluation of the newborn infant. Originally published in *Curr Res Anesth Analg*. 1953;32:260–7 reprinted *Anesth Analg*. 120:1056–9
[2] NHS vaccinations and when to have them

Newborn problems

BIRTH MARKS (Fig. 5.1)

(a) Neonatal urticaria (erythema toxicum) → *up to 50% infants*
- At 2–3 days age → resolves within 2w
- White pinpoint papules on erythematous base
- Concentrated on the trunk ± other areas

(b) Naevus simplex (stork bites) → *distension of capillaries*
- Fade over 1y
- Pink macules on upper eyelids, forehead & neck

(c) Strawberry naevus (cavernous haemangioma)
- Appear in first month – ↑ size for 3–15m, then regress
- Only treat if complications: ulceration/haemorrhage, vision disturbance

(d) Port wine stain (naevus flammus) → *vascular malformations of dermal capillaries*
- Grow with the infant – **don't disappear unless laser therapy**
- May associate with vascular abnormalities elsewhere
  ▸ intracranial = Sturge–Weber syndrome
  ▸ on limbs = Klippel–Trénauny syndrome

(e) Café au lait spots
- If >5 develop by age 5y, see GP → associates with **neurofibromatosis**

(f) Mongolian blue spots → *mostly Afro-Caribbean/Asian infants*
- Fade over 1–2y
- Blue/black macular discolouration at spinal base & buttocks
- **DDx: bruises**

(g) Congenital melanocytic naevi (moles)

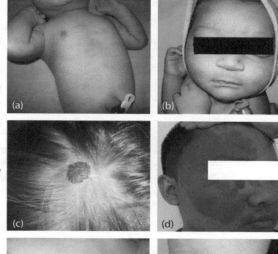

Fig. 5.1

BIRTH TRAUMA
- **Caput succedaneum** → *swelling (oedema & bruising) of presenting part*
  ▸ due to pressure against cervix during birth
  ▸ within skin → swelling crosses suture lines
  ▸ resolves in a **few days**
- **Cephalohaematoma** → *bleeding below periosteum*
  ▸ due to pressure on head during birth
  ▸ confined by margins of skull sutures
  ▸ resolves in a **few weeks**
- **Chignon** → *oedema & bruising due to ventouse delivery*
- **Erb palsy** → *brachial plexus (C5,6) injury*
  ▸ due to breech or shoulder dystocia
  ▸ **Sx:** limp arm, hand pronated, fingers flexed (waiter's tip)
  ▸ refer to orthopaedic surgeon if not resolved in 2–3m

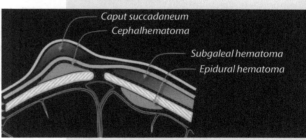

Fig. 5.2

STICKY EYE → *narrow/blocked tear ducts affecting 1 in 20 babies*
Sx: watery eyes ± sticky discharge
Mx: keep eyes clean (cotton swabs + saline)
→ if unresolved within a year, may need surgery to unblock ducts
*Safety-net for signs of infection**

HAEMORRHAGIC DISEASE OF THE NEWBORN → *presents in **weeks 1–8**, due to **vitamin K deficiency***
Symptoms
- **Mild:** bruising, haematemesis, melaena, prolonged bleeding
- **Severe:** intracranial haemorrhage → disability/death

Management
- Prophylactic vitamin K at birth (1x IM injection or PO course)

*****Signs of eye infection/conjunctivitis**
- Red/sore/puffy eye
- Greenish/yellow discharge
- Light sensitivity

Causes
- Strep/staph → topical neomycin
- Gonococcal → IV penicillin/ceftriaxone
- Chlamydial → PO erythromycin

→ *gonorrhoea/chlamydia can lead to permanent blindness*

Risk factors for haemorrhagic disease
- Wholly breast-fed (poor source of vit K)
- Mother taking anticonvulsants
- Neonates with liver disease

HYPOXIC ISCHAEMIC ENCEPHALOPATHY (HIE)   0.1% of infants

→ *perinatal asphyxia causes* $\downarrow O_2$, $\uparrow CO_2$ *and acidosis* → *poor tissue perfusion & hypoxic damage to organs*

Causes
- **Failed gas exchange at placenta:** prolonged contractions, placental abruption, uterine rupture
- **Interrupted umbilical blood flow:** cord compression/prolapse
- **Inadequate placental perfusion:** maternal hyper-/hypotension
- **Compromised fetus:** IUGR, anaemia
- **Failure of cardiorespiratory adaptation at birth**

Symptoms: immediately or up to 48h after asphyxia

Mild	Moderate	Severe
• Irritable / ↑ response to stimuli • Staring eyes • Hyperventilation • Impaired feeding	• Abnormal tone/movement • Inability to feed • Altered consciousness • Seizures	• No spontaneous movement/ response to pain • Hyper-/hypotonia • Prolonged seizures • Multi-organ failure

Management[3]
- Respiratory support
- Anticonvulsants (for seizures if correlated on aEEG)
- Fluids & inotropes (for hypotension)
- Monitor and treat hypoglycaemia & electrolyte imbalance
- Careful fluid monitoring (as transient renal impairment)
- **Therapeutic hypothermia: cool to 33°C for 72h** → reduces brain damage if **within 72h of birth**

Prognosis
Mild HIE: complete recovery expected
- If abnormalities >2w, full recovery is unlikely

Severe HIE: 30–40% mortality
- 80% of survivors have neurodevelopmental disabilities → esp. cerebral palsy

Neonatal jaundice

→ *>50% of newborns*

CAUSES
- **Physiological:** high rate of RBC breakdown & less efficient bilirubin metabolism

- **Haemolytic disorders:** likely if onset <24h from birth
  - Rh/ABO incompatibility between mother and baby
  - Inherited enzyme deficiencies e.g. G6PD deficiency, Crigler–Najjar syndrome
  - Abnormal RBCs e.g. spherocytosis
  - Congenital infection

- **Infection**

- **Biliary atresia:** #1 cause of prolonged jaundice*
  - **Pathogenesis:** progressive destruction/absence of bile ducts
  - **Sx:** normal BW but failure to thrive, pale stools/dark urine (hepatosplenomegaly may develop)
  - **Ix:** deranged LFTs & ↑ conjugated bilirubin

---

[3] EOE Neonatal (2021) *Guidelines for management of infants with suspected hypoxic ischaemic encephalopathy (HIE)*

Investigations for HIE

Amplitude-integrated EEG (aEEG): Detects abnormal brain activity in neonates to confirm early encephalopathy/seizures

---

most common cause

Jaundice noticed if: BR >80μmol/L (5mg/dl)

*Prolonged jaundice: >2w (>3w if preterm)

- ▸ **Dx:** cholangiography (imaging of bile duct)
- ▸ **Mx:** Kasi procedure (connect jejunum to porta hepatis to bypass ducts)
  → liver transplant if unsuccessful
- **Neonatal hepatitis syndrome:** consider if prolonged jaundice
  - ▸ **Signs:** liver inflammation with IUGR & hepatosplenomegaly at birth
  - ▸ **Sx:** N&V, abdo pain, lethargy
  - ▸ **Ix:** deranged LFTs
  - ▸ **Causes:** viruses (hep A/B/C, CMV, rubella), α1 antitrypsin deficiency, CF

Summary of causes of neonatal jaundice

<24h = Pathological	1–14d	>2w
Haemolysis: • Rh/ABO • Thalassaemia • G6PD **Infection:** • Sepsis • Congenital e.g. rubella **BLACK = unconjugated** **GREY = conjugated**	**↑ RBC turnover:** • Physiological • Polycythaemia **Enzyme deficiency:** • Crigler–Najjar/ Gilbert's • G6PD deficiency • Hypothyroidism **Other:** • Dehydration • Breast milk jaundice	**Enzyme deficiency:** • Crigler–Najjar/ Gilbert's • G6PD deficiency • Hypothyroidism **Hepatitis:** • Hep A, B, C • CMV, rubella, HSV • CF **Metabolic:** • α1 antitrypsin deficiency **Biliary atresia**

COMPLICATIONS

Kernicterus: encephalopathy resulting from deposition of unconjugated bilirubin in the brain

MANAGEMENT[4]: use chart to determine appropriate Tx

1. **Ensure hydration:** daily weighing & assess wet nappies
2. **Phototherapy:** blue-green band wavelengths → convert unconj. BR to water-soluble pigment → excreted in urine
3. **Exchange transfusion:** if very dangerous BR levels → replace twice the infant's blood volume with donor blood

Neonatal respiratory distress (NRD)

CAUSES

- **Respiratory distress syndrome (RDS)** = **surfactant deficiency**
  - ▸ **RFs:** preterm, maternal diabetes   ↳ surfactant only produced from 24w
  - ▸ **Prevention:** steroids 48h before delivery (if <34w)
  - ▸ **Mx:** artificial surfactant + ambient O_2
- **Transient tachypnoea of the newborn (TTN)*** = delayed reabsorption of lung fluid   ↳ 1% preterm
      ↳ 0.4% term
  - ▸ **RFs:** C-section delivery, preterm, maternal analgesics/ anaesthetics, maternal asthma/diabetes
  - ▸ **Ix:** Dx of exclusion (CXR for other causes)
  - ▸ **Mx:** ambient O_2 → resolves in 24h
- **Meconium aspiration** = follows meconium passing (may be triggered by hypoxia)
  - ▸ **RFs:** ↑ gestational age, fetal hypoxia
  - ▸ **Complications:** mechanical obstruction + chemical pneumonitis (lung irritant), infection, pneumothorax

[4]NICE (2010, updated 2016) *Jaundice in newborn babies under 28 days* [CG98]

Ix for specific causes

General
- Physical examination
- FBC
- LFTs, U&Es

Infection
- CRP/ESR
- Blood/urine culture

Haemolysis
- Blood group (mum & baby)
- Coombs test

Other
- G6PD levels
- Hep A/B/C antibodies
- Cholangiography

Unconjugated BR: prehepatic cause
- Haemolysis, infection, physiological
→ *normal stools & urine*

Conjugated BR: intra/post-hepatic cause
- Biliary atresia, hepatitis syndrome
→ *pale stools & dark urine*

Assess severity

- **Skin blanch test**
- **BR levels** (transcutaneous meter)
- **Bloods:** serum BR
  (conjugated vs. unconjugated)

Symptoms of jaundice: ↑ severity with ↑ BR levels

- Lethargic/irritable
- Muscular twitching
- Seizures/coma
- Poor feeding
- Opisthotonos (hypertonia & back arching)
- Death if untreated

Complications of kernicterus
- Cerebral palsy
- Learning difficulties
- Sensorineural deafness

---

*most common cause of NRD

Symptoms of NRD

- Tachypnoea (>60 breaths/min)
- Nasal flaring & chest wall recession
- Expiratory grunting
- Cyanosis (if severe)

---

*NB Infants may suffer **respiratory depression** if mother took **opiate** analgesics in labour*
Tx: naloxone

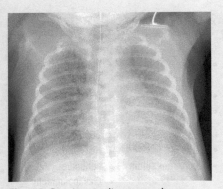

Fig. 5.3 Respiratory distress syndrome: bilateral, uniform hazy, 'ground glass' appearance; reduced lung expansion.

If RFs present give prophylactic ABX in labour

Bowel atresia/stenosis: congenital malformation
→ *often seen in polyhydramnios/Down's*

Meconium ileus: very thick meconium impacted in ileum
→ *90% have CF*

DDx bilious vomiting: always Ix with AXR to exclude obstruction
- Atresia/stenosis of small bowel
- Malrotation of bowel
- Volvulus
- Meconium ileus
- NEC (necrotising enterocolitis)

DDx poor feeding
- Neurological disorder e.g. cerebral palsy
- Cleft lip/palate
- Neck/head abnormalities
- Premature/LBW
- Respiratory problems
- GI problems

▶ **Ix:** CXR – overinflated, patches of collapse & consolidation
▶ **Mx:** mechanical ventilation

- **Pneumonia** = neonatal respiratory distress + signs of infection (fever, respiratory crackles)
  ▶ **RFs:** PPROM, chorioamnionitis, LBW
  ▶ **Ix:** CXR – consolidation
  ▶ **Mx:** broad-spectrum ABX + ambient O_2
- **Other**
  ▶ **pneumothorax:** spontaneous (2% births) or 2° to meconium aspiration, ventilation or RDS
  ▶ **diaphragmatic hernia:** usually LHS → confirmed on X-ray

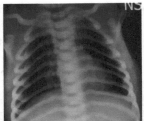

Fig. 5.4 Bilateral pneumothorax (dark air-fields).

Gastrointestinal disorders

CAUSES

- **Oesophageal atresia** = associates with other congenital malformations
  ▶ **RFs:** polyhydramnios
  ▶ **Sx:** persistent salivation/drooling, aspiration/choking on feeding
  ▶ **Mx:** surgery

- **Small bowel obstruction** = associates with Down syndrome, CF & prematurity
  ▶ **Causes:** duodenal atresia/stenosis, volvulus rotation, meconium ileus/plug
  ▶ **Sx:** persistent vomiting (bile-stained), slow/absent meconium passage, abdo distension
  ▶ **Ix:** X-ray & contrast studies
  ▶ **Mx:** surgery or dislodge meconium with contrast medium (gastrografin enema)

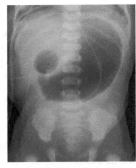

Fig. 5.5 'Double bubble' sign: indicates duodenal atresia (or stenosis).

- **Large bowel obstruction**
  ▶ **Causes:** Hirschsprung disease (absent rectal nerve plexus), rectal atresia
  ▶ **Sx:** same as for SBO
  ▶ **Mx:** surgery

- **Exomphalos/omphalocele** = protrusions of bowel through umbilicus (Fig. 5.6)
  ▶ Covered with transparent sac
  ▶ **Associates with other major congenital abnormalities (trisomies 13, 15, 18 & Beckwith–Wiedemann)**
  ▶ **Mx:** IV ABX & surgical repair

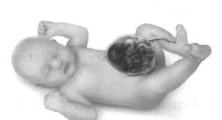

Fig. 5.6 Exomphalos.

- **Gastroschisis** = protrusions of bowel through abdominal wall (paraumbilical) (Fig. 5.7)
  ▶ No covering of bowel contents
  ▶ **Mx:** IV ABX & surgical repair within 4h

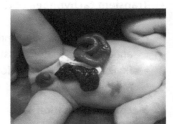

Fig. 5.7 Gastroschisis.

RFs of gastroschisis: maternal drugs, smoking, illness & younger maternal age

Congenital abnormalities

→ *structural or functional anomalies that occur during intrauterine life*

→ *detected prenatally, at birth or later in infancy*

RISK FACTORS

- Consanguinity
- Ethnic minorities with high prevalence of rare genetic mutations
- Low socioeconomic background
- Maternal exposure to pesticides, medications, alcohol, tobacco, radiation
- Congenital infections (rubella, syphilis, etc.)
- Maternal folate insufficiency (NTDs)

NEURAL TUBE DEFECTS (NTDs)

= *failed fusion of neural plate to form neural tube in* **first 28d after conception**

Risk factors

- Poor folate intake – all women advised to take folate preconception
- Previous baby with NTD – high risk women advised high dose folate preconception

400 micrograms OD from preconception to 12w

5mg OD from preconception to 12w

NTD	Definition	Complications	Mx
Anencephaly	Failed development of most of brain & cranium	• Stillbirth • Death shortly after birth	Terminate pregnancy (Dx: antenatal USS)
Encephalocele	Extrusion of brain & meninges through midline skull defect	Underlying cerebral malformations	Surgery
Spina bifida occulta:	Failed fusion of vertebral arch	Overlying skin lesion in lumbar region e.g. hair patch, lipoma, birth mark Underlying cord defect → bladder dysfunction / leg paralysis	Surgery
a) Meningocele	Protruding sac of CSF but **no neural tissue**		Surgery
b) Myelomeningocele	Protruding sac of CSF, and **neural tissue**	• Variable leg paralysis • Sensory loss • Muscle imbalance • Scoliosis • Bladder dysfunction • Hydrocephalus	Surgery ± physiotherapy ± catheterisation

VACTERL ASSOCIATION = *disorder affecting multiple organ systems (a group of associated congenital abnormalities)*
↳ **V**ertebral, **A**norectal, **C**ardiac, **T**racheo-o**E**sophageal, **R**enal, **L**imb
↳ **Cause:** sporadic/random

AMBIGUOUS GENITALIA = *external genitalia is neither definitely male or female*
Cause: hormonal imbalance in early embryonic development preventing differentiation of the genitalia
Ix: chromosome evaluation, USS (for uterus), endocrine studies
↳ **Female pseudo-hermaphroditism** = *females with male genitalia*
- ► **Cause:** congenital adrenal hyperplasia (CAH), maternal ingestion of hormones
- ► **Sx:** enlarged clitoris resembling a penis & wrinkled labia majora
- ► **Dx:** USS confirms presences of uterus & ovaries
↳ **Male pseudo-hermaphroditism** = *females with male genitalia*
- ► **Cause:** insensitivity of genitalia to testosterone, enzyme deficiencies, maternal ingestion of hormones
- ► **Sx:** hypoplastic penis resembling clitoris
↳ **Congenital adrenal hyperplasia (CAH)** = *autosomal recessive*
- ► **Cause:** lack of enzyme for cortisol synthesis = ↑ ACTH = ↑ androgen production & adrenal hyperplasia
- ► **Sx:** ambiguous genitalia, **adrenal crisis in 2nd–3rd w of life**
- ► **Ix:** U&Es, hormone screen (↑ serum 17-hydroxyprogesterone levels, ↓ 21-α-hydroxylase)

fail to feed, vomit, dehydration, ↓ BP, ↑ K⁺, ↓ Na⁺

CONGENITAL DIAPHRAGMATIC HERNIA = *defect in diaphragm*
so abdominal contents enter chest cavity   1 in 4000
    ↳ Results in **pulmonary hypoplasia** (inadequate lung development)

Signs/symptoms
- **Respiratory distress**/cyanosis shortly after birth → failure to respond to resuscitation
- Chest wall asymmetry
- Displaced apex beat (opposite side to herniation)
- Bowel sounds audible over chest wall

Investigations
- Antenatal USS – often detected before birth
- **CXR/CT**

Management
- NG tube + suction
- Surgical repair

POTTER SYNDROME = *typical physical characteristics due to oligohydramnios that is secondary to kidney agenesis*

Cause: fetal kidney agenesis/dysgenesis → low urine output → oligohydramnios → ↑ pressure on fetus

Features
- 'Frog-like face'
- Low-set ears
- Beaked nose
- Wide-set, down-slanting eyes

Complications
- Pulmonary hypoplasia → respiratory failure
- Death shortly after birth

TALIPES (CLUBBED FOOT) = *inverted feet* (M:F = 3:1)
- **Positional:** due to squashed feet in womb
- → **reassure parents:** resolves after birth → common
- **Structural:** muscles/bones do not grow straight
- → Tx with plaster cast & special footwear → 1 in 1000

Diagnosis: antenatal USS, but cannot tell which type until birth

Causes: idiopathic, familial, oligohydramnios, neuromuscular disorder

Associations: developmental dysplasia of the hip (DDH)

DEVELOPMENTAL DYSPLASIA OF THE HIP (DDH) = *congenital dislocation of the hip*

Risk factors
- Female (↑ × 6)
- FHx of DDH
- Breech birth
- Neuromuscular disorder

Diagnosis
Tested for on examination of the neonate
Management: specialist orthopaedic opinion
Early splinting in abducted position

CLEFT LIP & PALATE → *0.08% babies (1 in 700)*

Cleft lip: failed fusion of frontonasal & maxillary processes

Cleft palate: failed fusion of palatine processes & nasal septum

Causes
- Inherited polygenically (most)
- Chromosomal disorders
- Maternal anticonvulsants

Symptoms
- Poor feeding
- Secretory otitis media

- Dental problems
- Speech problems

Management
- Surgical repair

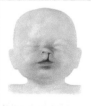 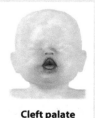

    Cleft lip   **Cleft palate**

Fig. 5.8

Infection

→ *neonatal period = highest risk for serious invasive bacterial infection*

0.3% of births

	Early onset sepsis <48h	Late onset sepsis >48h
Source	**Bacterial:** ascend from birth canal • Invade amniotic fluid & pass into fetal lungs **Viral:** via placenta	Infection acquired from environment
Organisms	• GBS • *Listeria monocytogenes* • **Gram –ve:** gonococcus, chlamydiae, *E. coli* • HSV, CMV, HIV, hepatitis B, toxoplasmosis	• Coagulase –ve staphylococcus • *Staphylococcus aureus* • Enterococcus • GBS • **Gram –ve:** gonococcus, chlamydia, klebsiella, *E. coli*
Presentation	• Respiratory distress & apnoea • Temperature instability • ↓HR/RR • Pallor/jaundice/mottled **Meningitis:** bulging fontanelle, hyperextended neck & back (opisthotonos)	• Failure to feed / gain weight • Fatigue, irritability, crying • Abdo distension / vomiting
Risk factors	• PROM / prolonged ROM (>24h) • Maternal fever in labour (chorioamnionitis) • Infected 2nd baby in multiple pregnancy • Maternal GBS in pregnancy / prev. GBS baby	• Parenteral nutrition (infected lines) • Tracheal tubes • Invasive procedures • Premature/LBW
Investigations	• CXR • Septic screen (FBC, U&Es, LFTS, **blood & urine cultures**, CRP, glucose, lactate) • **LP** & CSF culture (if signs of meningitis or raised CRP with no known source)	
Management[5]	Immediate broad-spectrum IV ABX e.g. penicillin & gentamicin + supportive Tx (fluids, O_2) + **senior review**	

GROUP B STREP
Source: 20% women = carriers → 10% of these will pass to baby
Presentation: respiratory distress/ pneumonia, sepsis, meningitis
Prevention: screen high risk mothers
→ intrapartum ABX

LISTERIA
Source: unpasteurised milk, soft cheese, undercooked poultry
Presentation: flu-like illness in mother, meconium-stained liquor, fetal rash
Complications: miscarriage, preterm delivery, neonatal sepsis

HSV
Source: active maternal infection → 40% of these will pass to baby
Presentation: herpetic lesions on skin/eye, encephalitis
Prevention: C-section if active at labour, aciclovir for flare-ups in pregnancy

HEPATITIS B
Prevention: screen high risk mothers
→ active immunisation: neonatal hep B vaccination shortly after birth
→ passive immunisation: hep B Igs given to neonate
→ do not breastfeed

CHLAMYDIA
Timing: 1–2w
Sx: purulent discharge + swollen eyelids
Tx: PO erythromycin

OPHTHALMIA NEONATORUM
Gonococcus/chlamydia
Timing: within 48h
Sx: purulent discharge + swollen eyelids
Complications: ulceration → blindness
Tx: IV penicillin/cephalosporin

High risk GBS:
Confirm with vaginal swab/MSU
• Previous GBS baby
• Maternal fever in labour
• Prolonged ROM
• Preterm labour/PPROM

prematurity = <37w

Antenatal steroids given if:

- maternal DM
- threatening labour <34w
- → helps pulmonary maturation
- → reduced risk of IVH & PDA

Periventricular leukomalacia (PVL)

= hypoxia damages white matter surrounding the ventricles
RFs: preterm, LBW, IVH

Problems of prematurity[6]

- **Respiratory distress syndrome (RDS)** → *within 4h of birth*
  - Increased risk of lung infection e.g. RSV, adenovirus (causing bronchiolitis)
  - Pneumothorax may occur 2° to artificial ventilation
  - **Mx:** artificial surfactant, respiratory support
- **Apnoea, bradycardia & desaturation**
  - Episodes are common <32w – cessation of breathing for 20–30s
  - Usually due to immature respiratory control – but need to exclude hypoxia, infection, anaemia, hypoglycaemia, HF
  - **Mx:** gentle physical stimulation, caffeine stimulants, CPAP
- **Bronchopulmonary dysplasia / chronic lung disease** → *still require O$_2$ therapy >36w corrected age*
  - **RFs:** artificial ventilation, oxygen toxicity, infection
  - **Complications:** recurrent infection, pulmonary hypertension
  - **Mx:** wean off artificial ventilation onto CPAP, then ambient O$_2$
    → corticosteroids may help
- **Hypothermia**
  - Due to large surface area to volume ratio, thin skin, little subcutaneous fat, cannot curl up/shiver
  - **Consequences:** ↑ energy consumption, hypoxia, hypoglycaemia, no weight gain
  - **Mx:** incubation / plastic wrap
- **Infection** → *Major cause of death*
  - IgG transferred across placenta in 3rd trimester – preterm infants have less
  - Usually nosocomial – catheters, ventilators
- **Intraventricular haemorrhage (IVH)** → *25% very low BW infants*
  - **RF:** very low BW, pneumothorax, RDS, perinatal asphyxia, CMV
  - **Sx:** apnoea, lethargy, hypotonia coma, bulging fontanelle
  - **Complications:** hydrocephalus, PVL, cerebral palsy
  - **Mx:** CSF drainage, ventriculoperitoneal shunting
- **Necrotising enterocolitis (NEC)** → *bacterial infection of ischaemic bowel wall*
  - **RFs:** preterm, very low BW, cow's milk (not breast milk)
  - **Sx:** feed aspiration, vomiting (may be bilious), abdo distension/pain, fresh bloody stools
  - **Complications:** shock, bowel perforation, post-surgical strictures
  - **Ix:** AXR ± USS
  - **Mx:** stop oral feeding, broad-spectrum ABX, parenteral nutrition, artificial ventilation → surgery if perforated bowel
- **Retinopathy of prematurity (ROP)** → *vascular proliferation at junction of retina*
  - **Complications:** retinal detachment, fibrosis, blindness
  - **RFs:** high conc. O$_2$ therapy, very low BW
  - **Mx:** laser therapy → screen high risk infants weekly (<1.5kg or <32w)
- **Hypoglycaemia**
  - **RFs**
    - preterm, IUGR (low glycogen stores)
    - diabetic mother (islet cell hyperplasia = hyperinsulinaemia)
    - LGA, hypothermia, polycythaemia, illness (↑ demand)
  - **Sx**
    - irritable/jittery
    - lethargic/drowsy/hypotonic
    - apnoea
    - seizures
  - **Mx: aim for BG >2.6mmol/L**
    - early, frequent feeding
    - regular BG monitoring
    - IV glucose

[6]NICE (2019) *Specialist neonatal respiratory care for babies born preterm* [NG124]

Genetics & syndromes

↳ **Syndrome: particular set of multiple** anomalies occurs repeatedly in a consistent pattern due to an **underlying mechanism**

Chromosomal abnormalities

TRISOMIES → *non-disjunction, translocation or mosaicism*

DOWN SYNDROME (trisomy 21)   **≥50% live over 50y**

Physical features
- round face
- small mouth/ears
- hypotonia
- flat nasal bridge
- protruding tongue
- single palmar crease
- epicanthic folds (upper eyelid)
- Brushfield spots (in iris)
- 'sandal gap' between toes

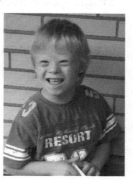

Fig. 5.9 Down syndrome.

Associated abnormalities: screen for these at birth e.g. ECHO, TFTs, vision & hearing screens
- congenital heart defects (40%)
- hearing impairments (otitis media)
- early onset Alzheimer's disease
- moderate learning difficulties
- visual impairments (cataracts, squint)
- epilepsy, coeliac disease, infections

Maternal age:	20	30	35	40	44	Overall
Prevalence:	1 : 1530	1 : 900	1 : 385	1 : 110	1 : 37	1 : 650

EDWARDS SYNDROME (trisomy 18)

Physical features
- IUGR / low BW
- Prominent occiput, small mouth
- Flexed, overlapping fingers
- Rocker-bottom/clubbed feet
- Cardiac & renal malformations

→**most die in infancy**

PATAU SYNDROME (trisomy 13)

Physical features
- Brain defects (microcephaly)
- Small eyes (microphthalmia)
- Cleft lip/palate
- Polydactyly
- Cardiac & renal malformations

→**most die in infancy**

OTHER CHROMOSOMAL SYNDROMES

TURNER SYNDROME (45,X) = **1 in 2500**

Physical features
- Short stature
- Spoon-shaped nails
- Lymphoedema of hands/feet
- Webbed neck

Associated conditions
- Congenital heart defects (aortic coarctation)
- Delayed puberty
- Hypothyroidism
- Ovarian dysgenesis = infertile
- Renal anomalies

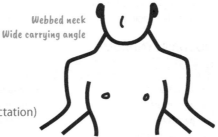

Webbed neck
Wide carrying angle

Fig. 5.10 Physical features of Turner syndrome.

→ 2% babies have congenital malformation
→ 5% babies have genetic disorder

Down syndrome affects 1 in 150 live births

Diagnosis of Down syndrome
- antenatal screening: combined/ triple test
- chromosome analysis (blood test): **FISH**

Investigations for Turner syndrome
- Blood karyotyping
- Buccal swab (for **Barr body** = inactive X chromosome)
- LH & FSH
- **For complications:** TFTs, urinalysis (for glucose etc.)

Tx for Turner syndrome
- Growth hormones
- Oestrogen replacement
→ develop 2° sexual characteristics **but still infertile**

KLINEFELTER SYNDROME (47,XXY) = 1 in 1000

Physical features

- hypogonadism/small testes = infertile
- gynaecomastia
- lack of chest/facial hair
- tall stature

Tx: testosterone therapy may help

Single gene/Mendelian disorders

AUTOSOMAL DOMINANT = 50% chance child inherits affected allele

TUBEROUS SCLEROSIS = 1 in 6000

Signs	Associated conditions
• 'ash-leaf' lesions (hypopigmented) • shagreen patches (rough patches) • ungual fibroma (nail tumour) • **angiofibromata** (benign nasopharyngeal tumour in butterfly distribution over nose)	• **benign tumours** (brain, skin, heart, eyes, lungs) • **infantile spasms** • autism • epilepsy

ACHONDROPLASIA (DWARFISM) = disorder of bone growth

→ Tx: growth hormones/surgery for spine

Signs	Associated conditions	
• short stature & limbs/digits • large head (macrocephaly) • large forehead & depressed nasal bridge	• apnoea • lordosis	• obesity • spinal stenosis

MARFAN SYNDROME = 1 in 5000 → **disorder of connective tissue**

(fibrillin-1 mutation)

Signs	Associated conditions
• tall & thin • hypermobility • scoliosis • long limbs • crowded teeth • sunken chest	• AAA, aortic dissection, valve regurgitation • glaucoma, cataracts, retinal detachment • lung collapse, asthma, sleep apnoea

NEUROFIBROMATOSIS = 1 in 3000–4000 → skin changes + tumours along nerves

Signs	Associated conditions
Type 1: • café au lait spots • axillary/groin freckles • Lisch nodules (benign growth in eye)	• neurofibromas (benign) • malignant peripheral nerve sheath tumours • hypertension • scoliosis
Type 2: (much rarer) • hearing loss / balance problems • juvenile cataracts	**CN VIII tumours** • vestibular schwannoma • bilateral acoustic neuromata

NOONAN SYNDROME = 1 in 1000

Signs	Associated conditions
• short stature • webbed neck • pectus excavatum • flat nasal bridge • wide-set eyes	• **mild learning difficulties** • congenital heart disease (pulmonary stenosis, ASD) • bleeding disorders • scoliosis

→ similar phenotype to Turner syndrome

Fig. 5.11 Angiofibromata.

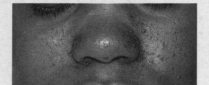

Fig. 5.12 Ash-leaf patch.

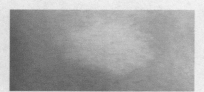

Fig. 5.13 Café au lait spots.

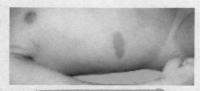

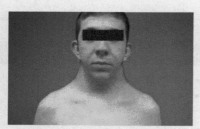

Fig. 5.14 Noonan syndrome.

AUTOSOMAL RECESSIVE = if both parents are carriers, 25% chance child is affected (all offspring = carriers)
↳ often affect metabolic pathways
↳ risk increased by **consanguinity**

Examples of autosomal recessive conditions	
• CF	• Tay–Sachs
• SCA	• Friedreich ataxia
• PKU	• Thalassaemiar

PHENYLKETONURIA (PKU) = very rare
= congenital enzyme deficiency (phenylalanine hydroxylase) → **phenylalanine accumulation**

Symptoms
- very fair hair/skin & eczema
- severe learning difficulties/ behaviour problems
- anxiety/depression
- epilepsy

Diagnosis
- blood phenylalanine levels **(heel-prick test)**

Treatment
- phenylalanine-restricted diet

X-LINKED RECESSIVE = males are affected, females are carriers (but may show mild disease)
↳ 50% chance son of female carrier is affected
↳ 50% chance daughter of female carrier is carrier
↳ All daughters of affected males are carriers
↳ Sons of affected males are unaffected

Examples of X-linked recessive conditions
• Colour-blindness
• Fragile X
• Haemophilia A/B
• DMD/BMD
• G6PD deficiency

FRAGILE X = very rare
→ due to ↑ CGG nucleotide repeats

Signs	Associated conditions
• macrocephaly	• **mod/severe learning difficulties** (mean IQ 50)
• large testes (post-puberty)	• autism
• long face & broad forehead	• hyperactivity
• large, everted ears	• mitral valve prolapse / joint laxity
• prominent mandible	• scoliosis

DUCHENNE MUSCULAR DYSTROPHY = 1 in 4000
→ loss of matrix protein dystrophin → abnormal cell signalling

Signs	Associated conditions	Management
• waddling gait (frequent falls) – climb stairs / run slowly	• **learning difficulties**	• exercise, stretching
• calf pseudohypertrophy – fat replaces muscle	• cardiomyopathies	• walking aids
• Gower sign – must turn prone to rise	• respiratory failure	**Scoliosis:** brace/surgery
• **progressive muscular atrophy** (cannot walk by 10–14y)	• scoliosis	**Respiratory:** CPAP
Diagnosis: clinical signs + markedly elevated serum CK	**Life expectancy:** late 20s	**Parental support groups**

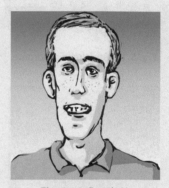

Fig. 5.15 Fragile X.

X-LINKED DOMINANT = **very rare** → both males & females affected
(males usually die)

RETT'S SYNDROME – **99% of cases are *de novo* mutations** (1% = X-linked dominant)

Symptoms: severe speech, learning & coordination problems
- **6–18m:** apparently normal development (may be delay in motor skills / signs of autism)
- **>1y:** repetitive hand/eye movements (wringing, clapping, blinking, staring), apraxia, slow growth

Other problems: seizures, scoliosis, muscle weakness, breathing abnormalities

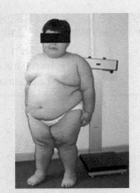

Fig. 5.16 Prader–Willi syndrome.

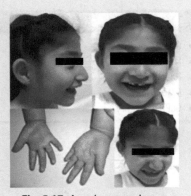

Fig. 5.17 Angelman syndrome.

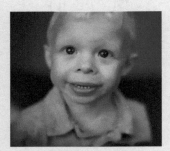

Fig. 5.18 Williams syndrome.

OTHER DYSMORPHIC CONDITIONS

PRADER–WILLI SYNDROME = no paternal copy of Chr. 15q11–13 (sporadic)

Signs	Associated conditions
<ul><li>**hypotonia**</li><li>neonatal feeding difficulties</li><li>insatiable appetite later in childhood</li><li>narrow forehead</li><li>almond-shaped eyes</li><li>triangular mouth</li></ul>	<ul><li>poor growth in childhood</li><li>developmental delay</li><li>obesity/T2DM</li><li>**learning difficulties**</li><li>behavioural problems</li></ul>

ANGELMAN SYNDROME = no maternal copy of Chr. 15q11–13 (sporadic)

Signs	Associated conditions
<ul><li>'coarse' facial features (rounded, heavy, thickened skin)</li><li>microcephaly</li><li>widely spaced teeth & wide mouth</li><li>prominent lower lip</li></ul>	<ul><li>**intellectual disability**</li><li>severe speech impairment</li><li>hyperactivity</li><li>ataxia</li><li>seizures</li></ul>

RUSSELL–SILVER SYNDROME = slow growth before & after birth **PLUS** dysmorphic features

Signs	Associated conditions
<ul><li>**LBW** / failure to thrive</li><li>head often disproportionate to small body</li><li>triangular face (prominent forehead, narrow chin)</li><li>curved 5th finger</li></ul>	<ul><li>**short stature**</li><li>delayed development</li><li>**learning disabilities**</li></ul>

WILLIAMS SYNDROME = may be auto dominant or *de novo*

Signs	Associated conditions
<ul><li>'elfin' appearance (wide mouth, small, upturned nose, short)</li><li>outgoing and friendly</li></ul>	<ul><li>mild **learning disabilities**</li><li>**hypercalcaemia**</li><li>ADHD</li><li>**aortic stenosis**</li></ul>

Growth and puberty

Stage of growth	% height grown	Dependent on*
1. Fetal	30%	Placental nutrition, maternal size/health
2. Infantile (<2y)	15%	**Nutrition**, thyroid hormones, *genes*
3. Childhood	40%	Nutrition, thyroid & **growth hormones**, *genes*
4. Puberty	15%	**Sex hormones** & growth hormones, *genes*

emotions/happiness also impact growth by affecting hormones

Role of hormones

- **Growth hormone:** at growth plate & stimulates ILGF to ↑ organ size
- **Thyroid hormones:** act at growth plate
- **Sex hormones:** cause growth spurt and fusion of growth plates
  (*oestrogen deficiency = delayed fusion = tall stature*)

Measuring growth

- **Weight, height****, head circumference   ***<2y measure length not height*
- Plot serial growth measurements on growth chart
- ± Bone age, pubertal stage, BMI

Short stature

→ *height **below the 2nd centile** (2 SDs below the mean)*

CAUSES
- **Non-pathological**
  - **familial** – short parents (consider genetic growth disorder – karyotype Ix)
  - **constitutional delay of growth & puberty** – late bone maturation & growth spurt (genetics, poor diet or ↑ exercise)
- **Pathological**
  - **IUGR / extreme prematurity** – may need GH Tx
  - **Chromosomal disorders** – Down's, Turner, Noonan, Russell–Silver
  - **Endocrine** – associated with ↑ weight (weight > height centile)
  - **Nutritional / chronic illness** – associates with ↓ weight (weight<height)
    e.g. coeliac, Crohn's, chronic renal failure

INVESTIGATIONS
- **Height velocity:** 2 measurements, 1y apart
- **Height comparison:**
  1. against weight   2. against expected/mid-parental height (MPH)

$$MPH = \frac{Height\ of\ father + height\ of\ mother}{2} \quad \begin{array}{l} +7cm\ for\ boys \\ -7cm\ for\ girls \end{array}$$

- **Hx, examination, hormone screen (GH, TFT, cortisol):**
  - dysmorphic features, features of chronic/endocrine illness, birth Hx

Growth hormone = peptide hormone

Indications for urgent specialist referral:
- **<0.4th** centile or **>99.6th** centile
- Height **markedly discrepant** from weight
- Measurements **cross centile line** after 1y
- Measurements **cross 2 centile lines** in 1st y

Remember to correct for prematurity:
- subtract no. of weeks premature
- correct up to 1y of age if born ≥32w
- correct up to 2y of age if born <32w

Endocrine causes of short stature
- **GH deficiency**
  - 1° deficiency
  - 2° to hypopituitarism e.g. craniopharyngioma
  - Laron syndrome = defective GH receptors
- **Excess corticosteroids**
  - Iatrogenic – alternate Tx days to ↓ risk
  - Cushing's syndrome = rare in children
- **Hypothyroidism**

Target height: MPH ± 2SDs
(±10cm in boys, 8.5cm in girls)

DDx of tall stature
- Familial
- Endocrine: hyperthyroidism, CAH, ↑ GH
- Precocious puberty
- Genetic syndromes: Marfan, Klinefelter

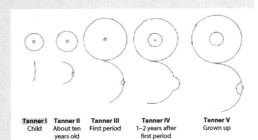

Tanner I
Child

Tanner II
About ten years old

Tanner III
First period

Tanner IV
1–2 years after first period

Tanner V
Grown up

Fig. 5.19

Stage 1 = no pubertal signs

precocious puberty is more common in females

prevent negative psychological impacts & conserve height potential (stop premature growth plate fusion)

Puberty

Females	Males
9–11y: 2° sexual characteristics: → breasts then pubic hair **10–12y:** growth spurt **11–13y:** menarche	**10–14y:** 2° sexual characteristics: → testicles ↑ >4ml then pubic hair **12–14y:** growth spurt (after 18m delay)

If pubic hair but no breast/testicle development, must Ix for CAH etc.

PRECOCIOUS PUBERTY → *development of 2° sexual characteristics <8y in females and <9y in males*
↳ **True/central:** gonadotropin-dependent (premature activation of hypothalamic axis)
↳ **False/pseudo:** gonadotropin-independent (excess sex steroids)

Causes
Females:
- **Central = majority** (idiopathic/familial) – ask about FHx
- Other = CAH, adrenal tumour, pituitary adenoma

Males: nearly always pathological
- Central = uncommon
- **Mainly tumours:** intracranial, adrenal, testicular

Investigations
- FHx, examination, hormone screen
- Growth chart
- X-ray hand – determine bone age
- Orchidometer – >4mm = puberty started
- USS ovaries/uterus – size/endometrial thickness
- MRI – hypothalamic tumours

Management*:
- **Central:** GnRH analogues
- **Pseudo:** identify & treat underlying cause of excess sex hormones

PREMATURE THELARCHE = *early breast development (6m – 2y) but no other 2° sexual features / growth spurt*
↳ of no consequence – do not need to intervene

PREMATURE ADRENARCHE = *pubic hair <8y (F) or <9y (M) but no other 2° sexual features / growth spurt*
↳ due to early maturation of androgen production in adrenal glands
↳ USS ovaries/uterus + bone age Ix to **r/o central precocious puberty or conditions like CAH**

GYNAECOMASTIA = *abnormal breast enlargement in males (in 50% boys during early adolescence → self-limiting)*
↳ **Causes:** Klinefelter, testicular feminisation, hypo-/hyperthyroidism, obesity, alcohol

DELAYED PUBERTY → *absence of pubertal development by 14y in females and 15y in males*

Causes
Constitutional delay in growth & puberty (most)
- short in childhood, long legs compared to back

Other causes
- **Hypogonadotropic hypogonadism** (↓ gonadotrophins)
  ► systemic disease: CF, anorexia, Crohn's, ↑ exercise
  ► intracranial tumours / pituitary damage
  ► syndromes: Kallmann's   *have ↓ smell*

- **Hypergonadotropic hypogonadism** (↑ gonadotrophins)
  ► syndromes: Turner's, Klinefelter's
  ► steroid hormone enzyme deficiency

Investigations
- FHx, examination, hormone screen (TFT, LH/FSH)
- Growth chart
- X-ray hand – determine bone age
- Pubertal staging: testicular volume/USS
- Karyotyping

Management
- r/o or treat underlying causes
- reassure puberty will occur (Tx not usually needed)
- IM testosterone/oestradiol

Diabetes mellitus

DM affects 2 in 1000 children (98% = T1DM)

TYPE 1 DIABETES MELLITUS → *autoimmune* destruction of pancreatic beta cells = *insulin insensitivity*
  ↳ GAD or islet cell antibodies

Risk factors
- **Genetics:** HLA-DR3/4, 30–40% if identical twin with T1DM, 2–5% if mum or dad with T1DM
- **Environmental triggers:** enteroviral infections, cow's milk, overnutrition

Symptoms
- Polydipsia, polyuria, weight loss, lethargy
- ± nocturnal enuresis, infections, signs of DKA

Diagnosis = symptoms PLUS
- Random blood glucose >11.1mmol/L
- Fasting blood glucose >7mmol/L (TFTs, coeliac screen, TPO to r/o other causes)

Management[7]:   MDT (paediatrician, specialist nurse, dietitian, support groups)

1. **Intensive education for child & parents**   Need to educate school too
   - Injection of insulin & blood glucose monitoring (finger-prick/continuous monitoring)
   - Diet & exercise: carb counting, low GI carbs, carb-free snacks, adjustment for activity, **alcohol**
   - 'Sick-day' rules: **do not stop insulin** (monitor glucose every 3–4h, may need ↑ insulin)
   - Signs of DKA/hypoglycaemia

2. **Insulin**
   - Subcutaneous pump = continuous infusion of rapid acting (NovoRapid)
   - Basal-bolus injection regimen = 2× LA breakfast & night **PLUS** SA before each meal

3. **Monitoring for complications: annual review**
   - Growth & pubertal development – risk obesity / delayed puberty
   - BP, renal function, eyesight, foot health
   - Associated autoimmune conditions: TFTs, coeliac screen, RA

Target blood glucose:

Pre-prandial: 4–7mmol/L
Post-prandial: 5–9mmol/L

LA = Long-acting   **SA** = Short-acting

Difficulties of glucose control in children
- Sugary foods/eat at odd times
- Infrequent/unreliable monitoring
- Poor family support
- Exercise
- Illness (↑ insulin need)

DIABETIC KETOACIDOSIS (DKA)
Symptoms
- 'Pear-drop' smelling breath
- Abdominal pain
- Vomiting
- Dehydration
- Hyperventilation (Kussmaul breathing)
- Drowsiness/coma

Think sepsis if:
Fever/hypothermia, hypotension, refractory acidosis, lactic acidosis

---

[7]NICE (2015, updated 2022) *Diabetes (type 1 and type 2) in children and young people* [NG18]

Management[8]: emergency → hospital admission

1. ABCDE
2. Fluid resuscitation & ongoing rehydration (cautiously)
3. Insulin therapy & potassium

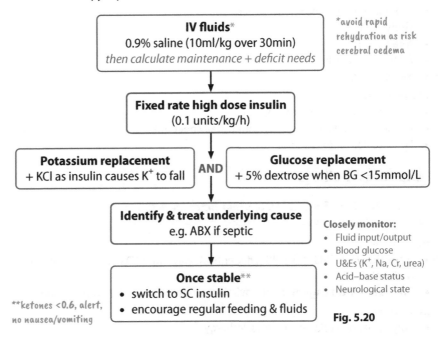

IV fluids*
0.9% saline (10ml/kg over 30min)
then calculate maintenance + deficit needs

*avoid rapid rehydration as risk cerebral oedema

Fixed rate high dose insulin
(0.1 units/kg/h)

Potassium replacement
+ KCl as insulin causes K^+ to fall

AND

Glucose replacement
+ 5% dextrose when BG <15mmol/L

Identify & treat underlying cause
e.g. ABX if septic

Closely monitor:
- Fluid input/output
- Blood glucose
- U&Es (K^+, Na, Cr, urea)
- Acid–base status
- Neurological state

Once stable**
- switch to SC insulin
- encourage regular feeding & fluids

**ketones <0.6, alert, no nausea/vomiting

Fig. 5.20

Complications

- Electrolyte imbalances (Na^+, K^+) – monitor U&Es
- Cerebral oedema – headache, agitation, ↓ GCS, eye palsies
- Aspiration

HYPOGLYCAEMIA = *blood **glucose <2.6mmol/L***

Symptoms

- Sweating, pallor, palpitations/tremor
- Headache / vision changes / confusion
- Hypotonia, poor feeding (in infants)
- Drowsiness, seizures, coma

<4.0 in diabetics
<2.0 in asymptomatic, term neonates

Investigations

- Careful Hx
- Physical examination
- **Blood glucose & ketones**
- FBC, CRP, U&Es, LFTs, TFTs, blood gases
- Hormones – insulin, C-peptide, GH, cortisol
- Urinalysis – pH, ketones, reducing substances

short/pigmentation suggest hormone issue
hepatomegaly suggests glycogen storage disease

Management[9]

1. **Oral fast-acting glucose:** sugary drink / Glucogel
2. **IV glucose:** 2ml/kg dextrose bolus then 10% dextrose infusion
3. **IM glucagon** if unconscious / fail to respond

DIABETES INSIPIDUS (DI) = *ADH (antidiuretic hormone) disorder causing polydipsia and polyuria*

- **Central DI:** insufficient ADH production → responds to desmopressin
- **Nephrogenic DI:** lack of kidney response to ADH → **more common type in children** → no response to desmopressin

[8] BSPED (2021) *Guideline for the management of children and young people under the age of 18 years with diabetic ketoacidosis*
[9] NICE (2015, updated 2022) *Diabetes (type 1 and type 2) in children and young people* [NG18]

Risk factors

Central: Head injury / brain surgery / brain tumour

Nephrogenic:

- Kidney disease / genetic mutation
- Nephrotoxic medications e.g. lithium

Investigation: high plasma osm, low urine osm

Management

- Drink more to prevent dehydration & low salt diet
- Medication review (nephrotoxics)
- Desmopressin* (antidiuretic hormone analogue)

THYROID DISEASE

Hypothyroidism

Congenital hypothyroidism = relatively common (1 in 4000)

- Most cases detected with heel-prick test ($\downarrow T_3/T_4$, $\uparrow$ TSH)
- Preventable cause of severe learning difficulties
- **Tx:** lifelong levothyroxine

Acquired hypothyroidism = usually autoimmune thyroiditis

- Girls > boys
- **RFs:** Down's, Turner's, other autoimmune disorders
- **Tx:** lifelong levothyroxine

Hyperthyroidism

Graves' disease = most common cause

- Investigations = antibodies (TPO, TSIs), TFTs ($\uparrow T_3/T_4$, $\downarrow$ TSH)
- Commonly presents in adolescent girls
- **Tx:** anti-thyroid meds, beta-blockers, thyroidectomy (if Tx-resistant)

CUSHING SYNDROME → *glucocorticoid excess*

Causes

- **Long-term glucocorticoid Tx** (most common cause in children)
  - ▶ **Uses:** nephrotic syndrome, asthma, bronchopulmonary dysplasia
  - ▶ **Sx:** Cushing syndrome + growth suppression + osteopenia (short & obese)
  - ▶ **Mx:** take in the morning on **alternate days**
- **Other causes** (rare in children)
  - ▶ pituitary adenoma, ACTH-secreting tumour, adrenal tumour

Investigations

- Serum cortisol levels – diurnal variation lost
- Dexamethasone suppression test – failed ACTH suppression

OBESITY → *obese children tend to become obese adults*

Risk factors

- Lack of exercise/poor diet/low socioeconomic status – tall/normal height & obese
- Endocrine disorder: hypothyroidism/Cushing's – short & obese
- Genetic syndrome: Prader–Willi – dysmorphic features & obese

Management[10]: weight maintenance = most realistic (BMI $\downarrow$s as height $\uparrow$s)

1. **Lifestyle:** diet, exercise, restricted screen time
2. **Medical*:** orlistat (lipase inhibitor)
3. **Bariatric surgery:** not recommended for children. May consider if sexually & physically mature & with complications.

[10]NICE (2014) *Obesity* [CG189]

---

*only DI of a central cause responds to desmopressin

Congenital	Acquired
• Initially asymptomatic • Feeding problems • Failure to thrive • Prolonged jaundice • Constipation • Pale, cold, mottled skin • Coarse facies, large tongue	• Short stature • Bradycardia • Dry skin, thin hair • Obesity • Constipation • Cold intolerance • Delayed puberty • ± goitre

Symptoms of hyperthyroidism = similar to adults except:

+ rapid growth in height
+ advanced bone maturity
+ learning difficulties/behavioural problems
− eye signs (uncommon in children)

Symptoms of Cushing syndrome

- Central obesity **but short stature**
- 'Moon face'
- Hirsutism (hair & acne)
- Hypertension
- Depression

	<12y	>12y
Overweight	BMI >91st centile	BMI >25
Obese	BMI >98th centile	BMI >30

*medical Tx only indicated if both of:
1. BMI >40 or >35 with complications (e.g. T2DM)
2. lifestyle changes have failed

Gastroenterology

Milk requirements <6m:
150ml/kg/day (across all feeds)

*1oz = 30ml

Nutritional requirements	Energy (kcal/kg/d)	Protein (g/kg/d)
0–6m	115	2.2
6m–3y	95	1.8–2.0
4–6y	90	1.5
7–10y	75	1.2

Non-organic causes of FTT (>95%) = associated with low socioeconomic status

1. **Feeding difficulties**
   - Poor technique / fussy baby
   - Incorrect formula preparation
   - Budgeting/shopping/cooking issues – lack of info on diet
2. **Psychosocial deprivation**
   - Maternal depression / poor bonding
3. **Neglect / child abuse**
   - Insufficient/irregular feeding

Organic causes of FTT (<5%)

1. **Inadequate intake**
   - Impaired suck/swallow: cleft palate, neuromuscular
2. **Inadequate retention**
   - Vomiting, severe GORD, diarrhoea
3. **Malabsorption**
   - Crohn's, coeliac, CF, lactose intolerance, post NEC
4. **Failure to utilise nutrients**
   - Premature, hypothyroidism
5. **Increased requirements**
   - Hyperthyroidism, malignancy, chronic infection, congenital cardiac disease

Management of FTT: most non-organic cases managed by MDT in primary care

GP: provide education, advice & **monitor child's growth**
Health visitor: assess eating behaviour & provide advice
Paediatric dietitian: recommendations to ↑ dietary intake *e.g. supplements*
Speech & language therapist: help with feeding difficulties / assess swallow

Nutrition

BREASTFEEDING: recommended exclusively for first 6m
→ first feed given within first hour of life
→ **>6m breast milk = nutritionally inadequate** → wean onto solids

Advantages	Complications
• **Ideal nutrient composition:** changes with baby's needs • **Rich in growth factors & immunoglobulins** • **Protects against infection:** gastroenteritis, necrotising enterocolitis • **Protects against later-life disease:** DM, obesity, IBD, HTN • **BONDING**	• **Transmission of** drugs, infection, toxins • **Breast-milk jaundice** • **Harder to measure intake** • **Less flexible:** harder with twins, etc. • **Can be difficult:** psychological distress

FORMULA-FEEDING: modified cow's milk → Do not start on unmodified cow's milk until 1y of age
→ **Specialised formula (hydrolysed):** if lactose intolerant/ CMP enteropathy / CF / liver disease
→ Gradual reintroduction of milk when >1y

Cow's milk protein allergy (most resolve by 5y)
Ix: skin prick
Sx: N&V, abdo pain, loose mucus stools ± blood, no ↑ weight
→ often rash / bad nappy rash

Failure to thrive (FTT) / faltering growth

↳ **Mild FTT:** fall over 2 centile lines   ↳ **Severe FTT:** fall over 3 centile lines

INVESTIGATIONS

1. **History & food diary** – clarify exact intake
   - Details of mealtimes / what happens?
   - Details of child's health/energy levels
   - Other Sx in child e.g. diarrhoea, cough, vomiting, infections
   - Hx of IUGR/ prematurity?
   - Maternal illness/smoking/alcohol in pregnancy
   - Medical conditions in child or family?
   - Growth in other family members?
   - Any psychosocial problems at home?
2. **Examination**
   - Signs of malabsorption
   - Signs of chronic lung disease
   - Signs of heart failure
   - Signs of nutritional deficiencies
   - Dysmorphic features
3. **Other tests** – **not usually needed**
   - FBC, CRP, ferritin – anaemia/immunodeficiency
   - LFTs – liver disease, malabsorption, metabolic
   - U&Es, Cr, calcium, phosphate – renal disorders
   - TFTs – thyroid disease
   - Urine dip/MCS – UTIs
   - Stool MCS – intestinal infection, parasites
   - Immunoglobulins – immunodeficiency
   - IgA transglutaminase antibodies – coeliac
   - Karyotype (girls) – Turner syndrome
   - CXR & sweat test – CF

Malnutrition

ASSESSING NUTRITIONAL STATUS
- **Food intake** – via food diary
- **Anthropometry** – weight for height, height for age, BMI, MUAC, STAMP chart PYMS
- **Laboratory Ix** – specific deficiencies (albumin, vitamins, minerals)

	Normal	Severe wasting	Severe stunting
Weight for age	100%	<70%*	<70%*
Weight for height	100%	<70%*	100%
Height for age	100%	100%	<84%

*<70% is ≥3 standard deviations below median

MANAGEMENT
- Correct electrolyte imbalances/hypoglycaemia
- IV fluids if dehydrated
- Keep warm (wrap up, especially at night)
- **Therapeutic feeding**
↳ **1. Enteral** (via GI tract) ⟶
  - **Short-term:** NG tube
  - **Long-term:** Gastrostomy

2. Parenteral: direct into circulation (IV)
  - **Short-term:** cannula in peripheral vein
  - **Long-term:** CVC

KWASHIORKOR: severe protein malnutrition
- Wasted appearance
- **Generalised oedema**
- Abdo distension / hepatomegaly
- Diarrhoea, hypothermia, bradycardia

MARASMUS: protein-energy malnutrition
- Wasted/skinny appearance
- **Weight for height <70%**
- **Fat & muscle wasting**

VITAMIN A DEFICIENCY
Complications
- Xerophthalmia, corneal ulceration & scarring
- **Blindness**, especially at night
- Increased susceptibility to infection – especially measles

Prevention
- Vit A dose/supplementation in developing countries

VITAMIN D DEFICIENCY: causes rickets → failed bone mineralisation
Risk factors
- Diet: vegan, low Ca/phosphorus
- Lack of sunlight
- Malabsorption: CF, coeliac, etc.
- Chronic liver disease
- Genetic conditions

Symptoms
- Bowing of bones (e.g. legs)
- Delayed dentition
- Craniotabes (soft skull)
- Harrison sulcus (soft ribs)
- FTT & misery

Diagnosis/investigations
- **Dietary Hx** – prolonged breastfeeding = risk factor
- **Bloods:** ↓ Ca, ↓ phosphorus, ↑ ALP, ↑ PTH
- **X-ray wrist:** widened epiphyseal plate & frying of metaphysis

Management
- Treat underlying risk factors
- Daily cholecalciferol (vit D3) & educate on balanced diet

9% of children <5y worldwide suffer from malnutrition

MUAC = Mid-Upper-Arm Circumference: constant from 1–6y
<11.5cm = severe malnutrition – **refer for Tx**
<12.5cm = moderate malnutrition – **refer for Tx**
>12.5cm = well nourished

PYMS = Paediatric Yorkhill Malnutrition Score Used in patients >1y old

→ most common cause of blindness in developing countries

Malabsorption

General symptoms:

- Abnormal stools – diarrhoea, steatorrhoea, foul-smelling
- Abdominal pain/distension
- FTT / poor growth / weight loss (not always)
- Specific nutrient deficiencies, e.g. anaemia

COELIAC DISEASE → *gluten provokes damaging immunological response in the proximal small intestine mucosa = **loss of villi***

Symptoms*:

- **FTT** ± weight loss / wasted buttocks
- **Diarrhoea**
- Abdo pain/distension
- Irritability/fatigue
- Anaemia

Investigations:

- Serological testing – IgA transglutaminase, anti-endomysial
- **Small intestinal biopsy = diagnostic**

Management: gluten-free diet for life

→ If diagnosed <2y, need gluten challenge later in childhood to confirm Dx

INFLAMMATORY BOWEL DISEASE

→ 25% cases diagnosed in childhood or adolescence (often mistaken for psychological problem)

→ **Symptoms:** poor general health, growth failure, psychological impact

---

Causes of malabsorption

- **Food intolerance*:** lactose intolerance, cow's milk protein allergy
- **Bowel disease (enteropathies):** coeliac, Crohn's, UC
- **Bowel resection**
- **Pancreatic dysfunction:** CF
- **Cholestatic liver disease / biliary atresia**

*Ix for intolerance/allergy: skin prick & IgE

*Sx begin after introduction of wheat into diet (8–24m)

	CROHN'S DISEASE	ULCERATIVE COLITIS
Pathogenesis	**transmural inflammation mouth → anus** (especially distal ileum & proximal colon)	**inflammatory ulceration of mucosa** (extends proximally from rectum)
Symptoms	<ul><li>abdominal pain</li><li>bloody or non-bloody diarrhoea</li><li>weight loss</li><li>fever/lethargy</li><li>mouth ulcers</li><li>perianal skin tags/fissures</li></ul> *children often lack the GI Sx*	<ul><li>abdominal pain (colicky)</li><li>bloody diarrhoea</li><li>weight loss (less than in Crohn's)</li><li>tenesmus/urgency</li></ul>
Associations	uveitis, arthritis, erythema nodosum, arthropathy	arthritis, erythema nodosum
Complications	bowel obstruction, fistulae, abscess	adenocarcinoma, toxic megacolon
Investigations	**Bloods:** ↑ CRP/ESR, platelets, ↓ Hb/Fe **Endoscopy + biopsy:** non-caseating granuloma & deep ulcers / wall thickening	**Bloods:** ↑ CRP/ESR, platelets, ↓ Hb/Fe **Colonoscopy/ileocolonoscopy + biopsy:** crypt abscesses & mucosal ulceration
Management[11,12]	1. **Induce acute remission:** liquid polymeric / elemental diet **plus** systemic steroids 2. **Maintain:** immunosuppressant 1) azathioprine 2) methotrexate 3) infliximab 3. **± Surgery:** especially if complications (colectomy + ileostomy)	1. **Induce acute remission:** → **mild:** topical aminosalicylates (mesalazine) ± topical steroid → **severe:** PO steroids + immunosuppressants (ciclosporin) 2. **Maintain:** aminosalicylate (topical or oral) ± PO azathioprine 3. **± Surgery:** can be curative (colectomy + ileostomy)

consider oral aminosalicylate if extensive disease

---

[11] NICE (2019) *Crohn's disease* [NG129]
[12] NICE (2019) *Ulcerative colitis* [NG130]

TODDLER DIARRHOEA (chronic non-specific diarrhoea) = **maturational delay in intestinal motility** = **rushed passage**   ~~Resolves by 5y~~

Symptoms: offensive, loose stools with undigested vegetables

Management: ↑ fat/fibre in diet to slow transit

Constipation

→ *infrequent passage of dry, hardened faeces ± straining & pain*

CAUSES
~~Diagnosis of exclusion~~

- Idiopathic
- Following febrile illness
- Due to dehydration / lack of fibre
- Medications, e.g. opiates
- Toilet-training issues
- Stress / psychological issues
- Food allergies/intolerances/diet changes
- **Underlying condition** (red flag Sx)

Red flag symptoms	Diagnostic concern
Fail to pass meconium in first 24h	Hirschsprung disease/CF/imperforate anus
Gross abdo distension	Hirschsprung disease
FTT/growth failure	Crohn's, coeliac, hypothyroidism
Abnormal lower limb neurology	Lumbosacral pathology
Sacral dimple/hairy patch	Spina bifida occulta
Perianal bruising	Abnormal anal anatomy
Perianal fistula/abscess/fissure	Crohn's

INVESTIGATIONS

- Careful history
  - ▸ recent illness, food/fluid intake
- Abdo palpation
  - ▸ soft, non-tender **but palpable mass**
- DRE (by specialist paediatrician)
  - ▸ **ONLY IF UNDERLYING PATHOLOGY SUSPECTED**

MANAGEMENT SUMMARY[13]

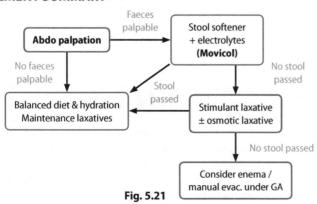

Fig. 5.21

Encopresis: faecal soiling by children >4y & toilet-trained

Pathology:
a) long-standing constipation
faecal holding → rectal dilation → lost reflex
(don't feel need to defecate)
b) behavioural – must consider child abuse as differential

Management: encourage & reassure child
1. **Evacuate overloaded rectum:**
   - ▸ stool softeners (polyethylene glycol = Movicol)
   - ▸ stimulant laxative (senna) ± osmotic laxative (lactulose)
2. **Maintenance therapy:**
   - ▸ stool softeners ± stimulant laxative (gradually ↓ dose)

---

[13]NICE (2010, updated 2017) *Constipation in children and young people* [CG99]

→ 1 in 5000 births
(4x more common in males)
RF = Down syndrome

→ 75% just rectosigmoid
→ 10% entire colon

Hirschsprung disease

→ *absence of ganglion cells in myenteric & submucosal plexuses of colon & rectum*

SYMPTOMS
- **Fail to pass meconium in first 24h** / constipation
- Abdominal distension
- Bilious vomiting

SIGNS ON DRE: one of the rare times a DRE is performed in kids
- **Narrowed segment of rectum/colon**
- Release of fluid/liquid stool on withdrawal

DIAGNOSIS
- AXR shows dilated bowel loops but isn't diagnostic
- **Suction rectal biopsy** – absence of ganglion cells
- **Barium enema** – shows constricted segment

MANAGEMENT
- **Colostomy** + anastomosis of bowel to anus

> **Complications of Hirschsprung disease**
> - Hirschsprung enterocolitis – *C. diff.* infection
> - Growth failure

Vomiting

Non-forceful return of milk:
1. **Posseting:** small amounts milk + swallowed air
   → *normal*
2. **Regurgitation:** larger amounts/more frequent
   → *suggests more significant reflux*

Forceful return of milk: VOMITING

Red flag symptoms	Diagnostic concern
Bile-stained	Intestinal obstruction
Haematemesis	Oesophagitis, peptic ulcer
Projectile vomit	Pyloric stenosis
Vomit after paroxysmal cough	Whooping cough
Abdo pain on movement	Surgical abdomen
Abdo distension	Intestinal obstruction
Blood in stool (needs stool culture)	Intussusception, gastroenteritis, dysentery (e.g. *E. coli*, shigella)
Severe dehydration/shock	Severe GE, systemic infection, DKA
Bulging fontanelle / early morning vomiting	Raised ICP
Failure to thrive	GORD, coeliac

DIFFERENTIALS OF VOMITING

Infants	Preschool	School/adolescent
GORD – most common cause **Overfeeding** **Dietary intolerances** **Infection** • Gastroenteritis, respiratory, UTI, meningitis **Intestinal obstruction** • Pyloric stenosis, duodenal atresia • Malrotation, volvulus, intussusception • Strangulated inguinal hernia	**Infection** • Gastroenteritis, respiratory, UTI, meningitis **Intestinal obstruction** • Malrotation, volvulus, intussusception • Foreign body **Appendicitis** **Coeliac disease** **Raised ICP** **Torsion of testes**	**Infection** • Gastroenteritis • Pyelonephritis • Septicaemia **Appendicitis** **DKA / renal failure** **Coeliac disease** **Raised ICP** **Torsion of testes** **Alcohol/drugs** **Bulimia nervosa**

GORD → *Functionally immature lower oesophageal sphincter relaxes inappropriately =* **VERY COMMON IN INFANTS**

Symptoms
- Recurrent regurgitation/vomiting (non-bilious)
- Epigastric pain (crying/distressed during feeds)
- → most cases are **otherwise well & gaining weight**

Complications
- FTT (if severe vomiting) → refer to paediatrician
- Oesophagitis = pain feeding, haematemesis, IDA
- Recurrent aspiration = cough/wheeze, pneumonia
- Dystonic neck posturing = Sandifer syndrome

Investigations: most cases diagnosed clinically → **r/o OVERFEEDING**
- Urine dip / bloods if concerned about infection
- 24h oesophageal pH monitoring
- Endoscopy + biopsy = r/o other causes / identify oesophagitis

Management[14]:

Mild/uncomplicated	More severe	Tx-resistant/complications
• Position upright after feeding • Antacids e.g. Gaviscon	• Feed thickeners e.g. Carobel/Nestargel • PPIs e.g. omeprazole	• Nissen fundoplication

OVERFEEDING
Symptoms: no red flags / normal examination
- Milk regurgitation / vomiting
- Foul-smelling diarrhoea & extreme flatulence
- Irritable / sleep disturbance
- May be over average weight for age

GASTROENTERITIS → *Affects* **10%** *of children <5y*
Symptoms
- Loose, watery stools
- Vomiting
- Dehydration & shock = dangerous complication

→ **Increased risk if:**
- <6m
- diarrhoeal stools ≥6× in 24h
- vomited ≥3× in 24h

Investigations: usually clinical Dx
- **Assess dehydration** (see *Emergency Paediatrics* section)
- Bloods: FBC, U&Es, glucose
- Capillary or venous blood gas
- Stool culture – if septic/bloody stools/recent travel

Management[15]: self-limiting
→ *Risk cerebral oedema/seizures*
- **Oral rehydration (IV if severe/shock → not too fast & monitor Na)**
- Adequate nutrition following diarrhoea
  (encourage breast/formula milk & reintroduce solids)

→ **No anti-diarrhoeals or ABX**
↳ *Unless confirmed sepsis, salmonella in <6m or immunocompromised*

Predisposing factors in infants:
1. Mostly fluid diet
2. Horizontal posture
3. Short intra-abdo portion of oesophagus

Nearly all resolve spontaneously by 1y

Risk factors for severe GORD
- **Neuro disorders** e.g. cerebral palsy
- **Preterm** especially if bronchopulmonary dysplasia
- **Post-surgery** (for oesophageal atresia / diaphragmatic hernia)

Reassure GORD will get better as grow

take thorough feeding Hx

RFs for overfeeding: newborns and bottle-fed babies

Normal feed volume
= 150ml/kg/day (over 5–8 feeds)
= 5oz/kg/day (30ml = 1oz)

Organisms causing gastroenteritis:

Viral: ROTAVIRUS (60% all cases), adenovirus, astrovirus, norovirus, coronavirus

Bacterial: *E. coli*, campylobacter, salmonella, shigella, *V. cholerae*

Parasites: giardia, entamoeba, cryptosporidium

Haemolytic uraemic syndrome (HUS)

HUS is a rare but serious complication of *E. coli* infection

Triad of symptoms:
- Microangiopathic haemolytic anaemia
- Thrombocytopenia
- Acute kidney injury

Management: fluid & electrolyte management ± red cell / platelet transfusion

---

Post-gastroenteritis syndrome

Watery diarrhoea & temporary lactose intolerance following a return to a normal diet

Ix: 'Clinitest' for sugar in stools

Mx: another 24h oral rehydration
→ severe cases: temporary parenteral feed

---

[14] NICE (2015, updated 2019) *Gastro-oesophageal reflux disease in children and young people* [NG1]
[15] NICE (2009) *Diarrhoea and vomiting caused by gastroenteritis in under 5s* [CG84]

> **Often associates with 1 of these Sx constellations:**
> - Abdominal migraine
> - IBS
> - PUD/dyspepsia/gastritis

conditions in bold in table = most common

DDx: appendicitis (mesenteric adenitis is often only diagnosed post-appendicectomy when appendix is found to be normal)

> **Infant colic**
> - **Up to 40% of babies**
> - Resolves by 4m
> - Suspected to be a GI cause

often worse in evenings

Recurrent (functional) abdominal pain

↳ no physical findings = Dx of exclusion

→ *pain that disrupts normal activities & lasts >3m*

Investigations: minimise but r/o serious causes
- Full Hx & examination – **r/o constipation**
- Check growth
- Urine MCS – for UTIs
- Abdo USS – gallstones/obstructions

Management: biopsychosocial (symptom relief + cognitive therapy + education / family support)

ABDOMINAL MIGRAINE → ususally personal/FHx of migraines

Symptoms: (last 12–48h then often weeks without)
→ midline abdo pain
→ ± vomiting & facial pallor

Management
1. Manage triggers e.g. stress, lack of sleep
2. Simple analgesics e.g. paracetamol

IRRITABLE BOWEL SYNDROME → Interaction of physical, psychological & environmental factors altering GI motility

Symptoms
- abdo pain relieved by defecation
- bloating
- explosive, loose or mucous stools
- constipation / feeling of incomplete emptying

PEPTIC ULCER/GASTRITIS → nodular antral gastritis is caused by *H. pylori*

Symptoms
- epigastric pain
- regurgitation/vomiting
- ± weight loss

Investigations
- 13C urease breath test

Management: triple therapy
- PPI + 7d ABX

Acute abdominal pain

→ *huge number of differentials*

Surgical*	Medical	Extra-abdominal
• **Acute appendicitis**	• **Gastroenteritis**	• Torsion of testes
• Intestinal obstruction	• **Urinary tract infection/** stones	• Lower lobe pneumonia
• Inguinal hernia		• Upper respiratory tract infection
• Peritonitis	• DKA	
• Inflamed Meckel diverticulum	• IBD/**constipation**	• Hip & spine
• Pancreatitis	• Hepatitis	• Migraine
• Trauma	• Henoch–Schönlein purpura	• Psychological/stress

*See *Paediatric surgery* section

MESENTERIC ADENITIS → *Non-specific inflammation of ≥3 mesenteric lymph nodes in RIF*
↳ *Occurs after an infection (esp. viral gastroenteritis)*

Symptoms
- Abdo pain – mainly in RIF
- N&V
- Diarrhoea
- Fever, malaise

INFANT COLIC → *Paroxysmal, inconsolable crying occurring several times a day*

Symptoms
- Paroxysmal, inconsolable crying
- Knees drawn up
- Excess flatus

Management

Reassure parents that it is benign & will pass

→ if persistent, need to r/o milk protein allergy & GORD

Signpost parents to support: online resources / helplines / support groups

Infection & immunology

NICE guidelines for managing fever in under 5s[16]

1. **Identify fever**
   - **<4w:** axilla electronic thermometer
   - **>4w:** electronic/chemical dot in axilla or tympanic thermometer in ear
2. **Identify RFs for infection**
   - Illness of family members
   - Unimmunised/immunodeficient
   - Recent travel abroad / contact with animals
3. **Assess severity of illness**
   - NICE traffic light system
4. **Examine for rash & focus of infection**
   - Can aid diagnosis & guide Tx
   - **If no focus** identified must consider **serious bacterial infection** especially UTI and septicaemia

Management of febrile child

- **Not seriously ill:** at home, with clear instructions/ safety-netting (± PO ABX)
- **Significantly ill:** further Ix (septic screen) & monitoring/Tx in hospital
- **Seriously ill:** immediate IV ABX (cefotaxime/ceftriaxone)

NICE traffic light system

	Green	Amber	Red
Colour	Normal skin, lip, tongue colour	Pallor	Pale/mottled/ashen/blue
Activity	• Responds normally • Smiles/content • Normal crying	• Not responding normally • Wakes if prolonged stimulation • Reduced activity • No smile	• No response • Appears ill • Unable to rouse • Weak, high-pitched cry
Breathing		• Nasal flaring • Tachypnoea • O_2 sats <95% on air • Crackles	• Grunting • Tachypnoea >60 • Chest indrawing
Hydration	• Normal skin & eyes • Moist mucous membranes	• Dry mucous membranes • Poor feeding • CRT >3 • Reduced urine output	Reduced skin turgor
Other		• Fever >5d • Swollen limb/joint • Non-weight bearing • New lump >2cm	• Fever >38°C (if <3m) • Fever >39°C (if >3m) • Non-blanching rash • Neck stiffness • Bulging fontanelle • Focal seizures • Bilious vomit

Infant <3m with fever:

ADMIT & MONITOR (+ Ix)
→ Low threshold for IV ABX

Key red flag features

- Fever >38°C if <3m
- Fever >39°C if 3–6m
- Pale/mottled/blue
- Capillary refill >3s
- Altered consciousness, seizures
- Stiff neck, bulging fontanelle
- Significant respiratory distress
- Bilious vomiting

Safety-netting:

- poor oral intake
- signs of dehydration
- abnormal movement
- breathing difficulties
- rash
- rigors/seizures

Give written advice if possible

Septic screen:

- Blood culture
- FBC (inc. WCC, Hb, plt)
- Urine MCS
- CRP
- VBG

Also consider:
- CXR
- LP
- Antigen screen
- U&Es/LFTs
- PCR (viruses or meningo-/ pneumococcus)

Contraindications for lumbar puncture

- cardiovascular shock
- focal neurological signs or seizures
- signs of raised ICP
- thrombocytopenia
→ *Indications = <1y or suspect meningitis*

Possible sources of infection in the febrile child

- **URTI** – very common
- **Otitis media** – examine tympanic membrane
- **Tonsillitis** – examine tonsils
- **Pneumonia** – fever, cough, tachypnoea, crackles, chest indrawing
- **Gastroenteritis** – diarrhoea, blood/mucus in stool
- **UTI** – urine sample if fever doesn't settle / no clear source
- **Osteomyelitis / septic arthritis** – painful joint / reluctant to move
- **Septicaemia** – may be hard to recognise (↑ HR, ↑ RR, poor perfusion)
- **Meningitis** – non-specific Sx if young (drowsy, seizures) → later = bulging fontanelle, papilloedema, opisthotonos

Sudden onset purpura in febrile child should be **assumed due to meningococcal sepsis** (however, any severe sepsis can cause non-blanching rash due to DIC)

[16]NICE (2019, updated 2021) *Fever in under 5s* [NG143]

Septicaemia

→ *infection of bloodstream causing release of cytokines & host response that results in **septic shock***

SYMPTOMS

- Fever, ↑ HR, ↑ RR, ↓ BP
- Purpuric rash (meningococcal)
- Poor feeding, vomiting
- Irritable (high-pitched cry) / lethargic
- Myalgia/arthralgia
- Shock & multi-organ failure

CAUSATIVE ORGANISMS

- Meningococcus = most common cause of septic shock ± meningitis
- Pneumococcus
- *Staphylococcus aureus*
- GBS ⎱ most common causes in neonates
- *E. coli* ⎰ (acquired from birth canal)

MANAGEMENT[17]: SEPSIS 6 within 1h

1. **IV ABX** – choice depends on age/organism
2. **High-flow O$_2$**
3. **IV access** – blood cultures, glucose & gases (+ FBC, lactate, CRP, U&E, clotting)
4. **Fluid resuscitation** – early & aggressive (20ml/kg bolus & repeat if necessary)
5. **Consider inotropes** – help cardiac contractility
6. **EARLY SENIOR INVOLVEMENT** – may need PICU/anaesthetist

> **Fluid overload** causes pulmonary oedema & respiratory failure
> Monitor fluid balance with central venous pressure & catheter

Meningitis

→ *inflammation of meninges (due to host response to bacterial or viral infection)*

TYPES

1. **Viral (²/₃ cases)** = less severe than bacterial
   = enterovirus, EBV, adenovirus, mumps

2. **Bacterial (80% cases are in <16y)** = 10% mortality, 10% morbidity

<3months	GBS, *E. coli*, listeria
1m–6y	*N. meningitidis, S. pneumoniae, H. influenzae*
>6y	*N. meningitidis, S. pneumoniae*

3. **TB** (rare in countries with low TB prevalence)

INVESTIGATIONS

- Lumbar puncture = confirm Dx, identify organism & sensitivity
- FBC, CRP, U&Es, LFTs, clotting
- Blood glucose & blood gases (for pH & lactate)
- Blood, urine, stool, throat swab culture
- Rapid antigen test (on CSF or blood)
- PCR (of blood or CSF)
- **If TB suspected:** Mantoux, sputum, urine

CSF RESULTS

	Appearance	Neutrophils	Lymphocytes	Protein	Glucose
Normal	Clear	WCC <5/mm³		0.15–0.4g/L	≥50% blood
Bacterial	Turbid	↑↑↑	↑ / normal	↑↑	↓↓
Viral	Clear	↑ / normal	↑↑↑	normal / ↑	normal / ↓
TB	Turbid/viscous	↑ / normal	↑↑↑	↑↑↑	↓↓↓

MANAGEMENT[18]

1. **IMMEDIATE IV ABX** 3rd generation cephalosporin covers most common bacteria: cefotaxime/ceftriaxone

   + dexamethasone if >3m & CSF purulent / white cells >1000 AND NOT TB

2. **Supportive therapy:** high flow O$_2$, fluids, antipyrexials, correct metabolic disturbance

→ ***notifiable disease** (chemoprophylaxis for contacts – rifampicin/ciprofloxacin)*

> **Symptoms of meningitis**
> - **FEVER**
> - **Non-blanching purpura** (meningococcal)
> - Neck stiffness, bulging fontanelle
> - Opisthotonos (arched back)
> - Focal neuro signs, seizures
> - Altered consciousness
> - +ve Brudzinski & Kernig sign
> - Signs of shock
>
> ↳ *NB In infants symptoms are often non-specific*
> *e.g. poor feeding, vomiting, irritability, crying*

> **Brudzinski:** flexion of neck causes hip & knee flexion
>
> **Kernig:** with hips & knees flexed there is pain extending knees

> **Complications of meningitis**
> - Septicaemia
> - Hearing impairment
> - Cranial nerve palsies
> - Seizures/epilepsy
> - Hydrocephalus
> - Cerebral abscess

> **IM benzylpenicillin & 999 if GP**

---

[17] NICE (2016, updated 2017) *Sepsis* [NG51]
[18] NICE (2010, updated 2015) *Meningitis (bacterial) and meningococcal septicaemia in under 16s* [CG102]

Childhood exanthems

EXANTHEM: eruptive skin rash associated with systemic symptoms such as a fever
ENANTHEM: eruptive lesion on the mucous membranes

Children commonly present with a rash. Rashes can be split into 3 broad categories:
1. **Possibly worrying** e.g. meningococcal petechiae
2. **Named rash** e.g. HSP, chickenpox, eczema
3. **Nondescript viral rash** e.g. erythema infectiosum, roseola exanthem

COMMON CHILDHOOD EXANTHEMS

Infection	Rash appearance	Location	Associated features	Duration of Sx	Infectivity	Management	Complications
Chickenpox (VZV)	Crops of itchy red macules which become raised, then **blister & crust**	Most prominent **trunk & face**	• Fever **If fever >4d suspect bacterial complication**	4–10d	Scabs not infectious	Symptomatic treatment Oral aciclovir if immunocompromised VZIG to neonates if mother develops rash 7d before or 7d after birth	• **Pneumonia** Can be severe/fatal if immunocompromised
Measles/rubeola (paramyxovirus)	Erythematous maculopapular rash (pink then red macules) • Oral 'Koplik's spots'	**First face,** then chest & abdomen, then arms and legs	• Preceding fever, **cough & red eyes** • Photophobia if older • Miserable, looks sick	4–7d	From prodromal symptoms to 4d after the rash onset	**NOTIFIABLE DISEASE** Symptomatic treatment Consider ABX if vulnerable/immunocompromised	• Otitis media • Bronchopneumonia • Encephalitis • Cardiac problems • Death
Scarlet fever (streptococcus)	• Fine papular rash (feels like sandpaper) • **Strawberry red tongue** • Perioral pallor	**Starts face & elbows, then spreads rapidly** to entire body in 24h	• Fever • Tonsillitis / sore throat	5–7d	5d if penicillin given, otherwise 10–21d	**NOTIFIABLE DISEASE** 10d penicillin V or erythromycin	• Sinusitis/mastoiditis • Meningitis • Pneumonia • Septicaemia • Glomerulonephritis • Rheumatic fever
Rubella / German measles (rubella virus)	• Pink macular rash • **Forchheimer spots** (pinpoint red petechiae on the soft palate)	**Starts face/neck** then onto trunk and limbs	Prodrome 1–5d before rash: • Mild fever • URTI • Conjunctivitis • Tender LNs	1w before rash until 4d after	7d after rash starts	**NOTIFIABLE DISEASE** Supportive care **AVOID PREGNANT CONTACTS**	• Conjunctivitis • Hepatitis • Pericarditis Congenital rubella if infected in pregnancy
Erythema infectiosum / fifth disease (parvovirus B19)	• **Slapped cheek appearance** → Surrounded by 'halos' (rash appears as fever fades) • Maculopapular rash on trunk & limbs 1–4d after red cheeks	**Red cheeks first**	• Low grade fever • Myalgia/arthralgia	Wax and wane over 1–2w	Not infectious once rash appears	Symptomatic treatment May need blood transfusion if aplastic crisis	If infected in pregnancy in 1st/2nd trimester can lead to hydrops fetalis
Roseola infantum / exanthema subitum (herpes virus 6 or 7)	Discrete, blanching, red macules & papules • **Nagayama's spots** (red papules on soft palate)	**First trunk,** then arms and neck, **very little on face and legs**	• **High fever for 3d** • Mild URTI & cough • Abdominal pain • Diarrhoea • Eyelid oedema	1–2d	Spread orally	Symptomatic treatment	Rarely encephalitis or encephalopathy

OTHER CHILDHOOD VIRAL ILLNESS

Infection	Symptoms	Duration of Sx	Infectivity	Management	Complications
Mumps (paramyxovirus)	**Bilateral parotid gland swelling** + fever, headache, malaise, myalgia, anorexia Children commonly asymptomatic	7–14d	2d before to 9d after symptoms **Off school/work for 5d from development of parotitis**	**NOTIFIABLE DISEASE** Symptomatic treatment No need for ABX Warm/cold packs to swollen parotid glands	• Epididymo-orchitis (can cause infertility if bilateral) • Aseptic meningitis • Transient hearing loss • Pancreatitis • CNS disorders e.g. transverse myelitis
Flu (influenza A, B, C)	Coryza, nasal discharge, cough, sore throat, headache, fever, malaise, arthralgia, myalgia	3–7d	From 1d before, and up to 10day after symptoms develop	Symptomatic treatment Only consider antivirals if high risk (immunocompromised, chronic heart/lung/kidney disease, <6m **OR** admitted to hospital)	• Acute bronchitis • Pneumonia • Asthma exacerbation • Otitis media • Sinusitis
HPV (human papilloma virus)	• Warts: around genitals, on skin • Juvenile recurrent respiratory papillomatosis	Virus and symptoms may persist >1y	**Transmission via skin-to-skin contact during:** • sexual intercourse • vaginal childbirth	May not need treatment of warts **Topical cream** e.g. podophyllotoxin **Physical ablation:** excision, cryotherapy	→ Cervical cancer = complication **PREVENT TRANSMISSION VIA VACCINATION PROGRAMME:** boys & girls 12–13y

CHILDHOOD FUNGAL INFECTION

Infection	Symptoms	Duration of Sx	Infectivity	Management
Nappy rash (*Candida albicans*)	Red plaques, satellite papules, superficial pustules ± itching, soreness **Occurs in skin creases / areas of irritant dermatitis**	7d	Spreads via direct contact to other areas of the body / other people	1. Leave nappy off as much as possible & keep dry 2. Topical emollients + barrier creams 3. Topical antifungals (nystatin, clotrimazole)
Oral thrush (*Candida albicans*)	White spots in mouth & on tongue which can progress to yellow/grey oral plaques ± soreness of the mouth	7d	Can be transmitted when breastfeeding to mother's nipples **so treat mother's nipples as well**	1. Oral hygiene advice (if using inhaled steroid for asthma advise rinse mouth after) 2. Topical antifungals (miconazole oral gel, nystatin suspension)

Kawasaki disease

→ *systemic small-to-medium vessel vasculitis (due to immune hyperactivity)*
↳ *Rare disorder but important to diagnose as potentially fatal complication of*
CORONARY ANEURYSMS

SYMPTOMS (see Fig. 5.22)
Fever ≥38°C for >5d PLUS 4 of:
- Non-purulent conjunctivitis (E)
- Red mucous membranes
- Red/swollen/peeling skin (A, B)
  - ▸ cracked lips
  - ▸ 'strawberry tongue' (D)

- Rash (C)
- Cervical lymphadenopathy

INVESTIGATIONS
- History & examination
- ↑ CRP, ↑ ESR, ↑ WCC, ↑ platelets
- **ECHO** – shows coronary   *Important*
  aneurysms

MANAGEMENT[19]: + supportive (antipyrexials)
- IV Ig within first 10d – reduces risk of aneurysms
- Aspirin – high dose until fever subsides then low dose for 6w   ↓ risk thrombosis
- Long-term warfarin – if giant coronary aneurysms
- Monoclonal antibodies (infliximab), steroids, ciclosporin – if recurrence

Infectious mononucleosis (glandular fever)

→ *syndrome of symptoms mainly caused by host response to EBV*

SYMPTOMS
- **Fever, malaise**   → { • Cannot eat/drink
- **Tonsillopharyngitis** = very sore throat   • Breathing may be compromised
- Cervical lymphadenopathy

OTHER SX
- Hepatosplenomegaly/jaundice
- Petechiae on soft palate
- Maculopapular rash (if <4y)

INVESTIGATIONS
- **Blood film:** atypical lymphocytes
- **Monospot test:** heterophile antibodies → may be negative in young children
- **EBV antibodies:** IgM & IgG

MANAGEMENT
1. **Symptomatic relief** – self-resolves in 1–3m
2. **Corticosteroids** – if airway compromise
3. ABX – **only** if confirmed tonsillitis (5% cases)

HIV/AIDS

→ *affects >2 million children (mainly in sub-Saharan Africa)*

CAUSE: majority by transmission from mother (transplacental, at birth, breastfeeding)
PRESENTATION: opportunistic infections – bacterial, candida, diarrhoea, PCP
LONGER-TERM PROBLEMS: failure to thrive, encephalopathy, malignancy

NB Infants may not present with all symptoms so must maintain high suspicion if prolonged fever

Risk factors for Kawasaki disease
- 6m–4y
- Asian or Afro-Caribbean
- Covid-19

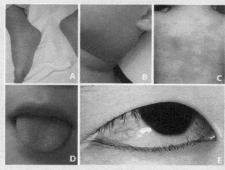

Fig. 5.22

Safety-net for glandular fever:
- Avoid close contact with others
- No contact sport
- No alcohol

AVOID AMOXICILLIN as causes rash in infective mononucleosis

Diagnosis of HIV

>18m: HIV Abs/antigen
<18m: HIV DNA PCR

All babies of HIV +ve mother need testing after ≥2w of ART to ensure not infected

[19]Eleftheriou D, Levin M, Shingadia D, *et al.* (2014) Management of Kawasaki disease. *Arch Dis Child*, 99:74–83

MANAGEMENT

1. **Anti-retroviral therapy (ART)** – started based on clinical status, viral load, CD4 count → infants **start ART ASAP**
2. **Infection prophylaxis** – co-trimoxazole (for PCP)
3. **Vaccinations** – flu, Hep A/B, VZV
4. **Regular follow-up** – monitor weight, neurodevelopment, signs of infection, adherence to Tx

Malaria

→ *700,000 child deaths in Africa every year*

CAUSE: *Plasmodium falciparum* parasite → transmitted by **female Anopheles mosquito**

SYMPTOMS: 7–10d post-infection
- Fever, malaise, myalgia
- V & D, abdo pain
- Jaundice
- **Anaemia** → children very susceptible
- Thrombocytopenia

DIAGNOSIS: thick blood film

MANAGEMENT: quinine

PREVENTION: nets, insect repellents, ABX prophylaxis

Typhoid

CAUSE: *Salmonella typhi* or *paratyphi* parasite

SYMPTOMS: 7–10d post-infection
- Worsening fever
- Headaches, malaise, myalgia
- Cough
- Abdo pain
- Anorexia, diarrhoea, constipation

SIGNS
- Rose-coloured spots on trunk

- Splenomegaly
- Bradycardia

MANAGEMENT
Azithromycin or ceftriaxone (3rd gen. cephalosporin)

COMPLICATIONS
- GI perforation
- Myocarditis
- Hepatitis, nephritis

Immunodeficiency

Suspect immunodeficiency in children with:
Severe Prolonged Unusual or Recurrent infections (SPUR)

PRIMARY: intrinsic defect of the immune system = often X-linked or autosomal recessive

Examples
- **T-cell defects:** DiGeorge, SCID, Duncan syndrome
- **B-cell defects:** agammaglobulinaemia, hyper IgM syndrome
- **Neutrophil defects:** chronic granulomatous disease

- **Leukocyte defects:** leukocyte adhesion deficiency

Investigations
- FBC (including WCC breakdown)
- Immunoglobulins
- Complement proteins
- Specific genetic/molecular tests

SECONDARY: due to another disease or treatment = more common

Examples
- Concurrent bacterial/viral illness
- HIV
- Malignancy
- Malnutrition
- Immunosuppressive therapy
- Splenectomy
- Nephrotic syndrome

Management options
- Antimicrobial prophylaxis
- Prompt treatment of infection (with prolonged ABX course)
- Ig replacement therapy
- Bone marrow transplant
- Gene therapy (for SCID)

School exclusion following infection

- Meningitis – until recovered
- Measles – 4d from rash onset
- Mumps – 5d from swollen gland onset
- Scarlet fever – 24h after ABX
- Impetigo – 48h after ABX
- Scabies – after treatment

Allergies/atopies

→ *40% UK children have allergic rhinitis, eczema or asthma* → ***can be fatal***

Cause: genetic susceptibility (FHx) PLUS environmental triggers

Pathophysiology: most are IgE-mediated
1. ***Early phase (immediate):*** mast cells & histamine → urticaria, angioedema, sneezing, bronchospasm
2. ***Late phase (4–6h):*** nasal congestion, bronchospasm, cough

FOOD ALLERGY → *6% children (many have other atopies)*

Triggers
- **Infants:** milk, egg, peanut
- **Older children:** peanut, tree nut, fish, shellfish

Symptoms
- **IgE-mediated:** urticaria/oedema 10–15min after ingestion → *severe = wheeze, stridor, abdo pain, shock, collapse*
- **Non-IgE-mediated (type IV delayed hypersensitivity):** D&V, abdo pain, failure to thrive *('intolerances')*

Investigations
- History & examination
- Total & specific IgE antibodies
- Skin-prick test
- Exclusion of food (+ careful reintroduction – 'food challenge')

Management
1. Avoid foods
2. **Mild reaction:** antihistamines
3. **Severe:** IM adrenaline (EpiPen) 'Allergy Action Plan'

ALLERGIC RHINITIS & CONJUNCTIVITIS → *20% children*

Types
- **Seasonal (hayfever):** related to grass/tree pollen
- **Perennial:** related to dust mites, pets, etc.

Symptoms
Sneezing, itchy eyes, runny nose
± cough, disturbed sleep, impaired concentration

Management[20]
- **Non-pharmacological:** allergen avoidance advice, nasal irrigation with saline
- **Pharmacological 1st-line**
  ▸ Non-sedating oral/intranasal antihistamines
  ▸ Topical nasal/eye corticosteroids
  ▸ Cromoglycate eye drops
- **Pharmacological 2nd-line**
  ▸ Nasal decongestants (max 7–10d at a time as **rebound effect**)
  ▸ Leukotriene receptor antagonists

Tolerance means Sx get worse

URTICARIA/ANGIOEDEMA

Acute (<6w): usually food allergy, drug reactions, infection

Chronic (>6w): usually non-allergic

Other causes: cold, heat, water, sunlight, sweating

Management: non-sedating antihistamines

e.g. dust mites/pollen/pet hair/mould, food items, insect stings, drugs, latex

NB *Secondary food allergies may develop later in childhood: due to similar proteins between plant pollen and fruit/veg plants = 'pollen–fruit syndrome'*

ECZEMA → see *Chapter 7*

Haematology

HbF: $2\alpha + 2\gamma \rightarrow$ higher O_2 affinity
HbA: $2\alpha + 2\beta \rightarrow$ lower O_2 affinity
So O_2 transfers from maternal Hb to fetal Hb

Haematological changes at birth

- **Haemopoiesis** switches from occurring in the **liver → bone marrow**
- **Fetal Hb (HbF) is replaced** so by 1y it is almost all **adult Hb (HbA)** → persistent high HbF suggests haemoglobinopathy
- **Hb levels are high in newborns** & drop over first few weeks

Anaemia

→ *Hb below the normal range for age*

↳ **Neonate:** <14g/dl
↳ **1–12m:** <10g/dl
↳ **1–12y:** <11g/dl

CAUSES

1. **↓RBC production (↓EPO** synthesis or RBC aplasia) e.g. IDA
2. **↑RBC destruction** e.g. SCD, thalassaemias, G6PD deficiency
3. **Blood loss** (rare in children) e.g. vWD, Meckel diverticulum

Age	Hb (g/dl)	WCC (×10^9/L)	Platelets (×10^9/L)
Birth	14.5–21.5	10.0–26.0	
2w	13.5–20.0	6.0–21.0	
2m	9.5–13.0	6.0–18.0	
1y	11.0–14.0	6.0–17.5	150–450
6y	11.5–13.5	5.0–17.0	
6–12y	11.5–15.5	4.5–14.5	
>12y (♀)	11.5–15.5	4.5–13.0	
>12y (♂)	13.5–17.5	4.5–13.0	

SYMPTOMS: if Hb <6–7g/dl
- Fatigue/weakness
- Pallor (conjunctiva & tongue)
- SOB/tachycardia
- Slow feeding / eating soil or chalk (pica)

PICA = consumption of non-nutritional substances

INVESTIGATIONS
- **FBC** – MCV (size of RBC) & MHC (Hb per RBC)
- **Iron studies** – serum iron & ferritin, TIBC
- **Blood film** – size, shape, colour
- **Serum bilirubin** – raised BR suggests haemolysis
- **Hb high performance liquid chromatography** OR **Hb electrophoresis**
  ▸ shows amount of each Hb type (HbS, HbA, HbF)

Anaemia from reduced RBC production

→ *Due to high iron requirement of growth*

IRON-DEFICIENCY ANAEMIA = #1 anaemia cause in children → *risk intellectual & behaviour difficulties if untreated*

Causes
→ **Inadequate intake** – if breastfeeding remains main nutritional source after 12m, iron-deficient diet
→ **Malabsorption** – coeliac
→ **Blood loss**

Breast milk: low Fe, 50% absorption
Cow's milk: low Fe, 10% absorption
Formula: high Fe, 10% absorption

Diagnosis
- **FBC:** ↓MCV & ↓MHC = microcytic, hypochromic
- **Iron studies:** ↓serum iron & ↓serum ferritin
- **Blood film:** abnormally shaped, small, pale RBCs

Management[21,22]
- Dietary advice
- Oral iron supplements e.g. Sytron/Niferex
  → Continue until Hb normal PLUS 3m

NB If no response to Tx consider Ix for other causes (esp. malabsorption)

DDx macrocytic anaemia: 'BCDEF'
- **B**12 deficiency
- **C**ompensatory reticulocytosis (blood loss)
- **D**rugs (cytotoxic)
- **E**ndocrine (hypothyroidism)
- **F**olate deficiency

DDx microcytic anaemia: 'TAILS'
- **T**halassaemia (α- or β-thalassaemia trait)
- **A**naemia of chronic disease e.g. renal failure
- **I**ron-deficiency anaemia
- **L**ead poisoning
- **S**ideroblastic anaemia

High-iron foods
- red meat, liver
- pulses, beans, peas
- leafy, green veg
- oily fish
- fortified cereals
- dried fruit/nuts
* Vit C (fruit & veg) helps Fe absorption

Foods to avoid
- Excess cow's milk (only 10% Fe is absorbed)

Full-term babies have iron stores sufficient to meet their needs until 4–6m, after which they depend on diet.

Premature infants have insufficient stores → infants <33weeks should receive iron from 4w of age.

---

[21] Paediatric BNF – *Anaemia, Iron deficiency*
[22] Journal of Paediatrics and Child Health (2007) *Policy statement on iron deficiency in pre-school-aged children*

B12 & FOLATE DEFICIENCY = rare in paediatrics

Causes
→ **Low dietary intake**
→ **Malabsorption** – e.g. Crohn's (↓ B12 absorbed from ileum)
→ **Low intrinsic factor** – e.g. pernicious anaemia (B12 needs to bind intrinsic factor to be absorbed in the stomach)

Diagnosis
- **FBC:** ↑ MCV = macrocytic
- **Iron & B12 studies:** ↓ serum folate, ↓ cobalamin (B12)
- **Blood film**

Management
- Dietary advice
- B12 & folic acid replacement

→ *B12 = eggs, fortified cereals, dairy*
Folate = broccoli, peas, brown rice

> **B12** = coenzyme needed for folate conversion
> **Folate** = needed for RBC synthesis

APLASTIC ANAEMIA = failure of blood cell synthesis

Causes
→ **Idiopathic**
→ **Transient erythroblastopenia** = triggered by viral infection
→ **Parvovirus B19** – can cause severe RBC aplasia in children with inherited haemolytic anaemia
→ **Inherited bone marrow failure syndromes** e.g. Diamond–Blackfan anaemia, Fanconi anaemia

> **Diagnosis of aplastic anaemia**
> - ↓ Hb, ↑ MCV
> - ↓ **reticulocytes**
> - Normal bilirubin
> - Coombs test −ve

Haemolytic anaemias (increased RBC destruction)

↳ **Clinical features**
- Anaemia
- Hepatosplenomegaly
- Jaundice

↳ **Investigations**
- **FBC:** ↓ Hb
- **Blood film:** ↑ reticulocytes → lilac colour, abnormal shape
- **Bilirubin:** ↑ unconjugated BR & urinary urobilinogen
- **Lactate dehydrogenase:** ↑ LDH

> **Further Ix**
> - Direct Coombs test
> - Hb electrophoresis

Summary of causes of haemolytic anaemias

Intrinsic	Extrinsic
- **RBC membrane abnormality** (hereditary spherocytosis)	- **Autoimmune**
- **Enzyme defects** (G6PD deficiency)	- **Infection** (malaria, CMV, EBV, *E. coli*, strep)
- **Hb abnormality** (thalassaemias, SCD)	- **Drugs** (nitrofurantoin, penicillin)
	- **Burns**

THALASSAEMIAS = *autosomal recessive disorders of α- or β-globin production causing ↓ HbA*

There are 2 beta-globin genes, 1 for each chain

Beta-THALASSAEMIA
→ **β-thalassaemia major:** both genes abnormal = no HbA = *very severe anaemia*
→ **β-thalassaemia minor:** 1 gene abnormal = *almost normal Hb with marked low MCV (60s)*

Clinical features (β-thalassaemia major)
- Severe anaemia from 3–6m (when HbF runs out) → transfusion dependent
- Jaundice & pallor
- Hepatosplenomegaly if untreated
- Characteristic facies (frontal bossing) if untreated

Management
- **Lifelong monthly blood transfusions**
- Iron chelation (prevent Fe overload of heart & liver from transfusions)
- Bone marrow transplant = only cure

> **RFs for thalassaemias:** Indian, Mediterranean, Middle Eastern

> **Prognosis (major):** 90% live >40y if Tx-compliant

> **Complications of long-term transfusion**
> 1. **Fe deposition**
>   - Heart = cardiomyopathy
>   - Liver = cirrhosis
>   - Pancreas = diabetes
>   - Skin = hyperpigmentation
> 2. **Antibody formation (in 10%)**
> 3. **Venous access problems** – may need CVC
> 4. **Infection** (HIV, hepatitis, etc.)

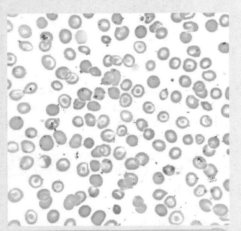

Fig. 5.23 Target cells & pale hypochromic cells.

Alpha-THALASSAEMIA

There are 4 alpha-globin genes, 2 for each chain

→ **Deletion of all 4 α-globin genes:** α-thalassaemia major/Hb Barts hydrops fetalis = *death* in utero

→ **Deletion of 3 α-globin genes:** HbH disease = *mild/moderate anaemia*

→ *may need transfusions*

→ **Deletion of 1–2 α-globin genes:** α-thalassaemia trait = *asymptomatic*

→ *marked low MCV*

INVESTIGATING THALASSAEMIAS:

1. **FBC & iron studies** – microcytic, hypochromic anaemia
2. **Blood film:** 'target cells' or nucleated RBCs
3. **Hb HPLC** – proportions of HbA, HbF, HbA$_2$

	HbA	HbA$_2$*	HbF	HbS
β-thalassaemia major	X	↑	↑	X
β-thalassaemia minor	✓	↑	↑↑	X
α-thalassaemia	Normal			
Sickle cell disease	X	✓	↑↑	✓
Sickle cell trait	✓	✓	↑↑	✓

*****HbA$_2$** = normal variant of Hb with levels higher than normal in thalassaemias

Sickle cell disease

→ *COMMON GENETIC DISORDER IN CHILDREN* → *1 in 2000* → *autosomal recessive*

CAUSE: mutation in β-globin gene which produces an **abnormal HbS chain*** rather than HbA

*If low O$_2$, infection or acidosis it polymerises and bends RBC into a sickle shape

PATHOGENESIS: sickle-shaped RBCs have ↓ lifespan → get stuck & occlude vessels causing infarction

Type	Hb	Symptomatic?
Sickle cell anaemia (HbSS)	Homozygous for **abnormal HbS**	**Yes** (no HbA)
HbSC disease (HbSC)	1 HbS gene + 1 **abnormal HbC**	**Yes** (less severe than SCA)
Sickle β-thalassaemia (HbSA)	1 HbS + β-thalassaemia trait	**Yes**
Sickle cell trait (HbSA)	1 HbS gene + 1 **normal HbA**	**No** (some HbA → carrier)

CLINICAL PRESENTATION OF HBSS

- **Moderate anaemia:** (6–10g/dl)
- **Jaundice** (clinically detectable)
- **Infection** (↑ susceptibility especially pneumococcus & *H. influenzae*)
- **Splenomegaly** – due to acute sequestration (children only) *due to hyposplenism from chronic infarction*
- **Painful vaso-occlusive crises**
  - ▸ hands & feet – dactylitis & swelling
  - ▸ bones of limbs – avascular necrosis of femoral head
  - ▸ lungs – acute chest syndrome = EMERGENCY (CPAP + exchange transfusion)
  - ▸ penis – priapism
- **Acute anaemia (aplastic crisis):** sudden ↓ Hb ± abdo pain ± hepatosplenomegaly
→ Triggers: infection, accumulation of sickle cells in spleen, parvovirus

DIAGNOSIS

→ NB Asymptomatic for 6—8w after birth due to persistent HbF

- **Screening:** pregnant women & neonates (Guthrie heel-prick test)
- FBC & iron studies = ↓ Hb, low MCV, normal Fe
- Blood film = sickle cells & target cells
- LFTs & bilirubin = raised
- Hb HPLC = HbS & ± HbA → **diagnostic**

MANAGEMENT[23,24]

1. **Infection prophylaxis:** vaccines + daily PO penicillin lifelong (for hyposplenism)
2. **Daily folate supplementation** (lifelong)
3. **↓ risk VO crises:** dress warmly, stay hydrated, avoid excessive exercise/stress
4. **Treat VO crises:** PO/IV analgesia (morphine + ABX/O_2 if need)
5. **Hydroxycarbamide to ↑ HbF:** if recurrent VO crises / acute chest
6. **Blood transfusion:** if acute complication (stroke, sepsis, aplastic crisis) & pre-operatively
7. **Bone marrow transplant:** only cure (for very severe cases)
8. **New treatments:** crizanlizumab
→ antibody binds p-selectin and stops RBCs sticking to endothelium

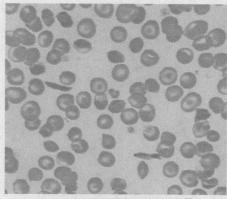

Fig. 5.24 Sickle cells & target cells.

Triggers of vaso-occlusive crises: cold, infection, dehydration, hypoxia/altitude, drugs

---

Mx of vaso-occlusive crises[25]

1. ABCDE – IV fluids, O_2 only if sats <93%
2. Analgesia*: IV/SC morphine AND paracetamol/ibuprofen (co-prescribe laxatives & anti-emetics)
3. FBC, reticulocytes, infection screen
4. X-match & transfusion
5. Enoxaparin

*Most patients have a 'pain plan'

Bleeding disorders

DIAGNOSTIC APPROACH

1. **History**
   - Age of onset
   - Bleeding Hx/pattern
     ▸ bleeds with previous surgery/dental work suggest inherited
     ▸ **mucous membranes:** platelet disorder/vWD
     ▸ **haemarthrosis:** haemophilia
   - Drug Hx
     ▸ anticoagulants

2. **Investigations**
   - FBC & blood film
   - **PT** (2, 5, 7, 10), **APTT** (2, 5, 8, 9, 10, 11, 12)
   - Thrombin time – fibrinogen deficiency/dysfunction
   - Mixing studies – determine if factor deficient or inhibitor present
   - D-dimers

---

[23] BSH (2018) *Guidelines for the use of hydroxycarbamide in children and adults with sickle cell disease*
[24] BSH (2016) *Guidelines for transfusion in sickle cell disease part I & II*
[25] NICE (2012) *Sickle cell disease: managing acute painful episodes in hospital* [CG143]

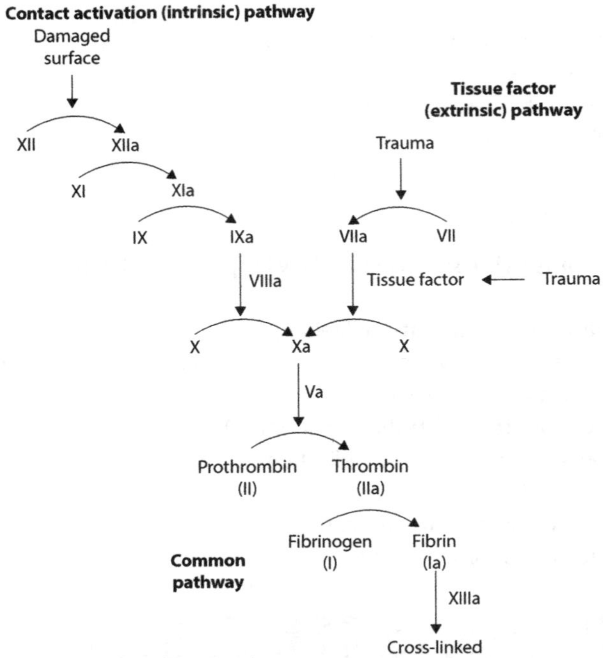

Fig. 5.25 Coagulation pathway.

INHERITED BLEEDING DISORDERS

↪ *Nearly always males*

1. HAEMOPHILIAS = *X-linked recessive* coagulation disorders

Clinical features

Mild: bleed after surgery

Moderate: bleed after minor trauma

Severe: ICH, spontaneous joint/muscle bleeds (haemarthrosis)

→ *Most present in first 18m*

→ *Commonly present when start to crawl/walk*

complication = arthritis

Investigations

- FBC, blood film, LFTs
- Coagulation screen: ↑ APTT & **normal bleed time**
- Clotting factor assays: low factor VIII or IX

Management: → Avoid NSAIDs & IM injections

- **For any acute bleeds:**
  → Elevation, compression & tranexamic acid
  → IV recombinant factor VIII/IX → given ASAP (parents taught how to administer at home)
- **For mild disease:** desmopressin (DDAVP) = antidiuretic that causes secretion of factor VIII & vWF into plasma
- **For severe disease or before major surgery:** regular prophylactic IV factor

A new monoclonal antibody Tx now available that is longer-acting: binds factor IXa and factor X → mimics activity of factor VIII

2. VON WILLEBRAND DISEASE (vWD) = *auto dominant* deficiency/defect in von Willebrand factor (vWF)

Clinical features

vWD = most common inherited bleeding disorder

- Bruising
- Prolonged bleeding
- **Mucosal bleeding** – epistaxis, menorrhagia

Diagnosis: mild ↑ APTT, **normal platelets & INR** → PROLONGED BLEED TIME

Haemophilia A: factor VIII deficiency (1 in 5000)

Haemophilia B (Christmas disease): factor IX deficiency (1 in 30,000)

Severity based on amount of clotting factor:

Mild: >5%
Mod: 1–5%
Severe: <1%

---

risk of hyponatraemia

Functions of vWF:
- facilitates platelet adhesion
- carrier protein for factor VIII preventing its degradation

Management: → avoid NSAIDs & IM injections
For all acute bleeds: elevation, compression & tranexamic acid
- **Mild (10–50%):** PO/IV tranexamic acid ± SC or nasal desmopressin (DDAVP)
- **Moderate/severe:** recombinant vWF

ACQUIRED BLEEDING DISORDERS

1. VITAMIN K DEFICIENCY = *causes haemorrhagic disease of newborn*
Causes: inadequate intake, malabsorption, warfarin   **Signs:** ↑ PT & & APTT
Prevention: recommended that all newborns have   excess bleeding
vitamin K after birth

Vit K needed for factors II, VII, IX, X

2. THROMBOCYTOPENIA = **platelets <150 × 10⁹/L**
Clinical features
- Bruising, petechiae, purpura
- Mucosal bleeding – epistaxis & gums
- **Less common:** GI haemorrhage, haematuria, intracranial bleed

	Plts × 10⁹/L	Symptoms
Severe	<20	Spontaneous bleeds
Mod	20–50	Excess bleeds in operations/trauma
Mild	50–150	Low risk of bleeding

3. IMMUNE THROMBOCYTOPENIC PURPURA (ITP) = *most common thrombocytopenia in childhood (4 in 100,000 per year)*
Cause: destruction of circulating platelets by IgG autoantibodies → *following viral infection*
Investigations: diagnosis of exclusion (child is well)
- Careful Hx & examination
- FBC & blood film – ↓ platelets = **only abnormality**
- Bone marrow examination – to exclude leukaemia/aplastic anaemia if ATYPICAL FEATURES & fail to respond to treatment

neutropenia/anaemia
hepatosplenomegaly
lymphadenopathy

→ **Peak age of ITP:** 2–10y
→ Onset 1–2w **post viral infection**

Management
A) **Benign, self-limiting (80%)** → resolves in 6–8w
- If major bleed / persistent minor bleed: oral prednisolone or IV Ig
- If life-threatening haemorrhage: platelet transfusion

General advice for ITP:
1. Avoid NSAIDs & IM injections
2. Avoid contact sports if platelet count is low

B) **Chronic ITP (20%)** → persistently low platelets >6m
- If major bleed / persistent minor bleed: oral prednisolone or IV Ig
- Persistent severe bleeding (rare): monoclonal antibodies, splenectomy

Thrombotic thrombocytopenic purpura (TTP)
= ↓ enzyme activity = ↑ clotting
= schistocytes on blood smear

4. DISSEMINATED INTRAVASCULAR COAGULATION
= *coagulation pathway activation* → *diffuse fibrin deposition & consumption of coagulation factors & platelets*

Causes
- Severe sepsis (infection)
- Trauma/burns
- Malignancy (especially AML)
- Toxins

Diagnosis: clotting screen
→ ↓ **platelets,** ↓ fibrinogen, ↑ D-dimers
→ ↓ antithrombin, ↓ proteins C & S
→ ↑ APPT & PT
→ **Blood film:** fragments (schistocytes)

Symptoms
Bruising, purpura, haemorrhage (can be life-threatening)

Management
1. **Treat underlying cause** e.g. sepsis
2. **Supportive:** FFP, platelets, cryoprecipitate (fibrinogen, vWF, other coagulation factors)

SPLENECTOMY
Pre-op: **vaccinations** (Hib, meningococcus, pneumococcus)
Post-op: lifelong low dose ABX (+ rescue high dose ABX on standby)
Complications:
Acute: bleeding, wound infection, VTE
Long term: infection from encapsulated bacteria e.g. streptococcus, Hib, meningococcus
Indications:
• Hereditary spherocytosis
• SCA
• ITP
• Lymphoma
• Trauma (splenic rupture)

Paediatric oncology

Red flags of lymphadenopathy:

- LNs >2cm in diameter
- No decrease in size after 4–6w
- Any supraclavicular node
- Abnormal CXR
- Systemic Sx (fever, weight loss, night sweats, hepatosplenomegaly)

Prognosis: approx. 90% cure rate

Before starting Tx: correct thrombocytopenia (+ severe anaemia), treat infections, renal protection (allopurinol)*

*prevents tumour lysis syndrome

Poor prognostic factors

Age <1y or >10y
WBC >50 × 10⁹/L
High risk genetic features of tumour cells
CNS involvement
Inadequate response to induction chemo

↳ **1 in 500 children** <15y develop cancer
↳ **82% 5-year survival rate** (most 'cured' by then)
↳ **2nd biggest killer of children 1–14y** (after infection)
↳ **Leukaemia & brain tumours** are most common

Leukaemia

→ *cancer of white blood cells*

ACUTE LYMPHOBLASTIC LEUKAEMIA (ALL) = *80% of childhood leukaemia*
→ *peak age 2–5y*
↳ *Rapidly proliferating lymphocytes resulting in accumulation of **abnormal, immature 'blast' cells*** *(B or T lymphocytes)*   RF = Down's

Symptoms: onset over several weeks
- **General:** malaise, anorexia, lymphadenopathy, hepatosplenomegaly
- **Anaemia:** lethargy, pallor, SOB
- **Neutropenia:** infections → risk of neutropenic sepsis
- **Thrombocytopenia:** bruising, petechiae, nose bleeds
- **Bone marrow infiltration:** bone pain
- **CNS infiltration:** headaches, vomiting

Investigations
- **FBC:** ↓ Hb, ↓ plts, ↓ neutrophils, ↑ or ↓ WCC
- **Peripheral blood film:** blast cells
- **Clotting screen:** 10% have DIC
- **Bone marrow biopsy** → diagnostic & prognostic
- **CXR:** mediastinal mass (characteristic of T-cell disease)

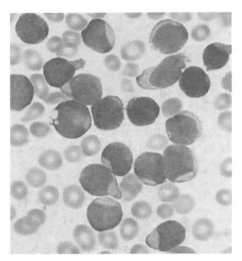

Fig. 5.26 'Blast' cells.

Cytotoxic drugs don't penetrate CNS, so **intrathecal chemo** (**methotrexate**) also given

Management[26]
1. **Chemotherapy:** including steroids and intrathecal chemotherapy
   → 2y for girls, 3y for boys
   → High risk patients receive more intensive chemotherapy
2. **Prophylactic co-trimoxazole:** given throughout treatment to prevent PCP infection
3. **Newer treatment options:** CAR-T cell therapy & monoclonal antibodies
4. **Relapse treatment:** consider bone marrow transplant ± CAR-T cell therapy

[26] Children's Cancer and Leukaemia Group (CCLG) (2017) *Acute lymphoblastic leukaemia*

Lymphoma

→ *solid malignancies of immune system* → ↑ *lymphocyte proliferation in LNs, spleen, thymus, bone marrow*

Investigations & diagnosis

- FBC & blood film
- Lymph node biopsy – RS cells in HL
- Bone marrow biopsy – for NHL
- ESR – helps staging of HL
- Lumbar puncture – helps staging of NHL
- MRI/CT/PET-CT – assess nodal sites
- CXR – check for mediastinal mass

Management

- **Chemotherapy** (± radiotherapy if HL)
- **PET** to monitor Tx response

Hodgkin lymphoma (HL) = Reed–Sternberg cells present
Non-Hodgkin lymphoma (NHL) = no Reed–Sternberg cells

Prognosis: >80% cure rate for both: Hodgkin (HL) slightly better than non-Hodgkin (NHL)

HODGKIN LYMPHOMA (20%) = Reed–Sternberg cells on LN biopsy → **more common in adolescents** (rare <5y)

Symptoms

- **Painless lymphadenopathy**
  - usually **cervical**
  - may cause **mass effects** (SVC/bronchial obstruction)
- B symptoms in 40%
  - fever, drenching night sweats, unexplained weight loss

Usually systemically well at presentation

Associates with EBV & altered immunity (need irradiated blood products)

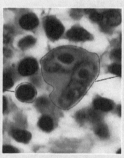

Fig. 5.27 Reed–Sternberg cells → binucleate 'mirror-cells'.

NON-HODGKIN LYMPHOMA (80%) = **no** Reed–Sternberg cells → **more common in childhood & males**

Symptoms

- **Painless lymphadenopathy**
  - **cervical, thoracic, or abdominal**
  - often cause mass effects – **mediastinal mass** (SVC/bronchial obstruction)
- Abdominal symptoms
  - palpable abdominal mass
  - pain from bowel obstruction / intussusception if ileum involved
- B symptoms in 20%

More likely to be systemically unwell at presentation

High grade lymphomas: divide rapidly
- Rapid onset lymphadenopathy
- Weight loss, fever, pressure effects

Low grade lymphomas: divide slowly
- More insidious onset of symptoms

Brain tumours

→ *#1 cause of childhood cancer deaths in UK* → *almost always primary*

Tumour	Location	Symptoms (depend on location & age)
Low grade astrocytoma (40%) benign	Cerebral hemispheres	Seizures, headaches, focal signs
Medulloblastoma (20%) malignant	Posterior fossa (cerebellum) spread via CSF	Ataxia, abnormal eye movements
Ependymoma (5–10%) malignant	Posterior fossa (cerebellum)	Ataxia, abnormal eye movements
Brainstem glioma (5–10%) malignant	Cranial nerve & pyramidal tract	Ataxia
Craniopharyngioma (4%) benign	From remnant of Rathke's pouch	Bitemporal hemianopia, pituitary Sx

MANAGEMENT

- Surgery + chemo ± radiotherapy
- Steroids (for pressure Sx)
- Anti-epileptics (for seizure Sx)
- **Rehab**

General Sx of raised intracranial pressure / hydrocephalus:
- Headaches
- Morning vomiting
- Drowsy/irritable
- Seizures
- Vision disturbance

most common in children <5y

Neuroblastoma

→ *tumour arising from neural crest tissue in adrenal gland or sympathetic nervous system*

SYMPTOMS
- **Abdominal mass:** usually adrenal gland BUT could be anywhere along sympathetic chain from neck → pelvis
- **Metastatic Sx:** pallor, weight loss, malaise, bone pain, cervical lymphadenopathy, constipation
- **Orbital disease:** proptosis, 'bruises' under eyes, eye movement disorders
- **Cutaneous:** 'blueberry muffin' rash

COMPLICATIONS
- **Spinal cord compression (if paravertebral):** paraplegia, Horner's
- **Adrenal tumour:** hypertension

MANAGEMENT[27,28]
1) **Low risk:**
   - Observation only (if subtype 'Ms disease' in children <18m, which can spontaneously regress)
   - Chemotherapy/surgery
2) **High risk: poor prognosis (40–50% survival)**
   - Induction chemo → surgery → high dose chemotherapy + radiotherapy + immunotherapy

---

> **Investigations**
> → FBC
> → Urine: ↑ catecholamines
> → USS, CT/MRI abdo
> → Biopsy: diagnostic
> → Bone marrow biopsy, MIBG scan: detect mets

Wilms tumour (nephroblastoma)

→ *tumour of embryonal renal tissue*

SYMPTOMS
- **Large abdominal mass:** often only symptom
± abdo pain, anorexia, anaemia, haematuria, HTN

INVESTIGATIONS
- **USS** – intrarenal mass
± CT/MRI – assess for mets (especially to lungs)

MANAGEMENT
Pre-op chemo → nephrectomy → post-op chemo ± radiotherapy

---

usually <5y (rare >10y)

> **5% present BILATERALLY →**
> suspect underlying genetic syndrome
> e.g. Beckwith–Wiedemann

20% already metastatic at presentation → lungs & liver

> **Prognosis for Wilms tumour:** approx. **85% cure rate** (60% if distal mets at presentation)

Soft tissue sarcomas

→ *tumours of connective tissue (muscles, tendons, fat, nerves, etc.)*

RHABDOMYOSARCOMA = most common → **highly malignant** cancer of **muscle & fibrous tissue**

Symptoms: can develop anywhere in body – symptoms depend on location (usually painless lump)

Most common locations in children:
- **Head & neck (40%):** proptosis, nasal obstruction / bloody discharge
- **Genitourinary:** dysuria, haematuria, urinary obstruction, scrotal/perineal mass, bloody PV discharge

Investigations
→ Biopsy
→ MRI/CT/PET to assess metastases → lung, liver, bone marrow
→ Bone marrow biopsy

Management
Chemotherapy ± surgery ± radiotherapy

> **Prognosis for soft tissue sarcomas:** approx. **65% cure rate** (worse if present with distal mets)

---

[27] CCLG (2020) *Low and intermediate risk neuroblastoma treatment guidelines*
[28] CCLG (2019) *Statement from CCLG Neuroblastoma SIG: Treatment and management of patients with high-risk neuroblastoma*

Malignant bone tumours

→ *osteosarcoma & Ewing sarcoma*

OSTEOSARCOMA = more common in older children
→ affects end of long bones (hip, shoulder, knee)

EWING SARCOMA = more common in younger children
→ usually affects legs, back, pelvis, ribs, skull

Symptoms
- Persistent, localised bone pain & limp
- Swelling & pathological fracture
- Mass on X-ray – often substantial soft tissue mass in Ewing's

Investigations
- **Bone X-ray** – destruction + new bone formation
- **MRI**
- **Chest CT** – assess mets
- **Biopsy** of lesion

Management
- Chemotherapy then surgery*   *limb-sparing surgery > amputation where possible
- Radiotherapy for Ewing sarcoma

M>F

Osteosarcomas = rapid growth & spread

Ewing: 'moth-eaten' appearance on radiograph

> **Red flags for bone tumours**
> - Progressive pain
> - Night pain / pain wakes child up
> - Reluctant to weight bear / stopped walking

Retinoblastoma

→ *malignant tumour of retinal cells*

CAUSE: *de novo* or **inherited (40%)** mutation in chromosome 13 → **all bilateral & 20% unilateral cases are inherited**

(autosomal dominant)

SYMPTOMS: 'SILVER'
Strabismus
Iris discolouration
Leukocoria → white pupillary reflex (instead of red)
Vision changes
Enlarged pupil
Red/sore/swollen eye

+ *systemic Sx if mets present*

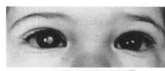

Fig. 5.28 Leukocoria.

INVESTIGATIONS
- MRI & examination under anaesthetic
- Lumbar puncture and bone marrow biopsy (for CSF spread)

COMPLICATIONS
- Severe visual impairment
- Cosmetic deformity
- 2° malignancy in future (bone/soft tissue, melanoma, breast/bladder)

MANAGEMENT
Chemo followed by local Tx e.g. surgery/radiotherapy

usually in children <3y

Nephrology

Bilateral hydronephrosis / suspected bladder obstruction in males needs urgent investigation with **MCUG to r/o posterior urethral valves**

Congenital abnormalities

1 in 300 births
- → most detected *in utero*
- → given prophylactic ABX at birth to prevent UTI

RENAL AGENESIS = absence of both kidneys
- **Result:** oligohydramnios (as no fetal urine)
- **Complications:** FATAL POTTER SYNDROME

MULTICYSTIC DYSPLASTIC KIDNEY (MCDK)
- **Cause:** failed union of ureteric bud & renal mesenchyme
- **Result:** non-functioning kidney with **variably sized fluid-filled cysts** & narrow ureter
- **Complications:** Potter syndrome if bilateral
- **Mx:** most involute by 2y (no Tx needed) → **nephrectomy** if remain large or HTN develops

POLYCYSTIC KIDNEY DISEASE (PKD) = always bilateral but some/normal renal function retained
- **Cause:** autosomal dominant (1 in 1000) or autosomal recessive
- **Result:** enlarged kidneys with **separate, discrete cysts**
- **Complications:** HTN, haematuria, renal failure

HORSESHOE/PELVIC KIDNEY = lower poles are fused in the midline
- **Complications:** ↑ risk infection or obstruction

DUPLEX KIDNEY = bifid renal pelvis or 2 complete ureters for 1 kidney
- **Complications:** reflux in lower ureter, ectopic drainage / prolapse of upper ureter (e.g. into vagina)

POSTERIOR URETHRAL VALVES = most common cause of outlet obstruction in male newborns
- **Cause:** abnormal flaps of tissue / membranes grow in urethras, obstructing drainage
- **Complications:** hydronephrosis / small, dysplastic, non-functioning kidney / ↓ amniotic fluid (Potter syndrome)
- **Mx:** cystoscopic ablation of valves

Assessing the urinary tract:

1. **eGFR** = low in newborns (rises rapidly in 1–2y)
2. **Plasma Cr** = ↑s through childhood with height & muscle
3. **USS** = visualise abnormalities, calculi & deposits
4. **DMSA scan** = static scan of renal cortex → shows functional defects e.g. scars*
5. **MCUG** (micturating cystourethrogram) = fill bladder with contrast medium to visualise anatomy & flow direction → shows vesicoureteric reflux & obstructions
6. **MAG3 renogram** = measure drainage of isotope-labelled MAG3 → shows vesicoureteric reflux & obstruction

NB Plain AXR not very useful to show stones/deposits

*false +ves if within 3m of UTI

Urinary tract infections

CLINICAL PRESENTATION → varies with age (non-specific in infants)

Infant	Child
• Fever	• Fever
• Vomiting	• Abdo/loin pain
• Lethargic/irritable	• Frequency/accidents
• Poor feeding / FTT	• Dysuria/haematuria
• Jaundice	• Lethargic
• Septicaemia	• Vomiting/anorexia
• Offensive urine	• Offensive urine

Pyelonephritis / upper UTI
1. fever >38°C + bacteriuria **OR**
2. fever <38°C + bacteriuria + loin pain

Cystitis / lower UTI
Bacteriuria without systemic Sx (fever)

Collecting urine samples
Infants in nappies
- **'Clean-catch'** – into prepared pot as nappy is removed → recommended method
- **Adhesive plastic bag** – applied to perineum after washing → contamination likely
- **Urethral catheter** – especially if need sample urgently
- **Suprapubic aspiration (SPA)** – needle into bladder via US guidance → invasive (↓ use)

Older children
- **MSU** – careful cleaning & collection avoids contamination

INVESTIGATIONS

1. **Urine dip** – screening test
→ **NITRITES** = SPECIFIC
→ **LEUKOCYTES** = SENSITIVE

2. **MCS** – ALWAYS NEEDED unless **BOTH** leukocytes & nitrites –ve
→ **To confirm diagnosis:** single org. >10^5 per ml
→ **To determine organism:** guides Tx

3. **Further investigations for cause** – ONLY if recurrent/atypical UTIs ────→
   - **USS:** shows structural abnormalities, renal defects, obstruction
   - **DMSA ± MCUG or MAG3:** for scarring, VUR or obstruction ↴

   NB If >3y & USS is normal then no further Ix

MANAGEMENT[29]
<3m: URGENT HOSPITAL ADMISSION
- IV ABX

>3m with upper UTI / pyelonephritis:
- PO ABX for 7–10d

>3m with lower UTI / cystitis:
- PO ABX for 3d

PREVENTION
- **Well hydrated** so high urine output (1–1.5L/day)
- **Regular voiding & complete emptying** – encourage double voiding
- **Prevent/treat constipation**
- **Perineal hygiene** – wipe front to back / foreskin hygiene
- **Probiotic** – *Lactobacillus acidophilus* = ↓ pathogens in gut

→ *Prophylactic ABX (trimethoprim/nitrofurantoin) – if age <2y with congenital abnormality or previous upper UTI or severe VUR*

Prevalence <6y:
Females: 3–7%　　**Males:** 1–2%

Causative organisms:
E. coli
Klebsiella
Pseudomonas
Strep. faecalis
Proteus

*Proteus causes **alkaline** urine & ↑ **risk phosphate stones***

Nitrites	Leukocytes	Interpretation
+	+	Confirms UTI
+	–	Start ABX & confirm with MCS
–	+	Only start ABX if clinical Sx of UTI
–	–	Repeat sample

SPECIFIC: +ve result = likely UTI, but –ve result does not rule out UTI

SENSITIVE: –ve result = unlikely UTI, but +ve result may be another cause (e.g. other febrile illness, balanitis/vulvovaginitis)

Atypical UTIs
- Severely ill or septicaemia
- Poor urine flow
- Abdo/bladder mass
- No Tx response in 48h
- ↑ creatinine
- Non-*E. coli* organism
- FHx urinary tract abnormality

IV antibiotics if:
→ Treatment-resistant pyelonephritis (no response in 48h)
→ **Urosepsis**

[29] NICE (2007, updated 2018) *Urinary tract infection in under 16s* [CG54]

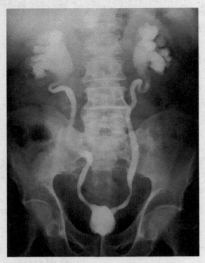

Fig. 5.29 Bilateral VUR showing dilated ureters and dilated, clubbed calyces.

Vesicoureteric reflux (VUR)

→ *developmental anomaly of vesicoureteric junctions*

CAUSE
- **Familial** = 30–50% risk if first-degree relative
- **Bladder pathology** – neuropathic bladder, urethral obstruction, post-UTI

TYPES
1. **Mild** – reflux into ureter only → usually not significant
2. **Severe** – reflux into kidney → grossly dilated ureter & renal scarring

INVESTIGATIONS
- **MCUS:** shows dilated ureters & direction of flow → **diagnostic (shows grade of reflux)**
- **MAG3:** shows direction of flow
- **USS:** show abnormalities/obstruction

MANAGEMENT
Mild: usually resolves within first few years of life
Severe: prophylactic ABX, surgery

COMPLICATIONS: (how it presents)
- **Incomplete bladder emptying** = risk of UTI
- **Intrarenal reflux** = risk of pyelonephritis → infection causes renal scarring
- **High voiding pressures** = transmitted back to kidneys → damaged renal papillae

Haematuria

CAUSES
Glomerular: brown urine, deformed RBCs, + protein
- Acute/chronic glomerulonephritis (+ proteinuria)
- IgA nephropathy
- Familial nephritis (Alport syndrome)
- Goodpasture syndrome (anti-basement membrane)
- Idiopathic/familial idiopathic

Non-glomerular: red urine, no protein
- Infection
- Trauma (to genitals/urinary tract/kidneys)
- Stones
- Tumours
- Renal vein thrombosis
- Sickle cell disease
- Bleeding disorders

INVESTIGATIONS

All patients with haematuria	If suspect glomerular haematuria
- Urine dip & MCS - FBC, ESR, platelets, clotting screen - Sickle cell screen - U&Es, Ca, phosphate, albumin - USS KUB	- Complement levels – often ↓ - Anti-DNA antibodies (ANCA present in vasculitis) - Throat swab + antistreptolysin O/anti-DNAse B - Hep B/C screen - Renal biopsy – if atypical features / severe Sx

Nephritic syndrome

→ *inflammation causes* ↑ *glomerular cellularity* → *restricts blood flow* = ↓ *filtration*

⎧ **1. HAEMATURIA** (>10 red cell casts)
→ ⎨ **2. OLIGURIA** (<0.5–1ml/kg/h)
⎩ **3. PROTEINURIA** (>3.0g/d)

Clinical features: volume overload
- Oedema (especially periorbital)
- Hypertension → seizures

Causes
- Post-infection (streptococcal)
- Vasculitis (HSP, SLE, Wegener granulomatosis)
- IgA nephropathy
- Membranoproliferative glomerulonephritis
- Goodpasture syndrome (anti-basement membrane antibodies)

Management
- **Diuretics** – maintain fluid & electrolyte balance
- **Treat infection if present** – ABX (penicillin)
- **If rapid ↓ renal function:** = renal biopsy, immunosuppression, plasma exchange

HENOCH–SCHÖNLEIN PURPURA (HSP): ↑ circulating IgA & IgG form
complexes that deposit in organs **(kidneys, skin, joints)**

ANCA antibodies

Clinical features
- **Palpable purpuric rash** – symmetrical over buttocks & extensor surfaces/ ankles
- **Arthralgia & periarticular oedema** (65%)
- **Colicky abdominal pain** (50%)
- **Glomerulonephritis** – micro-/macroscopic haematuria (80%)
- → **± fever & malaise**

Complications: rare
- **GI petechiae** → haematemesis/melaena
- **Intussusception** → redcurrant jelly stools
- **Nephrotic syndrome** – if severe proteinuria

Management: normally self-resolves in 6w
- Analgesia* – paracetamol   *avoid NSAIDs!
- Corticosteroids (immunosuppressants) – **ONLY if severe** gut/joint involvement

IGA NEPHROPATHY (BERGER'S DISEASE): similar pathology to HSP
(IgA vasculitis) **but only affects kidneys**
- → **RFs:** URTI, male, Asian, FHx
- → **Symptoms:** macroscopic haematuria, proteinuria, peripheral oedema, HTN
- → **Investigations:** bloods, urinalysis, **renal biopsy**
- → **Management:** same as HSP (analgesia, corticosteroids ± diuretics)

SYSTEMIC LUPUS ERYTHEMATOSUS (SLE): dsDNA autoantibodies
(+ others), ↓ complement
- → **RFs:** adolescent girls / young women, Asian/Afro-Caribbean
- → **Symptoms:** haematuria & proteinuria (+ malar rash, malaise, arthralgia)

Streptococcal nephritis:

7–21d after sore throat or skin infection
→ Low complement
→ Raised antistreptolysin-O (ASO)/anti-DNAse B

Risk factors for HSP
- 3–10y
- M>F (2:1)
- Winter
- Preceding URTI (strep)

prevalence of HSP = 1 in 5000

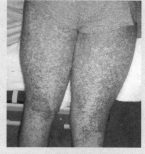

Fig. 5.30

HSP needs follow-up in 1y if renal involvement to ensure no CKD!

Glomerulonephritis: group of diseases causing immune-mediated inflammation of glomerulus (↑ permeability) → post-strep (HSP), other infections (malaria/staph/salmonella/candida), IgA nephropathy, SLE
Sx: nephrotic/nephritic syndrome
Tx: diuretics ± steroids ± ABX

Nephrotic syndrome

→ *inflamed basement membrane allows passage of proteins into nephron*

1. **Heavy proteinuria** (>200mg/d) = frothy urine
2. **Hypoalbuminaemia** (<25g/L)
3. **Oedema** – periorbital, legs, scrotal/vaginal

Clinical features
- Periorbital oedema (especially on waking)
- Leg, ankle, scrotal/vulval oedema
- Ascites
- Breathless (due to pulm. effusions)

Cause: unknown
→ may be 2° to systemic disease (HSP, SLE, infections, etc.)

Investigations
- Urine dip – protein ++
- FBC, ESR
- U&Es, albumin
- Urine MCS
- Complement levels
- Throat swab/anti-strep
- Hepatitis B & C screen
- Malaria screen

STEROID-SENSITIVE NEPHROTIC SYNDROME (85–90%)
Risk factors: male, Asian, 1–10y, PHx atopy, preceding respiratory infection

Features: minimal change disease
- No macroscopic haematuria
- Normal BP, complement levels & renal function
- **'Minimal change'** on histology

Management[30]
1. **Corticosteroids (8w PO)** – prednisolone
   - High dose oral steroids (then taper dose)
   - Tx-resistant cases need renal biopsy
   - Frequent relapses need high maintenance dose steroids

2. **Fluid balance**
   - Restrict intake ± diuretics
   - IV fluids if hypovolaemic

   Educate parents on how to do urine dip at home & on recognising signs of infection (risk of taking steroids)

3. **ABX prophylaxis (penicillin V)**
   - As loss of Igs leaves them susceptible to infection
→ **Refer to specialist if atypical features** →
   - <1y or >12y
   - HTN or impaired renal function
   - Gross haematuria
   - Hep B/C +ve
   - Tx-resistant

STEROID-RESISTANT NEPHROTIC SYNDROME (rare)
Causes
- Focal segment glomerulosclerosis – most common
- Membranoproliferative – haematuria & low complement
- Membranous nephropathy – associated with hepatitis B

Management: → early referral to paediatric nephrologist
1. **Fluid balance**
   - Restrict intake of water and salt
   - Diuretics, ACEis

2. **Pharmacological therapies**
   - Pulsed methylprednisolone
   - Other immunosuppressants (e.g. tacrolimus, cyclophosphamide)

Complications of nephrotic syndrome
- Hypovolaemia = abdo pain, faintness, low urine Na^+
- Thrombosis – exacerbated by steroid therapy
- Infection – especially pneumococcus (Igs lost in urine)
- Hypercholesterolaemia/hyperlipidaemia

Prognosis of nephrotic syndrome
$^1/_3$ resolve directly
$^1/_3$ have infrequent relapses
$^1/_3$ have frequent relapses

NB Relapses identified by parents doing urine dip

---

[30] NIDDK (2021) *Nephrotic syndrome in children*

Acute kidney injury (AKI)

→ *sudden, potentially reversible drop in renal function = oliguria <0.5ml/kg/h*

	Pre-renal	Renal	Post-renal
Causes	**Hypovolaemia** • Gastroenteritis • Sepsis • Burns • Haemorrhage • Nephrotic syndrome **Circulatory failure**	**Vascular** • HUS • Vasculitis • Embolus • Renal vein thrombosis **Tubular** • Acute tubular necrosis (ATN) • Ischaemic • Toxic *HUS & ATN = most common* • Obstructive *renal causes* **Glomerular:** glomerulonephritis **Interstitial** • Interstitial nephritis • Pyelonephritis	**Obstruction** • Congenital e.g. posterior urethral valves • Acquired e.g. blocked catheter
Symptoms	**Shock:** • Pallor • Cool peripheries • ↑HR, ↑RR	• Haematuria • Oedema • Metabolic acidosis (↑HR, ↑RR, confusion) • Hyperkalaemia (palpitations, weakness) • Hypocalcaemia (cramps, tingling, numb) • Hyperphosphataemia	• Bladder fullness & pain • Urinary dribbling
Management[31]		**Correct fluid and electrolyte balance / metabolic acidosis** Monitor weight + U&Es, record fluid input & output	
	Urgent • IV fluids • Circulatory support	**Fluid balance:** • Fluid restriction & diuretics **Prevent catabolism:** • High calorie, normal protein diet → *Immunosuppression if rapidly progressive glomerulonephritis*	**Urine drainage:** • Nephrostomy • Bladder catheterisation **Urology referral**

Haemolytic uraemic syndrome (HUS)

Triad of:

1. **Renal failure**

2. **Thrombocytopenia** → may have purpura/bruising

3. **Microangiopathic haemolytic anaemia** (damaged RBCs due to small vessel occlusion)

→ (95%) typical (diarrhoeal): good prognosis
→ (5%) atypical (non-diarrhoeal): poor prognosis

CAUSE
→ *Diarrhoeal prodrome*
→ 2° to gastroenteric infection with **verocytotoxin-producing *E. coli* 0157:H7** (from farm animals / uncooked beef)
→ toxin causes **intravascular thrombogenesis** in renal endothelial cells → clotting cascade activated
→ platelets are consumed & haemolytic anaemia occurs

INVESTIGATIONS
• FBC – ↓Hb, ↓plts, fragmented blood film
• U&Es
• Stool culture

MANAGEMENT: supportive → manage fluid balance
• Dialysis & plasma exchange
• **Follow up:** for persistent proteinuria, HTN, progressive CKD

Indications for dialysis
→ Failed conservative Mx
→ Hyperkalaemia or hypo-/hypernatraemia
→ Severe acidosis
→ Pulmonary HTN or oedema
→ Multisystem failure

---

[31] Cho MH (2020) Pediatric acute kidney injury: focusing on diagnosis and management. *Child Kidney Dis* 24:19–26

Chronic kidney disease (CKD)

→ *progressive loss of renal function* → *rare in kids (10 in 1 million)*

CLINICAL FEATURES

- Anorexia & lethargy
- Polydipsia & polyuria
- Hypertension
- Bone deformities →
  renal osteodystrophy
- FTT / poor or delayed growth
  (despite high GH levels)
- Anaemia (unexplained normochromic, normocytic) – due to ↓ EPO

CAUSES: most = familial/congenital

- Structural malformation (40%)
- Glomerulonephritis (25%)
- Hereditary nephropathies (20%)
- Systemic diseases (10%)
- Unknown (5%)

renal osteodystrophy = poor mineralisation due to renal failure → like rickets

MANAGEMENT[32]

→ By specialist paediatric nephrologist & MDT
→ **AIM: prevent metabolic complications & allow normal growth & development**

1. **Diet – combat losses from anorexia and vomiting**
   - Calorie supplements
   - NG tube / gastrostomy
2. **Prevent renal osteodystrophy**
   - Calcium & phosphate restriction
     – e.g. ↓ dairy
   - Vit D supplements if deficiency
3. **Salt & water balance**
   - Salt supplements

- Bicarbonate supplements
  if metabolic acidosis
4. **Anaemia**
   - Recombinant
     EPO / erythropoietic stimulating
     agent
   - Iron replacement
5. **Hormone abnormalities**
   - Recombinant human growth
     hormone

Dialysis & transplantation

- For end-stage CKD
- Ideally child gets transplant **before** dialysis is needed
- Needs immunosuppression with transplant

Hypertension

→ *BP >95th percentile for age, height & sex*

CAUSES: usually secondary in children

1. Renal
   - Renal parenchymal disease
   - Renal artery stenosis
   - PKD
   - Renal tumours
2. **Endocrine**
   - Congenital adrenal hyperplasia
   - Cushing's / steroid therapy
   - Hyperthyroidism

3. **Catecholamine excess**
   - Phaeochromocytoma
   - Neuroblastoma
4. **Coarctation of the aorta**
5. **Essential HTN** (diagnosis of exclusion)
6. **Obesity**

All children with a renal abnormality should have annual BP checks throughout their life

CLINICAL PRESENTATION

→ Failure to thrive
→ Vomiting
→ Headaches
→ Cardiac failure

→ Retinopathy
→ Facial palsy
→ Convulsions
→ Proteinuria

INVESTIGATIONS: for 2° cause

- 24h BP monitoring
- FBC, U&Es, renal function
- Blood glucose & fasting lipids
- TFTs
- Plasma renin & aldosterone
- Urinalysis
- Urine catecholamines

MANAGEMENT

- Tx underlying cause if possible
- Antihypertensives
- Regular BP monitoring
- Lifestyle advice if essential HTN

Further Ix to consider
ECHO, ECG, CXR, renal USS, renal artery Doppler

---

[32] NICE (2021) *Chronic kidney disease* [NG203]

Cardiovascular

Antenatal circulation

- **LA pressure low** as little return from lungs
- **RA pressure high** as receives all systemic blood (including from placenta)
- Keeps **foramen ovale open** & blood flows **from RA → LA**
- Blood also **bypasses lungs** by flowing through **ductus arteriosus**

CHANGES AT BIRTH

- **↓pulmonary resistance** means more blood into LA so **↑LA pressure**
- **Loss of placental circulation** causes **↓RA pressure**
- **Foramen ovale closes**
- **Ductus arteriosus closes** within first few hours/days

LA = left atrium
RA = right atrium

Fetal heart

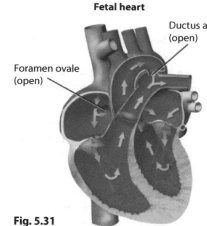

Ductus arteriosus (open)

Foramen ovale (open)

Newborn heart

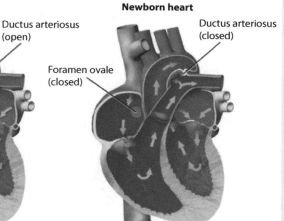

Ductus arteriosus (closed)

Foramen ovale (closed)

Fig. 5.31

Congenital heart disease

→ *1% of live births*

PRESENTATION

1. Antenatal cardiac USS diagnosis (at 20w)

2. Detection of a heart murmur (most common presentation)
- → *BUT 30% of children have an **innocent murmur** at some point, often during febrile illness/anaemia*

3. Heart failure   → *DDx = sepsis*

Symptoms: SOB, sweating, poor feeding, FTT, recurrent chest infections

Signs: ↑RR, ↑HR, murmur, crackles, enlarged heart, hepatomegaly, cool peripheries

Causes   Tx: diuretics, inotropes, treat cause

Neonates: duct-dependent (obstructed LHS)	**Infants:** high pulmonary flow (causing left → right shunt)	**Children/adolescents:** RHS or LHS heart failure
<ul><li>Hypoplastic left heart syndrome</li><li>Critical aortic valve stenosis</li><li>Severe coarctation of the aorta</li><li>Interrupted aortic arch</li></ul>	<ul><li>VSD</li><li>AVSD</li><li>Persistent ductus arteriosus</li></ul>	<ul><li>Eisenmenger syndrome (RHS heart failure)</li><li>Rheumatic heart disease</li><li>Cardiomyopathy</li></ul>

4. Cyanosis

Peripheral (hands & feet)**:** if cold, unwell from any cause or polycythaemia

Central (tongue)**:** if arterial O_2 tension drops

5. Shock & collapse

Symptoms: pallor, impalpable pulses, metabolic acidosis

DDx: congenital heart disease, infection, inherited metabolic disorder

Ix: Blood tests, blood & urine cultures, ECHO

SUMMARY OF CONGENITAL HEART DISEASE PRESENTATIONS

Symptoms	Type of lesion
Breathless (acyanotic)	**L→R shunts:** VSD, ASD, PDA
Blue (cyanotic)	**R→L shunts:** TOF, TGA
Collapse & shock	**Obstruction:** Coarctation, HLHS
Asymptomatic	**Obstruction:** Aortic/pulm. stenosis

} *May be mixed Sx in AVSD, complex congenital heart disease*

Blue = cyanotic conditions

Duct-dependent lesions: in severe left-sided obstructive lesions, blood flow through duct = critical for survival → dramatic deterioration in condition when duct closes

e.g. TOF, TGA, HLHS, aortic stenosis/ coarctation

Mx: prostaglandin to maintain duct patency

Features of innocent murmurs

- a**S**ymptomatic patient
- **S**oft blowing murmur
- **S**ystolic murmur only
- left **S**ternal edge

No parasternal thrill/radiation
May vary with posture

DDx of cyanosis in newborn PLUS respiratory distress (RR >60bpm)

- Cyanotic congenital heart disease
- Infection, e.g. GBS, septicaemia
- Respiratory disorder, e.g. RDS, meconium
- Persistent pulmonary HTN of newborn
- Inborn metabolic error = acidosis & shock

Persistent cyanosis in otherwise well infant = nearly always structural heart disease

---

PDA: Patent ductus arteriosus
TGA: Transposition of great arteries
HLHS: Hypoplastic left heart syndrome
TOF: Tetralogy of Fallot

↪ more flow in RHS = large heart & wet lungs (chest infections & inc. HR)

Left → right shunts

→ *acyanotic*

ATRIAL SEPTAL DEFECT (ASD)

Types
- **Secundum ASD** (80%) – defect in centre of atrial septum, *involving foramen ovale*
- **Primum ASD/partial AVSD** (20%) – defect of AV septum, allowing *communication between the atria & AV valves*

Left AV valve has 3 leaflets & tends to leak

Symptoms
- **Normally asymptomatic**
- Recurrent chest infections, wheeze, SOB
- Arrhythmias (from 40y onwards)

Signs
- Ejection systolic murmur – at ULSE (↑ blood through pulmonary valve)
- Fixed, widely split 2nd heart sound
- Pansystolic murmur – at apex (in AVSD due to AV valve regurgitation)

Investigations
- **CXR** – cardiomegaly, enlarged pulmonary arteries, ↑ pulmonary vascular markings
- **ECHO** – visualise abnormal anatomy
- **ECG**

Management
Small defects: monitor – often close spontaneously
Secundum ASD: cardiac catheterisation to insert occlusion device
Partial AVSD: surgical correction at 3–5y

VENTRICULAR SEPTAL DEFECT (VSD) = *defect anywhere in ventricular septum (30% cases of congenital heart disease)*

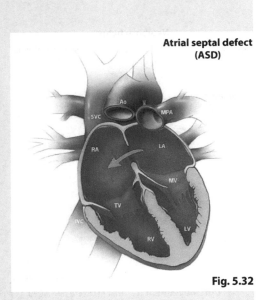

Atrial septal defect (ASD)

Fig. 5.32

ECG findings in ASD

- **Secundum ASD:** partial RBBB (RSR pattern) & right axis deviation (due to RV hypertrophy)
- **Partial AVSD:** superior QRS axis (= –ve AVF deflection due to displaced sinoatrial node)

	Small (<3mm)	**Large (>3mm)**
Symptoms	Asymptomatic	• **Heart failure:** ↑ HR, ↑ RR (SOB & active precordium), hepatomegaly • Failure to thrive • Recurrent chest infections
Signs	• **Loud pansystolic murmur** • At LLSE • Quiet 2nd pulmonary sound	• **Soft pansystolic / no murmur** • Mid-diastolic murmur – at apex • Loud 2nd pulmonary sound (due to ↑ pulm. aorta pressure)
Ix	• **CXR** = normal • **ECG** = normal • **ECHO** = visualise defect	• **CXR** = cardiomegaly, ↑ pulm. artery/markings, pulm. oedema • **ECG** = biventricular hypertrophy (T upright in V1, inverted in V6) • **ECHO** = visualise defect
Mx	Often close spontaneously but may persist to adulthood (if asymptomatic, no Tx needed)	**Heart failure:** diuretics + ACEi **Failure to thrive:** additional calorie intake **Surgery before 1y**

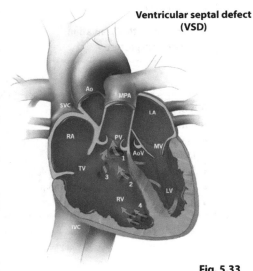

Ventricular septal defect (VSD)

Fig. 5.33

Louder murmur = smaller defect

PERSISTENT DUCTUS ARTERIOSUS → *failure of duct closure **by 1m after***
EDD (not pathological if preterm)

↳ So blood still able to flow from **aorta → pulmonary artery**

Symptoms
- **Normally asymptomatic**
- Heart failure & pulmonary HTN (if duct is large)

Signs
- Continuous murmur – below left clavicle/ULSE
- Collapsing/bounding pulse
- Swinging O_2 saturations

Investigations
- **ECHO** – readily shows patent duct
- **CXR & ECG** = usually normal

Management
- Ibuprofen / surgical tying
- Closure with coil or occlusion device (via catheter at 1y)

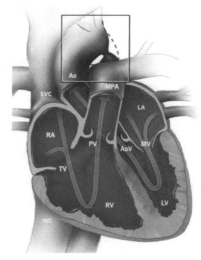

RF = preterm

Fig. 5.34 Persistent ductus arteriosus.

Right → left shunts

→ *CYANOSIS in 1st week of life*

blue, O_2 <94%, collapse

TETRALOGY OF FALLOT (TOF)
Four cardinal features

1. **Large VSD**
2. **Aorta overriding** the ventricular septum (receives blood from both ventricles)
3. **Subpulmonary stenosis** = RV outflow obstruction
4. **RV hypertrophy** as a result of RV outflow obstruction

> **TOF = most common** cyanotic congenital heart disease (10%)

Signs
- Cyanosis in 1st week – usually diagnosed before cyanosis is obvious
- Loud, harsh ejection systolic murmur – at LLSE

↳ (antenatally or due to early murmur)

Investigations

1. **ECHO:** shows cardinal features
2. **CXR:**
   - Small 'boot-shaped' heart
   - Pulmonary artery 'bay'
   - ↓ pulmonary markings
3. **ECG:** RV hypertrophy (upright T in V1 & no S)

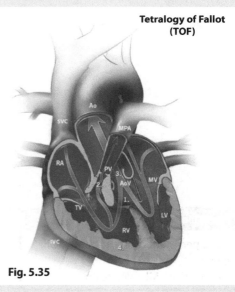

Tetralogy of Fallot
(TOF)

Fig. 5.35

Management
- **Maintain duct patency:** prostaglandin infusion
- **Surgery at 6m:** close VSD & relieve RV outflow obstruction
- **Blalock–Taussig shunt:** between subclavian artery & pulmonary artery to ↑ pulmonary flow (if very cyanosed)
- **Tx hypercyanotic spells >15min 'TET SPELLS'**
  - ▸ Knees to chest + sedation & pain relief (morphine)
  - ▸ O_2 ± ventilation
  - ▸ IV propranolol (relaxes right ventricle)
  - ▸ IV fluids (+ HCO_3^- for acidosis)

> **'TET SPELLS'** = worsening of right to left shunt during exertion/crying/agitation causing increased pulmonary resistance = **cyanotic episodes**
> *If severe = drowsy, seizures, death*

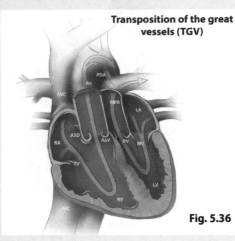

Transposition of the great vessels (TGV)

Fig. 5.36

TRANSPOSITION OF THE GREAT ARTERIES (TGA) = *5% of congenital heart disease*

Aetiology
- Aorta connected to RV & pulmonary artery connected to LV
- Incompatible with life unless blood can mix (e.g. via VSD/ASD)

Signs
- **CYANOSIS** – on day 2 when ductus arteriosus closes
- Loud, single 2nd heart sound
- May be murmur if another abnormality present

Investigations
- **ECHO** – visualise abnormalities
- **ECG** = usually normal
- **CXR:** 'egg-on-a-side' heart outline, ↑ pulmonary markings

Management
- **Maintain duct patency** – prostaglandin analogue
- **Balloon atrial septostomy** (needed in 20% as emergency procedure)
  - ▶ catheter with balloon passed through umbilical/femoral vein → RA → foramen ovale → LA
  - ▶ balloon inflated & pulled back to tear hole in atrial septum & allow blood mixing
- **Arterial switch procedure** – pulmonary artery & aorta transected above valves & switched over (must be <4w)

EISENMENGER SYNDROME

Aetiology
- High pulmonary blood flow due to L→R shunt causes **thickening of pulmonary artery walls = ↑ resistance**
- L→R flow will gradually decrease due to the ↑ resistance until eventually **the shunt reverses**

Symptoms
10–15y: become blue as shunt reverses (progressive if untreated)
40–50y: heart failure & death

Management
Prevent condition: early intervention for conditions with ↑ pulmonary flow

SUMMARY OF CYANOTIC CONGENITAL HEART DISEASE

	Signs/symptoms	Management
Tetralogy of Fallot	• Loud murmur ULSE • Hypercyanotic spells • Clubbing of fingers/toes	• Surgery 6–9m
Transposition of great arteries	• No murmur • **Severe cyanosis early on**	• Prostaglandin infusion • Balloon atrial septostomy • Arterial switch
Eisenmenger syndrome	• No murmur • Right heart failure (later)	• Manage causes early

Hypercapnia (resulting from cyanosis)

Signs: persistent crying, irritable, SOB, pallor
Complications: MI, CVA, death

Outflow obstruction in the sick child (shock/collapse)

COARCTATION OF THE AORTA
Aetiology
- Arterial duct tissue surrounds aorta at point of duct insertion
- Duct closure causes constriction of aorta = **LV outflow obstruction**

Signs/symptoms: present at day 2 when duct closes
- Sick with severe heart failure / renal failure
- Absent femoral pulses
- Severe metabolic acidosis
- **Ejection systolic murmur** between shoulder blades

Investigations
- **ECG** – normal unless older (LV hypertrophy)
- **CXR** – cardiomegaly

HYPOPLASTIC LEFT HEART SYNDROME (HLHS)
Aetiology: underdeveloped left side of the heart (including aorta)

Signs/symptoms: often detected antenatally so Sx prevented
- Profound acidosis & cardiovascular collapse
- Weakness of ALL peripheral pulses

Management: Norwood procedure (3-stage surgery)

Outflow obstruction in the well child (asymptomatic)

AORTIC STENOSIS

Aetiology: partial fusion of aortic valve leaflets

Signs
- **Ejection systolic murmur** at URSE → radiates to neck
- **Carotid thrill**
- Apical ejection click
- Small volume, slow rising pulses (globally poor perfusion)

Investigations
- **ECG** – LV hypertrophy (inverted T wave V6)
- **CXR** – prominent LV & post-stenotic dilation of aorta

PULMONARY STENOSIS

Aetiology: partial fusion of pulmonary valve leaflets

Signs
- **Ejection systolic murmur** at ULSE
- ± Carotid thrill
- Ejection click at ULSE
- RV heave

Investigations
- **ECG** – RV hypertrophy (upright T wave V1)
- **CXR** – post-stenotic dilation of pulm. artery

Management:
1. **Resuscitation**
2. **Prostaglandin infusion**

Management:

Only if symptoms on exercise or resting high pressure gradient
- Balloon valvotomy (valve dilation)
- Later may need valve replacement

Syndromes associated with congenital heart defects

Down syndrome – **ASDs/AVSDs**
Noonan syndrome – **pulmonary stenosis**, ASDs, hypertrophic cardiomyopathy
Marfan syndrome – mitral valve prolapse, aortic aneurysm
Turner syndrome – **aortic stenosis, coarctation** of the aorta
DiGeorge syndrome – TOF
Williams syndrome – pulmonary stenosis, aortic stenosis

Bold = key associations to remember for exams

Other important paediatric cardiac conditions

SUPRAVENTRICULAR TACHYCARDIA (SVT) = HR 250–300bpm

NB Sinus arrhythmia = normal in children
- acceleration in inspiration
- slowing on expiration

Signs/symptoms
- Dizziness, palpitations, chest pains, SOB → collapse
- Tachyarrhythmia (abnormal, fast HR)
- Heart failure (pulm. oedema, SOB, ↑RR)
- Hydrops fetalis (abnormal fluid accumulation) → intrauterine death

Investigations
- **ECG:** 250–300bpm & narrow QRS (P waves often hidden)
- **ECHO:** to r/o structural problem

Management[33]
Acute
- **Circulatory & respiratory support** – ventilation, correct acidosis
- **DIVING REFLEX** – dunking infant in water causes reflexive apnoea & bradycardia
- **Vagal manoeuvres** – carotid sinus massage / ice pack on face / blow into syringe

- **IV adenosine** – induces AV block
- **Electrical cardioversion with synchronised defib shock** – if adenosine fails

Maintenance
- Flecainide or sotalol
- Radiofrequency ablation / cryoablation

MYOCARDITIS = inflammation of myocardium (usually due to **infection**, but also drug reaction/chemicals/radiation)

Signs/symptoms
- Fever, malaise
- Non-specific Sx of heart failure: SOB, cough, chest pain, oedema, pallor

Management: usually resolves spontaneously
1. Diuretics
2. ACEis
3. Beta-blocker – carvedilol
→ *Severe cases may need heart transplant*

Investigations
- ECHO
- CXR – enlarged heart borders

SUBACUTE BACTERIAL ENDOCARDITIS (SBE) = slowly developing infection of endocardium

↳ Congenital heart defects = BIG RISK FACTOR (esp. VSD, PDA, coarctation)

Symptoms
- **Fever, malaise**
- **New murmur**
- Anaemia/pallor
- Arthritis/arthralgia

Signs
- **Microscopic haematuria**
- ± splinter haemorrhages
- ± Osler nodes, Janeway lesions, Roth spots

Investigations
- **BLOOD CULTURES** – before starting ABX
- **ECHO** – visualise vegetations
- **Bloods** – anaemia, ↑ ESR/CRP
- **Urine dip** – microscopic haematuria

Management
- **ABX** – high dose IV penicillin + gentamicin for 6w
- May need to remove prosthetic material

DDx = SEPSIS

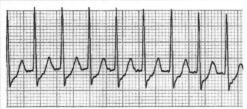
Fig. 5.37 SVT.

Common viral causes: parvovirus, influenza, adenovirus, rubella, HIV

SUSPECT SBE in anyone with: sustained fever, malaise, ↑ ESR, unexplained anaemia or haematuria

α-haemolytic strep (*Strep. viridans*) = most common cause of SBE

[33] Resuscitation Council UK (2021) *Paediatric cardiac arrhythmias algorithm*

Respiratory

Respiratory changes at birth

FETAL RESPIRATION
- Fetal **lungs are filled with fluid** & pulmonary vessels are constricted
- Blood is oxygenated via **gas exchange at the placenta**
- Most blood bypasses lungs via ductus arteriosus & flows straight into aorta

NB Fetal Hb has higher O_2 affinity & better O_2 dissociation

NEONATAL RESPIRATION
- During birth, fetal chest is squeezed → some lung fluid drains
- ↓ temperature, ↑ catecholamines & tactile stimuli initiate breathing*
- Most of remaining fluid is absorbed into lymphatic & pulmonary circulation
- **Pulm. resistance falls → ↑** LA filling & LA pressure **→ foramen ovale closes**

*6s after birth

Respiratory infections

→ Pre-school kids have **6–8 per year**
→ **80–90% are viral:** rhinovirus, parainfluenza, RSV, adenovirus
→ **Bacterial:** *Strep. pneumoniae, H. influenzae, M. catarrhalis,* pertussis, mycoplasma

RFs for respiratory infections
- Parental smoking
- Poor nutrition
- Overcrowded/damp living
- Chronic lung disease
- Immunodeficiency
- Male
- Premature
- Syndromes

Upper respiratory tract infections

Common symptoms: nasal blockage & discharge, fever, sore throat, earache

CORYZA (COMMON COLD) → *most common childhood infection*
Cause: rhinovirus, coronavirus, RSV
Symptoms: nasal blockage & discharge (clear or mucopurulent) ± fever, cough
Management: paracetamol/ibuprofen for symptom control → reassure parents it is self-limiting / ABX of no benefit

PHARYNGITIS (SORE THROAT)
Cause: rhinovirus, adenovirus, enterovirus, group A β-haemolytic strep.
Symptoms: sore throat + cervical lymphadenopathy

TONSILLITIS (FORM OF PHARYNGITIS)
Cause: EBV, group A β-haemolytic strep.

Symptoms
- Very sore throat & difficulty swallowing
- Enlarged tonsils + white exudate
- Cervical lymphadenopathy
- Headache, fever, malaise, apathy
- Abdominal pain

Management[34]: admit if severe dysphagia/dehydration
- Analgesia & fluids
- 5 days ABX only if bacterial*
- Tonsillectomy if indicated[35]

*CENTOR/ FeverPAIN score to assess likelihood of group A strep

Return to school 24h after start ABX

CENTOR score: 1 point each
C: absence of Cough
E: tonsillar Exudates
N: tender cervical Nodes
T: >38°C Temperature

$^0/_1$: no ABX
$^2/_3$: throat culture/ delayed script
4: ABX (penicillin or erythromycin)

FeverPAIN score: 1 point each
Fever
Pus on tonsils
Attends within 3d
Inflammation of tonsils = severe
No cough

Indications for tonsillectomy

- **Recurrent tonsillitis**
  - ► 7× in 1y
  - ► 5× in each of 2y
  - ► 3× in each of 3y
- **Peritonsillar abscess**
- **Obstructive sleep apnoea**

[34] NICE (2018) *Sore throat (acute)* [NG84]
[35] ENT UK (2020) *Commissioning Guide – Tonsillectomy*

> In any child with fever, must examine tympanic membranes

Start ABX immediately if: *bilateral <2y or systemically unwell, suspected complication*

Complications of OME
- Delay in speech development
- Difficulties at school

Indications for adenoidectomy
- Recurrent OME
- OSA

Mx of upper airway obstruction:
contact anaesthetist

- **DO NOT EXAMINE THROAT** → KEEP CHILD CALM
- Monitor for hypoxia/deterioration – O₂ sat.
- Dexamethasone/prednisolone
- Nebulised adrenaline – if severe
- Urgent tracheal intubation – if respiratory failure

ACUTE OTITIS MEDIA (AOM) → *most commonly at 6–12m*
Cause: RSV, rhinovirus, pneumococcus, *H. influenzae*, *M. catarrhalis*

Symptoms: inflammation of middle ear
- Fever & malaise
- Ear pain (tugging at ear)
- Bulging red tympanic membrane & absent light reflection

Complications
- mastoiditis
- meningitis

Management[36]
- Analgesia – regular paracetamol/ibuprofen for pain
- Delayed use of ABX (amoxicillin) → *give prescription to start if no improvement in 2–3d or Sx rapidly worsen*

OTITIS MEDIA WITH EFFUSION (OME) = 'GLUE EAR' → *most commonly at 2–7y*
Cause: middle ear infection, enlarged adenoids, nasal abnormalities

Symptoms: fluid collection in middle ear **without signs of inflammation**
- **No pain/fever**
- Middle ear fluid & dull, retracted TM
- Conductive hearing loss (20–30db)
  - type B tympanogram (flat line)
  - ↓ air conduction on PTA (if >4y)

Management[37]: 50% resolve spontaneously
If no improvement in 3m / complications: grommets **or** hearing aids ± adenoidectomy **if indicated**

Laryngeal & tracheal infections

→ *mucosal inflammation & swelling can cause **life-threatening obstruction***

SYMPTOMS
- **Stridor** (rasping inspiration)
- Hoarseness
- Barking cough
- Variable SOB

If severe: ↑ RR & HR, cyanosis, drowsiness

Classifying severity of stridor

Mild: only when active/upset, normal RR, minimal WOB
Moderate: some stridor at rest, ↑RR, ↑WOB
Severe: biphasic stridor at rest, ↑ or ↓ RR, & HR, ↑WOB, hypoxaemia

DDx upper airway obstruction / stridor

Acute infection	Mechanical obstruction	Congenital
• Croup (very common)	• Anaphylaxis	• Laryngomalacia (floppy larynx)
• Epiglottitis	• Smoke inhalation	• Laryngeal polyps (congenital HPV)
• Bacterial tracheitis	• Inhaled foreign body	• Acquired subglottic stenosis

[36]NICE (2018, updated 2022) *Otitis media (acute)* [NG91]
[37] NICE (2008) *Otitis media with effusion in under 12s* [CG60]

TYPES OF LARYNGEAL INFECTIONS

	Viral croup (laryngotracheobronchitis) >95% of laryngotracheal infections	Acute epiglottitis >99% reduction in cases since Hib vaccine	Bacterial tracheitis = rare but dangerous
Age group	6m to 6y (peak at 2y) → winter outbreaks	1–6y	3–5y
Pathogens	• **Parainfluenza 1&2** • Metapneumovirus • RSV • Influenza	• *H. influenzae* B	• *Staph. aureus*
Onset	3–5d	Hours	1–3d
Symptoms	• **Barking cough** • Preceding coryza • Worse at night • **Looks unwell**	• Very sore throat • Drooling saliva • Difficulty speaking • Sits still, upright, open mouth • **Looks toxic / very ill**	• Similar to viral croup **PLUS** • High fever • **Looks toxic/very ill**
Signs	• **Harsh stridor** • Hoarse voice • Fever <38.5°C	• **Soft stridor** • Muffled voice • Fever >38.5°C	• **Harsh stridor** • Hoarse voice • Fever >38.5°C
Management[39]	**Mild:** • Consider PO dexamethasone + **supportive:** paracetamol, fluids **Moderate:** • PO dexamethasone **or** • Budesonide nebs + **supportive:** paracetamol, fluids **Severe: ADMIT & ABCDE** + Adrenaline nebs + O$_2$ ventilation ± tracheal intubation	EMERGENCY: URGENT ADMISSION → involve paediatrics, ENT surgeons, senior anaesthetist • Examination & intubation under general anaesthetic → for 24h • IV ABX (cefuroxime) → 3–5d course • Prophylaxis for close contacts (rifampicin)	**ADMIT** • IV ABX • Airway intubation

> **Classifying severity of croup:**
>
> **WESTLEY CROUP SCORE[38]**
> • Air entry   • Stridor
> • Retractions   • Cyanosis
> • Consciousness level

Bronchitis

→ *inflammation & swelling of the bronchi*

Symptoms:
Cough – for ≥2w
Fever

WHOOPING COUGH (PERTUSSIS)

Symptoms
• Coryza (1w preceding other Sx)
• **Spasmodic cough followed by 'inspiratory whoop'** (for 3w)   = paroxysm
  ▸ worse at night
  ▸ may cause vomiting/epistaxis/subconjunctival haemorrhage
  ▸ face becomes red or blue (cyanotic episode)
  ▸ oral & nasal mucus

Investigations
• Nasal swab & culture
• PCR
• FBC = leucocytosis

Management[40]
• Azithromycin/clarithromycin Tx (reduces Sx if given early & reduces transmission risk)
• Antibiotic prophylaxis for close contacts
• **Stay off school until 48h ABX completed**

> **Prevention of whooping cough**
>
> Vaccination at 4m
> (does not guarantee immunity)

> Pertussis = notifiable disease!

[38] Westley CR, Cotton EK, Brooks JG (1978) Nebulized racemic epinephrine by IPPB for the treatment of croup. *Am J Dis Child* 132:484–487.
[39] NHS Children's Acute Transport Service Clinical Guideline (2020) *Upper airway obstruction*
[40] NICE (2021) Clinical Scenario: *Management of whooping cough*

Causes: 80% = RSV
20% = metapneumovirus, para/influenza, rhinovirus, adenovirus, *M. pneumoniae*

feeding difficulties are often the reason for admission — may need NG tube

Admit if:

- Apnoea/grunting
- RR >70bpm
- O_2 <90% on air
- **Fluid intake <75% of norm**
- **Food intake <50% of norm**
- Severe chest recessions

Bronchiolitis obliterans: rare inflammatory condition causing **permanent damage/ scarring** to bronchioles

Causes: Chemicals/irritants, infections
Symptoms: persisting LRTI Sx (cough, wheeze, crackles)

Causative organisms	
Newborns	GBS, *E. coli*
<5y	RSV, *S. pneumoniae*, Hib (pertussis, chlamydia)
>5y	*M. pneumoniae*, *S. pneumoniae*, *C. pneumoniae*

Complications of pneumonia
- Lobar collapse
- Atelectasis
- Empyema

Atypical pneumonia = new O_2 requirement & bilateral changes on CXR, **but child appears well**

Bronchiolitis

→ *infection of bronchioles (no SM so bronchodilators no help)*
↳ *2–3% of all infants admitted during annual winter epidemic*
↳ *most common serious paediatric respiratory infection*
↳ ***90% aged 1–9m** (rare if >1y)*
↳ ***Prematurity = #1 risk factor***

SYMPTOMS
- Preceding coryza – very congested
- **Sharp, dry cough (chesty)**
- **Feeding difficulties***
- Cyanosis/pallor
- Subcostal & intercostal recession
- Hyperinflated chest (prominent sternum & liver displaced downwards)

SIGNS
- **Fine end-inspiratory crackles**
- **High-pitched wheeze**
- Nasal flaring, recessions
- ↑HR & ↑RR

INVESTIGATIONS
- **Pulse oximetry**
- **PCR** of nasal swab = diagnostic
- CXR unnecessary in most cases

MANAGEMENT[41]: supportive (most recover in 2w)
- Humidified O_2 – via nasal cannulae or headbox if sats <90%
- Fluids/nutrition – nasogastric or IV if inadequate oral intake
- **If severe:** assisted ventilation – CPAP or mask
→ **infection control measures** (very contagious)

Prevention: monoclonal antibody to RSV → to high-risk preterm infants

Pneumonia

→ ↑ *incidence in infants*

SYMPTOMS
- Preceding URTI
- High fever >39°C
- SOB/difficulty breathing
- Cough: purulent
- Lethargy
- Poor feeding
± neck, chest, **abdo pain**

SIGNS
- ↑ **RR** = most sensitive sign in children (if persistent ↑ RR consider CXR)
- ↓O_2 sats
- Nasal flaring, chest indrawing
- **Coarse end-inspiratory crackles**
  ↳ *NB Dull percussion, bronchial breathing, ↓ breath sounds often absent in young children*

INVESTIGATIONS
- **CXR** – can confirm diagnosis – **but not needed if well enough to discharge with ABX**
- FBC, CRP/ESR
- Nasal swab PCR – identify viral causes
- Blood and sputum cultures

MANAGEMENT[42]
- **Supportive:** O_2 (if SpO_2 <92%), analgesia/antipyretics (paracetamol), fluids (if inadequate PO intake)
- **ABX:** depends on age, severity, organism, CXR
  → newborns = broad-spectrum IV ABX
  → older infants = PO amoxicillin/erythromycin
  → atypical pneumonia = PO azithromycin or amoxicillin
→ *If recurrent pneumonia, consider underlying immunodeficiency / CF*

---

[41] NICE (2015, updated 2021) *Bronchiolitis in children* [NG9]
[42] BTS (update 2011) *Guidelines for the management of community acquired pneumonia in children*

Tuberculosis

→ *droplet transmission*

SYMPTOMS

1° infection symptoms: non-specific in children

→ *may appear as Tx-resistant pneumonia*

- Prolonged fever
- Anorexia & weight loss
- Peri-bronchial lymphadenopathy – airway obstruction
- **Persistent, productive cough** & SOB
  - ↳ *50% infants & 90% older children = asymptomatic*
    - → *inflammatory response limits disease progression*
    - → *remains latent*

Reactivation symptoms

- Localised lung symptoms
- Effects on CNS (**TB meningitis**) = likely in children
- Effects on kidneys, joints, bones, heart

INVESTIGATIONS: difficult to diagnose in children

- **CXR**
  - ► hilar/paratracheal lymphadenopathy
  - ► may be pleural effusion
  - ► areas of consolidation/calcification
- **Mantoux test**
  - ► no BCG vaccine: >10mm suggests active infection
  - ► BCG vaccine: >15mm suggests active infection
- **Interferon gamma release assays (IGRA)**
  - ► also +ve in latent infection
- **Gastric washings:** 3× morning samples
  - ► MSC = acid-fact bacilli
  - ► important to identify resistant strains

MANAGEMENT[43]

- Triple/quadruple Tx for 2m: rifampicin, isoniazid, pyrazinamide, ethambutol
- Double Tx for another 4m: rifampicin, isoniazid
- Dexamethasone for 1m: if TB meningitis
- **Contact tracing:** screen family members → BCG or chemoprophylaxis

Inhaled foreign body

→ *right bronchial tree most common*

SYMPTOMS

often history of sudden onset / onset follows playing or eating

- Persistent cough / choking
- SOB
- ± **fever** due to secondary chest infection

SIGNS

- ↑ RR
- Wheeze
- Unilateral ↓ breath sounds / chest expansion
- Bronchial breath sounds

MANAGEMENT: immediate referral to paediatric ENT

- Removal of foreign body with bronchoscopy & forceps

Risk factors for TB
- Crowding / close contacts
- Immunodeficiency (especially HIV)

Latent TB
- **CXR:** usually normal
- **Mantoux test:** +ve

Prevention of TB

BCG at birth if high risk (from high prevalence area)
→ do not give BCG vaccine to immunosuppressed/HIV +ve

Mantoux test: inject purified protein derivative (PPD) under skin & measure induration after 48h
NB May be +ve due to BCG vaccine

[43] NICE (2016, updated 2019) *Tuberculosis* [NG33]

Consider CF in any child with recurrent chest infections, loose stools or failure to thrive

Complications of CF

Newborn	• Meconium ileus
Infant	• Prolonged jaundice • Faltering growth • Recurrent chest infections • Malabsorption/steatorrhoea
Young child	• Bronchiectasis • Nasal polyps / sinusitis • Rickets
Older child/ adolescent	• Allergic bronchopulmonary aspergillosis • Diabetes mellitus • Premature osteopenia • Cirrhosis & portal HTN • Renal stones / gallstones • Pneumothorax/haemoptysis • Male sterility • Rectal prolapse

Possible examination findings

- Coarse inspiratory crepitations
- Expiratory wheeze
- Finger clubbing

Other investigations

- Bloods – FBC, LFT, U&Es, CRP, clotting, amylase, glucose
- CXR
- Sputum cultures
- Spirometry = obstructive
- USS abdo – fatty liver, cirrhosis

Cystic fibrosis

→ *autosomal recessive* condition *affecting 1 in 2500* live Caucasian births
→ *1 in 25 = carriers*

AETIOLOGY

- Defective CF transmembrane conductance regulator (CFTR) = **abnormal Cl⁻ transport across epithelial cells**
- Mutation on chromosome 7 **(ΔF508)** = most common
- Causes **thickened mucus secretions** and **ciliary dysfunction**

SYMPTOMS

Lungs: impaired ciliary function & mucopurulent secretions
- **Recurrent chest infections** – *Staph. aureus, H. influenzae, Pseudomonas, burkholderia*   *Particularly hard to treat*
  →Persistent cough with purulent sputum
  → **Complications:** bronchiectasis, abscess

Intestine: thick, viscous meconium
- **Meconium ileus (10–20%)** = intestinal obstruction
  → Vomiting & abdominal distension
  → Fail to pass meconium in first few days of life

Pancreas: pancreatic duct blocked = enzyme insufficiency
- **Malabsorption & maldigestion**
  → Large, pale, offensive, greasy stools = steatorrhoea
  → **Complications:** failure to thrive / faltering growth

Skin: abnormal sweat gland function
- **Excessive Na & Cl in sweat** (very salty)

DIAGNOSIS

- **Screening with heel prick:** ↑ immunoreactive trypsinogen (IRT)
- **Genetic screen for CFTR mutations:** if ↑ IRT
- **Sweat test:** if 2 CFTR mutations to confirm diagnosis → Cl >60mmol/L

MANAGEMENT[44]

MDT: paediatrician, dietitian, physio, specialist nurse, child, parents, teachers

Respiratory

1. **Regular lung function review:** spirometry
2. **Chest physio:** 2× daily for 20–30min
   - **Younger:** parents perform percussion & positional drainage
   - **Older:** controlled deep breathing & physical exercise
3. **Prophylactic daily ABX:** + rescue stash for exacerbations
   - Daily flucloxacillin PO up to 3y, maybe 6y
   - Regular azithromycin (macrolide) nebulised   *Bilateral lung transplant = only option for end-stage CF lung disease*
4. **Tx of persisting symptoms:** 14d IV ABX via PIC line
5. **DNAse / hypertonic saline:** reduce viscosity of secretions

Nutrition

- **Regular dietary status assessment:** vitamins + high calorie diet (150% of normal)
- **Pancreatic insufficiency Tx:** oral enzyme replacement tablets with all food (Creon)

[44]NICE (2017) *Cystic fibrosis* [NG78]

Regular monitoring: review at least once a year (more frequently when new diagnosis)
- **Respiratory function**
- **Nutritional status & growth monitoring**
- **For complications:** DM, liver disease, bowel obstruction, pneumothorax, sterility, etc.

Psychological & emotional support: for child & parent → consider impact on school

Transient/viral-induced wheeze

→ *those with smaller airways = more likely to obstruct when inflamed*

Cause: triggered by viral infections (Hx coryzal symptoms)
Risk factors: maternal smoking, prematurity, male
Management: similar to acute asthma (O$_2$/back-to-back nebs & **send home with SABA inhaler**)

> Resolves by age 5 when airways widen

Asthma

→ *most common chronic respiratory disorder in childhood (15–20% of children)*

CAUSES
- **Genes:** FHx of asthma/atopies
- **Atopies**: eczema / rhino-conjunctivitis / food allergy often coexist
- **Environmental triggers:** allergens, URTIs, smoking, cold air, exercise, emotion

SYMPTOMS: exacerbated by triggers
- **Polyphonic expiratory wheeze**
- **Cough** – worse at night / early morning / with exercise
- **SOB causing ↑WOB**
  - ▸ intercostal & subcostal recessions
  - ▸ Harrison's sulci
  - ▸ tracheal tug
  - ▸ head bobbing & nasal flaring

INVESTIGATIONS
- **History & examination** – other Ix not usually needed
- **Spirometry: 1st line if >5y**
  - ▸ PEFR – diurnal & daily variability
  - ▸ BDR – FEV$_1$ improves >12% after bronchodilator
- **Skin prick test** – for common allergens
- **CXR** – to r/o other conditions → rarely needed

> **Consider asthma in any child with wheezing on >1 occasion**

Signs of poorly controlled asthma
- ↑ cough, wheeze, SOB
- difficulty walking/talking/sleeping
- ↓ relief from SABA

Abbreviations

BDR – bronchodilator reversibility
FEV$_1$ – forced expiratory volume in 1 second
FVC – forced vital capacity
ICS – inhaled corticosteroid
LABA – long-acting beta agonist
LTRA – leukotriene receptor antagonist
PEFR – peak expiratory flow rate
SABA – short-acting beta agonist

LONG-TERM MANAGEMENT[45]: EDUCATE CHILD & PARENTS
Stepwise approach (see below)
- PEFR monitoring
- **Check inhaler technique**/compliance – consider spacer
- Monitor growth – normal unless very severe
- Medication review – step up or down
- **Safety-net** – **personal action plan** for acute exacerbation

Fig. 5.38 Long-term asthma Mx.

1: Regular preventer	2: Add-on preventer	3: Add-on therapies	4: High dose therapies	5: Oral steroids
Very low dose ICS (<5y **without** interval Sx = oral LTRA)	+ oral LTRA review in 6w & switch to LABA if needed	↑ dose **ICS to low dose** review in 6w & ↑ dose **ICS to med dose**	↑ dose **ICS to high dose** Consider adding 4th drug (theophylline) Refer to specialist care	Alternate-day **PO steroids** at lowest effective dose Refer to specialist care

Regular reliever: SABA *(ipratropium bromide in infants)*

ACUTE ASTHMA MANAGEMENT[46]
Features of acute asthma

Severe	Life-threatening	
• SpO$_2$ <92% • PEFR 33–50% • RR raised • HR raised • Audible wheeze • Accessory muscles	• SpO$_2$ <92% • PEFR <33% • RR reduced = **EXHAUSTION** • **SILENT CHEST** • Cyanosis • Altered consciousness / confusion	Cyanosis Hypotension Exhaustion Silent chest Tachycardia

Mild/moderate: poor response = admission
- SABA via spacer (up to 10 puffs 30–60s apart)
- Consider PO prednisolone 20mg

Severe: poor response = admission
- O$_2$ via facemask (if O$_2$ sat <94%)
- SABA via nebuliser (every 20–30min)
- PO prednisolone (20mg if aged <5y, 40mg if >5y)

Life-threatening: urgent admission
- O$_2$ via facemask for 94–98% sat
- SABA + ipratropium via nebuliser (every 20–30min)
- PO prednisolone (1–2mg/kg) or IV hydrocortisone (50mg)
  - ↳ *No response = admit to PICU*
    - *CXR, blood gases*
    - *IV SABA or aminophylline (ECG monitoring)*
    - *IV magnesium sulphate*

Discharge when: off nebs & ≥4h between inhalers & PEF/FEV$_1$ >75% of best
• continue SABA PRN (4-hourly and taper dose over 3–4d) • continue prednisolone 3–5d • **GP follow-up in 48h**

Safety-netting for parents

Return to hospital if:
- Increased work of breathing
- Need SABA more than 4-hourly
- Need >10 puffs SABA at a time
- Any other concerns

[45] NICE (2017, updated 2021) *Asthma: diagnosis, monitoring and chronic management* [NG80]
[46] SIGN 158 (2019) *British guideline on the management of asthma* (2019)

Neurology

Seizures

→ *sudden disturbance of neurological function resulting in a change in behaviour*

Epileptic seizure: transient occurrence of signs and/or symptoms due to **abnormal, excessive, or synchronous neuronal activity** in the brain

Non-epileptic seizure: seizures that are not caused by abnormal electrical activity in the brain

Epileptic seizures	Non-epileptic seizures

• **Idiopathic** (70–80%) – presumed genetic
• **Secondary**
  ► cerebral dysgenesis
  ► cerebral vascular occlusion
  ► cerebral damage e.g. hypoxia/infection
  ► cerebral tumour
• **Epilepsy syndromes**
  ► Dravet syndrome
  ► West syndrome
  ► Rasmussen syndrome
• **Neurocutaneous syndromes**
	• **Febrile seizures**
	• **Dissociative seizures**
	• **Metabolic**
	  ► hypoglycaemia
	  ► hypocalcaemia, hypomagnesaemia
	  ► hypo-/hypernatraemia
	• **Head trauma**
	• **Meningitis/encephalitis**
	• **Poisons/toxins**
	• **Hypoxia/anoxia**
	  ► reflex anoxia
	  ► vasovagal
	  ► cardiac arrhythmia

INVESTIGATING SEIZURES

Beware of misdiagnosing epilepsy!

1. **History** = most important
   - Frequency, triggers, length, symptoms
   - Any impairments, educational/psychological/social impacts
   - **Video seizure if possible**

2. **Examination**
   - CNS & PNS examination
   - CVS & respiratory examination
   - Skin markers for neurocutaneous syndromes

3. **EEG (electroencephalogram)**
   - Can show neuronal hyperexcitability in epilepsy (sharp waves/complexes)
   - If normal consider **sleep-deprived EEG/24h ambulatory**

4. **Imaging**
   - MRI/CT – if <2y or neuro signs between seizures → r/o tumour or CVD
   - PET/SPECT – detect areas of hypo-/hypermetabolism

5. **Tests to r/o other causes**
   - ECG – cardiac causes
   - Bloods – metabolic disturbances (FBC, U&Es, LFT, CRP, culture GLUCOSE)
   - CSF analysis (lumbar puncture) – infection, metabolic disturbance

Consider screening for syndromes / neurological problems associated with epilepsy
e.g. tuberous sclerosis, cerebral palsy, autism

EEG may be normal in epilepsy or abnormal in non-epilepsy

Epilepsy

→ *chronic neurological disorder characterised by recurrent, unprovoked seizures*
→ *1 in 200 kids*

TYPES OF SEIZURE

1. **Generalised: discharge from BOTH hemispheres**
   → No warning
   → Always have LOC

2. **Focal: discharge from ONE part of ONE hemisphere**
   → May have preceding aura
   → May or may not have LOC
   → May lead to generalised tonic–clonic seizure if LOC

Complications of epilepsy
→ Many have **learning difficulties**
→ Continuation into adulthood
→ Medication side-effects
→ Sudden unexplained death in epilepsy (SUDEP)

Rare but must discuss with parents → ↓ risk by minimising seizures

Advice for parents during a seizure

DO: place pillow under head, move nearby objects, note time seizure began, place in recovery position afterwards
DO NOT: restrict/move child, give food/drink until complete

STATUS EPILEPTICUS = seizure >30min or repeated seizures for 30min with no recovery of consciousness

Generalised	
Tonic–clonic	**Tonic phase:** • May fall to ground • Hold breath → cyanosis **Clonic phase: secs-mins** • rhythmical jerking • irregular breathing, cyanosis, salivation • tongue-biting, incontinence → post-ictal sleep/LOC (up to several hrs)
Absence	• 'Blanking-out'/staring • May have 'lip-smacking' → brief onset & termination
Myoclonic	Repetitive, jerky movements
Tonic	Generalised increased tone → fall
Atonic	Loss of muscle tone ± jerking → fall

Focal	
Temporal	**AURA: fear / déjà vu** • Smell, taste, sound distortions • Lip smacking / chewing
Frontal	Clonic movements spread proximally* ***Jackson march**
Occipital	Visual disturbance
Parietal	• Contralateral sensory disturbance • Tingling/numbness

INVESTIGATIONS: see above
• **EEG** indicated if epilepsy suspected → *can help determine type & severity*

MANAGEMENT[47]: → depends on likelihood of recurrence, severity & impact on life of seizures

1. **Education & advice** – for parents & children
   • Specialist epilepsy nurse
   • Adaptation & lifestyle issues
     ‣ Avoid deep baths / swimming alone
     ‣ Avoid alcohol & sleep deprivation
     ‣ Only drive if no seizures for 1y
     ‣ Conception counselling
     ‣ Association with **learning difficulties** – liaise with school
2. **Anti-epileptic drugs:** until seizure-free for 2y
   • Drug depends on seizure type
   • Aim for **monotherapy** at **lowest effective dose**
   • Counsel on side-effects   *A single seizure does not indicate starting AEDs*
3. **Rescue therapy (benzodiazepines)**
   • Given to terminate prolonged seizures (>5min)
4. **Other options**
   • Vagal nerve stimulation
   • Surgery e.g. lobectomy

AED	Indication	Side-effects
Valproate	1st line generalised	• Weight gain • Hair loss • **Teratogen**
Carbamazepine	Focal	• Rash • Hyponatraemia • Ataxia • CYP140 inducer
Levetiracetam	Focal	• Irritability
Lamotrigine	2nd line generalised	• Rash (SJS) • Insomnia
Ethosuximide	Absence	• N&V

[47] NICE (2012, updated 2021) *Epilepsies* [CG137]

EPILEPSY SYNDROMES OF CHILDHOOD

	Age	Seizure pattern	Associations
West syndrome (infantile spasms + hypsarrhythmia)	4–6m	**Infantile spasms** • Violent spasms lasting 1–2s • Often on waking **Tx:** steroids/vigabatrin **DDx:** • Benign sleep myoclonus • Reflux (occurs with feeding)	• ↓IQ / developmental regression • Poor social interaction • **Hypsarrhythmia EEG** = *chaotic/no pattern/high amp* **Fig. 5.39** Hypsarrhythmia.
Lennox–Gastaut syndrome	1–3y	• Drop-attacks • Tonic–clonic seizures • Atypical absence	• Neurodevelopmental arrest • Behaviour disorder
Benign occipital	1–14y	**Younger:** • Unresponsive, eye deviation **Older:** • Headache, hallucinations • Visual disturbances	• Occipital EEG changes • Remits in childhood
Childhood epilepsy + centrotemporal spikes (15%)	4–10y	Tonic–clonic seizures in sleep	• Remits in adolescence
Childhood absence (2% → ⅔ girls)	4–12y	• Stop & stare for <30s • Eyelids twitch	• Interferes with school • Hyperventilation is a trigger • **EEG shows 3s spike**
Juvenile myoclonic	Adolescence	• Myoclonic jerks • After waking ('clumsy eating cereal')	• Remission unlikely

Non-epileptic seizures

FEBRILE SEIZURE: *seizure accompanied by* **fever** *caused by* **infection of extra-cranial origin**
↳ Affect **3%** of children
↳ **6m–6y**
↳ Genetic predisposition

Features
• Onset = early in viral infection
• Brief (<10min), generalised tonic–clonic
• **Rapidly rising temperature** ± other signs of infection
→ no need for Ix if obvious source of infection (1st-line Ix would be urine dip)

Management [48]
1. **Reassurance** – usually no long-term complications, but chance of recurrence
2. **Education** – high chance of another, seizure first aid, rescue Tx
3. **May give rescue Tx if >5min** – buccal midazolam or PR diazepam
4. **Manage underlying infection** – antipyrexials, fluids, etc.

REFLEX ANOXIC SEIZURES: *due to* **vagal inhibition** *causing temporary* **cardiac asystole**
Features: brief (10–15s) **& quick recovery**
• Becomes pale & falls to floor
• LOC & jerking (generalised tonic–clonic seizure)

CARDIAC ARRHYTHMIAS/SYNCOPE: *prolonged QT causes collapse or syncope* → may be **exercise-induced**

PSYCHOGENIC NON-EPILEPTIC SEIZURES (PNES): *triggers = stress/emotions* → more common in adolescent girls

BENIGN SLEEP MYOCLONUS: *myoclonic jerks during* **non-REM sleep**
→typically age <**6m** → **no EEG changes**

> *DDx: sepsis, meningitis, brain abscess, gastroenteritis*

> **Complications of febrile seizure**
> → Further febrile seizures
> → ↑risk epilepsy **if complex seizure***
> *Lasts >10min, focal signs, recurs in 24h, <18m

> **Triggers of reflex anoxic seizures***
> • pain • fear
> • cold food • fever
> *Grow out of these seizures by 4–5y

Paroxysmal disorders

→ *sudden onset symptoms mimicking seizures ('funny turns')*

BREATH-HOLDING ATTACKS: in some toddlers when they are upset
→ **Features:** hold breath, go blue, ± LOC → rapid spontaneous recovery (<1min)
→ **Mx:** behaviour modification therapy / distraction

NEURALLY MEDIATED SYNCOPE/FAINT: LOC due to abnormal autonomic response & temporary ↓ blood supply to brain
→ **Features:** nausea, sweating, pallor, **transient LOC ± clonic movements**
→ **Triggers:** hot/stuffy room, standing for long periods, fear

MIGRAINE
→ **Features:** headache with unsteadiness/light-headedness ± visual & GI upset

BENIGN PAROXYSMAL VERTIGO: recurrent **episodes of vertigo** lasting **one to several minutes**
→ **Features:** unsteadiness, falling, nystagmus

Headaches

PRIMARY HEADACHES
- **Tension-type:** symmetrical 'band' of pressure, gradual onset (usually evening)
- **Cluster:** one-sided, excruciating attacks of pain, often around eye
- **Migraine:** headache associated with other symptoms → common in kids

SECONDARY HEADACHES
May be due to raised ICP / space-occupying lesion → look for RED FLAG FEATURES → **need MRI**

> RED FLAG FEATURES:
> - Worse lying down
> - Morning vomiting
> - Night-time waking
> - Altered mood/behaviour

Other possible features
- Visual field defect
- Cranial nerve abnormalities
- Abnormal gait
- Torticollis
- Papilloedema
- Growth failure

MANAGEMENT OF HEADACHES[49]

1. **Thorough Hx** – triggers, onset, duration, symptoms, substance use, analgesia overuse → Ask about red flag features
2. **Physical examination** – vision, sinus tenderness, pain on chewing, BP, CNS & PNS
3. **Education & advice**
   - **reassure** that recurrent headaches are common & cause no long-term harm
   - **no cure** but can help symptoms
4. **Migraine prophylaxis: if >2 per month**
   - 5-HT antagonist e.g. pizotifen/topiramate
   - Beta-blockers e.g. propranolol
5. **Rescue Tx**
   - Analgesia: paracetamol & NSAIDs
   - Anti-emetics: prochlorperazine & metoclopramide
   - Serotonin agonists: sumatriptan (if >12y)
6. **Psychological support**
If headaches triggered by particular stressor *e.g. bullying, exams etc.*
→ *relaxation techniques can help*

---

[49] NICE (2012) *Headaches in over 12s* [CG150]

> **Migraine triggers:** stress, exercise, tiredness, bright lights, cheese/chocolate, hormones (menstruation)

> **Features of migraines**
>
> →**without aura (90%):** bilateral, pulsatile headache + N&V, abdo pain, photophobia, phonophobia → last 1–72h
> →**with aura (10%):** preceding visual disturbance (hemianopia/scotoma/zigzag lines) → last several hours

> **Other causes of 2° headaches:** head/neck trauma, IC haemorrhage, toxins (alcohol/drugs etc.), acute sinusitis

Cerebral palsy

→ *disorder of* **movement & posture** *due to* **non-progressive disturbance** *in developing brain <2y*

    ↳ Often accompanied by disturbed cognition, communication, vision, perception, sensation, behaviour

    ↳ Associated with seizures & secondary MSK problems

> #1 cause of motor impairment in kids = **2 in 1000 live births**

CAUSES

1. Antenatal (80%)
- Vascular occlusion – cord prolapse, APH, maternal shock, rhesus disease, **placental insufficiency** (pre-eclampsia)
- Cortical neurone migration disorder / structural maldevelopment – genetic syndromes, maternal drugs/alcohol
- Congenital infection – STIs, CMV, rubella

2. Perinatal (10%)
- Hypoxic-ischaemic injury – **prolonged labour/delivery**, breech, C-section, PROM

3. Postnatal (10%)
- Periventricular leukomalacia (PVL)* – **hypoxic injury**
- Intraventricular haemorrhage*
- Infection* – **meningitis, encephalitis**
- Metabolic disturbance – hypoglycaemia, **hyperbilirubinaemia (kernicterus)**
- Head trauma

*increased risk if preterm, therefore PREMATURITY = BIG RF FOR CEREBRAL PALSY

CLINICAL PRESENTATION → *although* **non-progressive damage,** *Sx often emerge over time during development*
- Abnormal posture & tone
- Delayed motor milestones – abnormal gait when do walk
- Feeding difficulties – gagging, vomiting, aspiration
- Asymmetric hand function – abnormal if <12m

> **Common comorbidities**
> - impaired vision/hearing/sensation
> - disturbed behaviour / learning difficulties
> - seizures

TYPES OF CEREBRAL PALSY

Spastic (90%) = damaged UMN (corticospinal/pyramidal) pathway → **spastic, hyperreflexia,** positive Babinski	**a) Hemiplegic** • Unilateral arm & leg (face spared) • Fisted hand, flexed & pronated forearm • Tiptoe walking	**b) Diplegic** • All 4 limbs (legs > arms) • Abnormal walking → *associated with prematurity (PVL)*	**c) Quadriplegic** • All 4 limbs severely affected • Opisthotonos • Poor head control
Fig. 5.40			
Dyskinetic (6%) = damaged basal ganglia or extrapyramidal tracts → **involuntary, uncontrolled movements**	**Chorea** = irregular, brief, fidgety movements **Athetosis** = slow writhing movements in distal muscles e.g. fanning of fingers **Dystonia** = abnormal tone & muscle contraction causing twisting appearance → Intellect may be unimpaired → *associated with kernicterus & perinatal hypoxic ischaemic damage*		
Ataxic/hypotonic (4%) = damage to cerebellum (genetic or injury) → **cerebellar signs,** hypotonia	• Poor balance – positive Romberg's • Uncoordinated movements – dysdiadochokinesia, dysmetria • Intention tremor • Ataxic gait – broad base, poor coordination		

MANAGEMENT OF CEREBRAL PALSY[50]: → MDT as wide range of associated medical, psychological & social problems

Therapies

- **Physiotherapy:** improve strength, balance, motor development
- **Occupational therapy:** improve independence at home, school and in the community → walking aids etc.
- **Speech & language (+ dietitian):** speech, eating, swallowing → communication aids

Medications

- **Botulinum toxin injections:** improve specific muscle tightness, stop drooling
- **Muscle relaxants:** baclofen (intrathecal), diazepam (PO)   *short-term only*
- **Glycopyrronium bromide / hyoscine hydrobromide:** reduce salivation

Surgery

- **Selective dorsal rhizotomy:** cut nerves to spastic muscles → may cause numbness
- **Orthopaedic surgery:** lengthen muscles, correct limb position

Continue to monitor

- Growth & nutrition
- Vision/hearing
- Learning difficulties
- Pressure sores
- GI problems (reflux)
- Osteopenia

→ **Investigate cause of CP as part of Mx:** MRI by 3y, metabolic screen, genetic testing

Ataxia

→ *incoordination of muscle movement* (gait, speech, posture) *due to cerebellar / posterior pathway problems*

Causes

- Medications/drugs
- Infection – varicella
- Posterior fossa lesions
- Genetic & degenerative disorders (Friedreich ataxia, ataxia telangiectasia)

Symptoms

- Unsteady, wide-based gait
- Dysdiadochokinesia & dysmetria (past pointing)
- Intention tremor
- Nystagmus

	FRIEDREICH ATAXIA = *autosomal recessive trinucleotide repeat (frataxin gene)*	**ATAXIC TELANGIECTASIA** = *autosomal recessive DNA repair disorder (ATM gene)*
SYMPTOMS	→ Worsening ataxia → Absent lower limb reflexes → Dysarthria → Distal leg muscle wasting → Pes cavus (high-arched feet)	→ Delay in motor & oculomotor development → Poor balance & coordination → Dystonia (most need wheelchair by adolescence) → Telangiectasia in conjunctiva/neck/shoulders
COMPLICATIONS	Kyphoscoliosis & cardiomyopathy = death at 40–50y	↑ risk infection (IgA defect) Malignancy (ALL)
DIAGNOSIS	genetic testing	genetic testing, ↑ AFP (alpha fetoprotein)

Subdural haematoma

→ *due to tearing of bridging veins as they cross the subdural space*

Causes

- **Non-accidental injury (NAI)** – due to shaking / direct trauma
- Direct trauma to head e.g. fall from height

Symptoms

- Altered mental state / seizures
- Apnoea / breathing difficulty
- → **retinal haemorrhages often present**

} If a child presents like this consider NAI & safeguarding

---

[50] NICE (2017) *Cerebral palsy in under 25s* [NG62]

Anterior horn cell disease

SPINAL MUSCULAR ATROPHY = 2nd most common cause of neuromuscular disease (after DMD)

→ **Cause:** autosomal recessive degeneration of anterior horn cells

→ **Sx:** progressive weakness & wasting of skeletal muscle

Type 1 (Werdnig–Hoffmann disease): severe progressive form presenting in infancy

- ↓ fetal movements in pregnancy & deformities at birth
- Absent deep tendon reflexes
- Intercostal recessions   *Type 2 & 3 are less severe*
- Tongue fasciculations

→ *death by age 1y from respiratory failure*

Peripheral neuropathies

GUILLAIN–BARRÉ = **autoimmune demyelination** of peripheral nerves **following infection** (URTI or campylobacter)

↳ *2–4w later*

SYMPTOMS

- **Ascending symmetrical weakness** (over days–weeks)
- Loss of reflexes
- Distal paraesthesia
- Difficulty chewing/swallowing – if bulbar muscles affected
- Difficulty breathing – if respiratory muscles affected
- **Autonomic dysfunction** – ↑ or ↓ HR, HTN, urinary retention

INVESTIGATIONS

- **Lumbar puncture** – ↑ protein, normal WCC
- **Nerve conduction studies** – slowed
- **± spinal cord MRI** to exclude spinal cord lesion

MANAGEMENT

Supportive: may need artificial ventilation

→ *Reassure 95% recover fully (may take 2y)*

CHRONIC INFLAMMATORY DEMYELINATING POLYNEUROPATHY (CIDP) = thought to be **autoimmune cause**

SYMPTOMS: similar to above but slower progression (over >8w)

MANAGEMENT: supportive as above **plus high dose corticosteroids** (prednisolone)

HEREDITARY MOTOR SENSORY NEUROPATHIES (HMSN)

= demyelination & attempted remyelination of nerves

Type 1 (Charcot–Marie–Tooth) = most common (dominant inheritance)

SYMPTOMS

- **Progressive symmetrical distal muscle wasting** → bilateral foot drop
- ± distal sensory & reflex loss
- Physical deformities – stork leg, **pes cavus**, hammer toes

MANAGEMENT: long-term physio & OT to improve symptoms / prevent decline

→ no cure

BELL'S PALSY = isolated LMN paresis of CNVII (facial)

- **Cause:** post-infectious (HSV), nerve trauma/tumour, ear pathology
- **Symptoms:** complete hemiparalysis of face
- **Complication:** conjunctivitis as cannot close eye
- **Differentials:** compression lesion at cerebellopontine angle
- **Prognosis:** usually full recovery in several months
- **Management:** corticosteroids in first week, eye patch

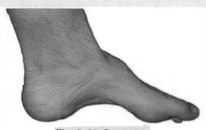

Fig. 5.41 Pes cavus.

DDx of the 'floppy' infant (hypotonia)

Cortical: hypoxic-ischaemic damage, malformation

Genetic: Down's, Prader–Willi

Metabolic: hypothyroidism, hypocalcaemia

Neuromuscular: check creatine kinase (CK)

- spinal muscular atrophy
- myasthenia gravis
- myopathy
- myotonia

Muscular dystrophies

DUCHENNE MUSCULAR DYSTROPHY = #1 neuromuscular disease
→ **1 in 4000 male infants**
Cause: X-linked or *de novo* **mutation**
→ deletion at Xp21 = reduced dystrophin protein (result = myofibre necrosis)

Symptoms: progressive muscle atrophy

Infants:
- **Gower's sign** – must turn prone to rise
- Waddling gait
- Climb stairs 1-by-1
- Language delay

Children:
- Slow running & clumsiness – fatigue quickly
- Pseudohypertrophy of calves – fat replaces muscle
- **Non-ambulatory by 10–14y**

Investigations: avg. age of diagnosis = 5½y
- **Serum CK (creatine kinase)** = RAISED
- Genetic testing
- Muscle biopsy

Management[51]
1. **Physiotherapy** – maintain muscle power & delay scoliosis, stretching to prevent contractures
2. **Orthoses** – scoliosis brace, foot & ankle boots/splints
3. **Medication** – corticosteroids (often intermittent dosing e.g. 10d on, 10d off)
4. **Surgery** – lengthen Achilles tendon, correct scoliosis
5. **Respiratory support** – CPAP/NIPPV overnight
6. **Nutritional support** – PEG may be needed once swallow becomes unsafe
7. **Education & support groups**

Complications: life expectancy = early 20s
→ Respiratory failure – nocturnal hypoxia
→ Cardiomyopathy
→ Scoliosis

→ if child is ambulatory, to delay scoliosis & preserve mobility

BECKER MUSCULAR DYSTROPHY = less common → **some functional dystrophin produced = SLOWER PROGRESSION**
→ Average onset = 11y
→ Non-ambulatory by late 20s
Life expectancy = late 40s – normal

CONGENITAL MUSCULAR DYSTROPHIES = present at birth/early infancy
→ **mostly autosomal recessive**
Cause: lack of an extracellular matrix protein
Symptoms: weakness, hypotonia, contractures ± learning difficulties

Myotonic dystrophies

→ *'myotonia' = delayed relaxation after sustained muscle contraction*
  ↳ e.g. difficulty releasing grip after handshake
DYSTROPHIA MYOTONICA = **autosomal dominant inherited trinucleotide repeat** → Sx worsen down generations

Symptoms
Newborns: hypotonia → feeding & breathing difficulties (tent-shaped mouth)
Children: myotonia, facial weakness, learning difficulties
Adults: cataracts, baldness, testicular atrophy, cardiomyopathy
Cause of death

Investigations
- **Clinical Sx** of child
- **Clinical Sx** of mother (myotonia)
- **Electromyography**

[51] BMJ (2021) Best Practice – *Muscular dystrophies*

Head growth

HYDROCEPHALUS = accumulation of CSF in the brain

Types   Part of brain extends into spinal canal
- **Non-communicating** = obstruction in ventricular system e.g. aqueduct stenosis, Chiari malformation, tumour
- **Communicating** = failure to reabsorb CSF or overproduction e.g. SAH, pneumococcal or TB infection (meningitis)

Presentation
- **Disproportionately large & rapidly increasing head circumference**
- Bulging fontanelles, distended scalp veins
- Fixed downwards gaze
→ **will develop signs of raised ICP:** headaches, seizures, irritability/drowsiness

Investigations: may be diagnosed on antenatal USS
- **Cranial USS** (infants) or **CT/MRI**
- Monitor head circumference

Management
- **Ventriculoperitoneal shunt** – drains fluid from brain into peritoneal cavity
- **Ventriculostomy**

MACROCEPHALY = head circumference >98th centile

Causes   *Rapidly increasing circumference needs urgent Ix
- Tall stature   via USS or CT/MRI
- Familial macrocephaly
- Raised ICP* – brain tumour, chronic subdural haematoma, hydrocephalus
- CNS storage disorders – Hurler syndrome
- Neurofibromatosis

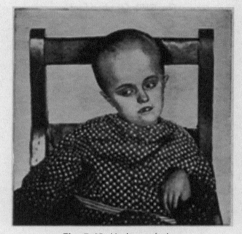

Fig. 5.42 Hydrocephalus.

MICROCEPHALY = head circumference <2nd centile

Causes
- Familial = present from birth
- Autosomal recessive condition = with developmental delay
- Congenital infection
- Acquired after insult to developing brain e.g. perinatal hypoxia, hypoglycaemia, meningitis

CRANIOSYNOSTOSIS = **premature fusion** of one or more sutures leading to **distorted head shape**

Types
- **Localised:**
  - ▸ sagittal suture → long, narrow skull = most common
  - ▸ coronal suture → asymmetrical skull
  - ▸ lambdoid suture → asymmetrical & flattened skull
- **Generalised:**
  - ▸ multiple sutures → microcephaly & developmental delay

Musculoskeletal

→ most resolve without Tx
→ refer if severe, progressive, painful or asymmetrical

Abnormal posture

PES PLANUS (FLAT FEET)

NB 20% adults have non-pathogenic flat feet

<4y = normal
→ due to flat medial longitudinal arch
→ standing on tiptoe / extension of big toe demonstrates arch

>5y = abnormal (fixed flat foot)
→ often painful, stiff & no arch on tiptoeing
→ **DDx:** Achilles contracture, tarsal coalition, juvenile idiopathic arthritis, infection
→ **Ix:** X-ray, MRI/CT
→ **Mx:** specialised footwear / arch support ± surgery (for tarsal coalition)

FOREFOOT ADDUCTION (IN-TOEING) → usually resolves by age 5y
Types
- **Metatarsus varus** = highly mobile foot causes adduction deformity
- **Medial tibial torsion** = lack of lateral rotation of tibia
- **Anteverted femoral neck** = at hip → twisted forward more than normal ('W-sitting')

DEVELOPMENTAL DYSPLASIA OF THE HIP (DDH)
= *spectrum from dysplasia of the joint to subluxation (partial dislocation) to frank dislocation* → due to **shallow acetabulum**

1 in 1000

Diagnosis
1. **Newborn examination / 6–8w postnatal check → identifies most cases**
   - Barlow & Ortolani test
   - If suspected or high-risk factors refer for hip USS
2. **Later presentation with abnormal limp/gait**
   - ± shortened leg (Galeazzi sign) or **limited abduction**
   - ± asymmetrical skin folds

Management[52]
<6m: hip abduction orthoses* (e.g. Pavlik harness)
→ maintains hip flexion & abduction until 12–18m of age
→ monitor progress with USS/X-ray

*Complication: femoral head necrosis

>6m or Tx failure
Surgery – closed or open reduction + 3m cast

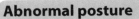

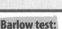

Fig. 5.43 Clubbed foot.

Tarsal coalition: lack of segmentation of small bones of feet → rigid & limit motion → **recurrent strains in adolescence**

Risk factors for DDH
- Female
- FHx
- Oligohydramnios
- Breech
- 1st-born

Barlow test:
Posterior dislocation out of acetabulum

Ortolani test:
Abductive relocation into acetabulum

Indications for hip USS:
- Breech after 36w
- Twin was breech
- 1st-degree relative had DDH
- Positive Barlow/Ortolani test

DDH is associated with co-existing talipes equinovarus & torticollis

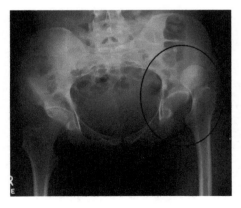

Fig. 5.44 DDH.

[52] BMJ (2021) Best Practice – *Developmental dysplasia of the hip*

STRUCTURAL SCOLIOSIS = Lateral curvature of spine

Causes

- **Idiopathic (85%)** → most often starts in girls at pubertal growth spurt (10–14y)
- **Congenital** → spinal defect e.g. VACTERL, spina bifida
- **Secondary** → to cerebral palsy, muscular dystrophy, neurofibromatosis, Marfan's, JIA

Investigations

1. **Examination of back**
   - Irregular skin creases, different shoulder heights
2. **X-ray** if more severe to assess & monitor progression

Management

- **Mild:** asymptomatic & resolve spontaneously
- **Severe:** bracing
- **Very severe or associated complication:** surgery

If scoliosis disappears on leaning forward = postural scoliosis

chest deformity → cardiorespiratory failure

TORTICOLLIS (WRYNECK) = tilted head/neck position **towards affected muscle**

Causes

- **Acute**
  - ▸ sleep in unusual position
  - ▸ neck sprain
- **Chronic**
  - ▸ SCM tumour
  - ▸ muscle spasm
  - ▸ ENT infection
  - ▸ spinal tumour
  - ▸ cervical spine arthritis

Management: treat underlying cause!
- **Conservative:** analgesia, heat packs, passive stretching
- **Medical:** muscle relaxants e.g. diazepam

SCM tumour = benign, mobile, non-tender nodule
→ resolves in 2–6m
→ common cause of torticollis in infants

SKELETAL DYSPLASIA = genetic mutations (inherited/*de novo*) causing generalised developmental disorders of bone

Features	Diagnosis	Management
• ↓ growth (short stature)	• Antenatal USS	• Bisphosphonates, vit D
• Abnormal bone shape	• Growth chart	• Enzyme replacement
• Intelligence usually normal	• X-ray	• Limb straightening/ lengthening
		• Scoliosis/kyphosis surgery

Types

1. **Achondroplasia (dwarfism)** – see *Genetics & Syndromes* section
2. **Thanatophoric dysplasia** – causes stillbirth of infant with **large head, short limbs, small chest**
3. **Cleidocranial dysostosis**
   - Absence of part/all clavicles (can bring shoulders together in front of chest)
   - Short stature
4. **Osteogenesis imperfecta (brittle bone disease)** = disorders of collagen metabolism causing bone fragility
   - **Sx:** bowing, frequent fractures
   - **Mx:** bisphosphonates, splinting of fractures

Type I: most common → + blue sclera, hearing loss
Type II: lethal → multiple fractures before birth → stillborn

Causative organisms

- *Staph. aureus*
- Streptococcus
- *H. influenzae*
- TB (rare)

Bone & joint infection

AETIOLOGY: spread from blood infection (haematogenous), adjacent soft-tissue infection or penetrating wound

→ *NB Osteomyelitis can spread to cause septic arthritis*

RISK FACTORS: immunosuppressed, DM, extremes of age (**50% children are <3y**), recent operation/injection, wounds

	OSTEOMYELITIS = infection of the *long bones*	SEPTIC ARTHRITIS = infection of the *joint space*
SYMPTOMS	• **PAIN** • **Immobile limb** (pseudoparesis) • **Fever** • Swelling, tender, warmth • Erythema over bone *15% have coexistent septic arthritis*	• **PAIN** (on passive movement) → **non-weight-bearing** • **Immobile limb** (pseudoparesis) • **Fever** • Swelling, tender, warmth, erythema over joint ± joint effusion ± limp
INVESTIGATIONS	**Bloods:** ↑WCC, CRP, ESR **Blood culture:** positive **X-ray:** radiolucent area with hypodense border (due to new bone formation) **USS:** identify if coexistent joint effusion (septic arthritis) **MRI:** subperiosteal pus **Bone scintigraphy:** ↑ radionucleotide uptake	**Bloods:** ↑WCC, CRP, ESR **Blood culture:** positive **Joint aspiration & culture:** diagnostic **X-ray:** normal (may be widened joint space / soft tissue swelling) **USS:** shows joint effusion **MRI / bone scintigraphy:** show if there is coexistent osteomyelitis
MANAGEMENT[53,54]	1. **IMMEDIATE IV ABX** then PO switch For minimum of 4w total 2. **SUPPORTIVE:** analgesia, bedrest, immobilise/splint then physio 3. **SURGICAL DECOMPRESSION/ASPIRATION** → of subperiosteal space if **abscess** or **Tx failure**	SEPSIS PROTOCOL IF SYSTEMIC INVOLVEMENT 1. **IMMEDIATE IV ABX** For minimum of 2w IV then PO switch 2. **SUPPORTIVE:** analgesia, bedrest, immobilise/splint then physio 3. **JOINT DRAINAGE & WASHOUT (lavage)** → if deep-seated or Tx failure
COMPLICATIONS	• Bone/cartilage necrosis • Chronic infection	• Limb deformity • Amyloidosis

NB Hip pain can be referred to the knee (obturator nerve)

Age (y)	Likely Dx
0–2	DDH
2–4	Irritable hip
5–10	Perthes
10–15	SUFE
Any age	Infection

The limping child

DDX OF LIMP IN A CHILD

Acute	Chronic
• Infection (OM/SA) • Transient synovitis • Trauma / overuse injury • Malignancy (leukaemia, neuroblastoma) • Complex regional pain syndrome • Slipped capital femoral epiphysis • Reactive arthritis / JIA	• Congenital problem (DDH, talipes) • Tarsal coalition • Neuromuscular (cerebral palsy, DMD) • JIA • Perthes disease • Slipped capital femoral epiphysis

[53] BMJ (2021) Best Practice – *Osteomyelitis*
[54] BMJ (2021) Best Practice – *Septic arthritis*

TRANSIENT SYNOVITIS (IRRITABLE HIP) → #1 cause of acute hip pain

in children   *Peak age = 4–10 years*

Cause: follows/accompanies **viral infection**

Symptoms
- Pain on movement (not at rest)
- ↓ range of movement (esp. internal rotation)
- **Afebrile / not ill**

→ there will be **fluid in hip joint**

Management: improves by 1w
- Bed rest & analgesia
- **Safety-net**: fever, unwell, non-weight-bearing   *NB 3% develop Perthes disease*

PERTHES DISEASE   *Peak age = 5–10 years*

→ **interrupted blood supply** to femoral head (cause unknown)

→ causes **avascular necrosis** of capital femoral epiphysis then **revascularisation & reossification**

Symptoms: insidious onset (days)
- Limp or hip/knee pain 80–90% = unilateral

Investigations
- X-ray (AP & frog lateral views)
- Bone scan
- MRI

Management

Early/mild: avoid intensive exercise
- Bed rest & traction + **analgesia**

Late/severe:
- Plaster/calipers to maintain hip in abduction
- Femoral/pelvic osteotomy

SLIPPED CAPITAL FEMORAL EPIPHYSIS (SCFE) → Postero-inferior

displacement of epiphysis   *Peak age = 10–15y*

Symptoms: acute (post-trauma) or insidious
- Limp or hip/knee pain – often bilateral
- Restricted abduction & internal rotation of hip

Investigations
- **X-ray** (AP & frog-lateral views) → *lost Klein's line, widened growth plate*

Management: ASAP to prevent avascular necrosis
- **Conservative:** analgesia, crutches
- **Surgical:** pin fixation *in situ*

Important to differentiate from septic arthritis

Ix findings in irritable hip are normal:
Bloods: WCC = normal
Culture: negative
X-ray: normal

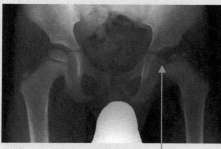

Fig. 5.45

Femoral epiphyseal head:
- Flattened & fragmented
- Increased density

Poor prognostic factors of Perthes: >5y, >50% epiphysis involved, deformed femoral head → *later complication = osteoarthritis*

Risk factors for SCFE
- Adolescent males (growth spurt)
- Obesity
- Hypothyroidism
- Hypogonadism

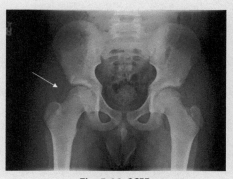

Fig. 5.46 SCFE.

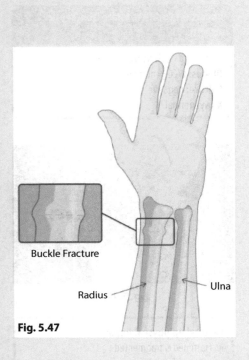

Buckle Fracture

Radius

Ulna

Fig. 5.47

Most common fracture sites in kids
• Distal radius & hand (FOOSH) • Clavicle • Tibial shaft, ankle & foot • Radial shaft & elbow

Fractures

INCOMPLETE FRACTURES
→ Common in children due to softer/more flexible bones
→ Bones bend/compress rather than break

- **Greenstick fractures** = **partial break in one side causes other side to bend**
  ▸ common mid-shaft of forearm and lower leg

- **Buckle/torus fractures** = **compression on one side of the bone causing bulging cortex**
  ▸ commonly involve distal metaphysis of radius
  ▸ following FOOSH
  ▸ appears as 'base of pillar'/ bulge & often no fracture line seen

- **Hairline (stress) fractures** = **small 'cracks' that do not traverse entire bone**
  ▸ usually from overuse / repetitive stress-bearing motions
     e.g. track runners, gymnasts, dancers

COMPLETE FRACTURES
- **Comminuted fracture** = **bone broken into >2 pieces / crushed into fragments**
- **Bucket-handle fracture** = **fragmentation of corner of metaphysis**
→ **indicates non-accidental injury**

GROWTH PLATE FRACTURES
→ Unique to children (common in growth spurt when physes are weakest)
→ Typically caused by great force during sports or playground accidents
→ Classified with **Salter–Harris System** → determines Tx options

Salter–Harris type	Treatment
I	Splinting or casting
II	
III	Open reduction & internal fixation
IV	
V	Surgery

Most common   *Likely to affect bone growth*

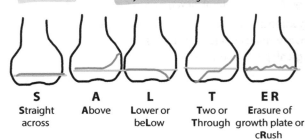

S	**A**	**L**	**T**	**E R**
Straight across	**A**bove	**L**ower or be**L**ow	**T**wo or **T**hrough	**E**rasure of growth plate or c**R**ush

Fig. 5.48

Management options for fractures

1. Simple cast/splint
2. Brace/boot   } + analgesia
3. Surgical fixation with metal pins/screws

Arthritis

JUVENILE IDIOPATHIC ARTHRITIS (JIA)   1 in 1000
= persistent joint swelling (>6w) presenting before 16y in **absence of infection or other defined cause**

Monoarthritis: 1 joint e.g. septic, gout
Oligoarthritis: ≤4 joints e.g. reactive, psoriatic
Polyarthritis: >4 joints e.g. rheumatoid, SLE

Classification: based on number of joints affected in first 6m

Subtype	Onset age & sex ratio	Articular pattern	Extra-articular features	Lab findings
Persistent oligoarthritis (50%)	**1–6y** F:M = 5:1	Max 4 joints (knee, ankle, wrist)	• Chronic anterior uveitis (20%) • Leg-length discrepancy	ANA ±
Extended oligoarthritis (8%)	**1–6y** F:M = 5:1	>4 joints after first 6m **= ASYMMETRICAL** → large & small joints	• Chronic anterior uveitis (20%) • Asymmetrical growth	ANA ±
Rheumatoid factor –ve polyarthritis (16%)	**1–6y** F:M = 5:1	**SYMMETRICAL** → large & small joints → marked finger involvement → ± TMJ or cervical spine	• Low grade fever • Chronic anterior uveitis (5%) • Late reduced growth	
Rheumatoid factor +ve polyarthritis (3%)	**10–16y** F:M = 5:1		• Rheumatoid nodules (10%) (similar to adult RA)	Rheumatoid factor +
Systemic arthritis (9%)	**1–10y** F:M = 1:1	• Oligo- or polyarthritis • Arthralgia/myalgia • Initially no arthritis	• Malaise, daily fevers • **Salmon-pink macular rash** • Lymphadenopathy	Anaemia ↑ CRP/ESR ↑ platelets
Psoriatic arthritis (7%)	**1–16y** F:M = 1:1	**ASYMMETRICAL** → large & small joints → dactylitis	• Psoriasis (nail pitting) • Chronic anterior uveitis (20%)	
Enthesitis-related arthritis (7%)	**6–16y** F:M = 1:4	Large joints mainly (lower limbs, lumbar spine, sacroiliac)	**Enthesitis** – inflammation at tendon/ligament insertion	HLAB27 +
Undifferentiated arthritis (1%)	**1–16y** F:M = 2:1	Overlapping patterns of subtypes		

General symptoms: → *poor mood or ↓ activity = indicators in infants*
- **Joint gelling** – stiffness after rest
- **Joint stiffness/pain** – in mornings
- **Joint swelling** – may appear later

Management[55]: MDT with rheumatology specialist

1. **NSAIDs** – relieve symptoms during flares

2. **Steroid injections**
   - 1st line for oligoarthritis
   - Bridging Tx for polyarthritis

3. **Methotrexate (tablet, liquid, injection weekly)**
   - 1st line for polyarthritis
   - SE: nausea, liver damage, bone-marrow suppression

4. **Systemic corticosteroids**
   - Sx relief in severe systemic JIA while DMARDs work
   - Avoid if can as growth suppression / osteoporosis

5. **Immunotherapy (e.g. anti TNF-a)**
   - If methotrexate-resistant

6. **Prevent / monitor for complications**
   - Physiotherapy – encourage activity
   - Ophthalmology, dentistry, orthopaedic reviews

Complications of JIA
- Bone/joint deformities
- Chronic anterior uveitis
- Flexion contractures
- Growth failure
- Osteoporosis
- Amyloidosis – proteinuria & renal failure (rare)
- **Side-effects of Tx** – growth suppression, immunosuppression

→ 1/3 have active disease into adulthood
→ may need joint replacements

[55]BMJ (2021) Best Practice – *Juvenile idiopathic arthritis*

Infectious triggers

- **Post-dysentery:** shigella, salmonella, campylobacter
- **Post-STI:** chlamydia, gonococcus
- **Post-viral**
- **Other:** mycoplasma, Lyme disease, rheumatic fever

REACTIVE ARTHRITIS = transient (<6w) joint swelling following extra-articular infection

Symptoms
- **Reiter's syndrome:**
  - ▸ joint swelling (often knees/ankles)
  - ▸ conjunctivitis (painful, red eyes)
  - ▸ urethritis (dysuria)
- **Dactylitis** (swollen 'sausage' fingers/toes)
- **± Mild fever**

Investigations: rule out other conditions
- **Bloods:** normal or mild ↑ ESR
- **Rheumatoid factor:** negative
- **Urine & stool MCS & PCR:** bacterial/viral infections
- **Joint aspiration & culture:** no organisms (r/o septic arthritis)
- **X-ray:** normal

Management
- **NSAIDs** – reduce inflammation
- **Steroid injections** – if severe

Other causes of polyarthritis

1. **Infection**
   - Bacterial e.g. septic arthritis
   - Viral e.g. rubella, mumps, adenovirus, HSV, Lyme disease
   - Reactive e.g. post-GI infection
2. **Inflammatory bowel disease:** Crohn's/UC
3. **Vasculitis:** HSP, Kawasaki
4. **Haematological:** haemophilia, sickle cell disease
5. **Malignancy:** leukaemia, neuroblastoma
6. **Connective tissue disorders**
   - JIA
   - SLE – butterfly rash, fatigue, kidney problems
   - Dermatomyositis – rash + Gottron's papules
   - Polyarteritis nodosa
7. **Other:** cystic fibrosis

Growing pains

- Wake in night with pain → no daytime Sx
- Often worse after activity
- Eased with massage
- **No abnormal physical signs**

Idiopathic pain syndromes: no identifiable cause

Types
- Chronic fatigue syndrome (myalgic encephalomyelitis)
- Fibromyalgia
- Diffuse idiopathic pain
- Localised idiopathic pain

Features
- Chronic pain
- Impacts ADLs
- Average age 9–12y
- F > M

Surgery

The acute abdomen

Surgical	Medical	Extra-abdominal
• **Acute appendicitis** • Intestinal obstruction • Inguinal hernia • Peritonitis • Inflamed Meckel diverticulum • Pancreatitis • Trauma	• **Gastroenteritis** • **Urinary tract infection**/stones • DKA • IBD/**constipation** • Hepatitis • Henoch–Schönlein purpura	• **Torsion of testes** • Lower lobe pneumonia • Upper respiratory tract infection • Hip & spine • Migraine • Psychological

conditions in bold in the table = most common

PERITONITIS = infection of the peritoneum

Causes in children

- Primary/spontaneous peritonitis – infection not directly related to another intra-abdominal abnormality
- Perforated appendix – most common cause in children
- Perforated bowel (e.g. Crohn's disease)
- Post abdominal surgery
- Post trauma to the abdomen

Symptoms

- Diffuse abdominal pain + guarding
- Vomiting/diarrhoea
- Fever
- Shock

Investigations

- Bloods
- Exploratory laparotomy
- CT/MRI
- Ascitic tap for MCS – if ascites

Management

IV ABX ± surgery (to fix the cause)

ACUTE APPENDICITIS → most common cause of surgically acute abdomen in childhood (>3y) → **10% morbidity**

Symptoms

- Anorexia & vomiting
- Fever
- Abdominal pain
  - ▶ central colicky → sharp in RIF
  - ▶ worse on movement
- Tenderness & guarding in RIF   may be absent if appendix = rectocaecal
  - ▶ +ve McBurney's test

Investigations

- **Hx & examination**
- **Bloods:** ↑ WCC & CRP
- **Urine dip:** +ve WBCs without blood
- **CT/USS abdo:** visualise appendix/abscess & exclude other causes

Management[56]

1. **Acute:** O_2, IV fluids, analgesia, NG tube
2. **Consider ABX:** if septic / suitable for conservative management
3. **Appendicectomy** ideally within 24h

> **Appendix mass/abscess:** palpable mass in RIF
> → IV ABX then delayed appendicectomy
> **Appendix perforation:** generalised guarding & pain
> → IV ABX, IV fluids, laparotomy

---

[56] Di Saverio SD, Podda M, De Simone B, *et al*. (2020) Diagnosis and treatment of acute appendicitis. *World Journal of Emergency Surgery* 15(1):27

MECKEL DIVERTICULUM → remnant of vitello-intestinal duct containing gastric or pancreatic mucosa

Symptoms: asymptomatic unless complication
- **Obstruction:** pain, vomiting, constipation
- **Haemorrhage:** bright red bloody stools
- **Diverticulitis:** mimics appendicitis

Investigations
- **Technetium scan:** ↑ uptake by gastric mucosa

Management
- Surgical resection

NECROTISING ENTEROCOLITIS (NEC) → bacterial infection of bowel wall (see *Neonatology* notes)

Symptoms
- Feed aspiration
- Bilious vomiting
- Abdo distension/pain
- ± blood in stools
→ complications = bowel perforation & shock

Investigations
- Bloods (show infection)
- **AXR ± USS**

Management
- NBM (nasogastric feeding)
- Broad-spectrum ABX
± surgical removal of necrotic bowel

> **Risk factors for NEC**
> - Preterm
> - Very low BW
> - Cow's milk diet

Intestinal obstruction

INTUSSUSCEPTION → *most common cause of obstruction after neonatal period*

Pathogenesis
→ invagination of proximal bowel into distal segment (often ileum via ileocaecal valve into caecum)   ↳ *Peak age: 3m—2y*
→ restricted venous blood flow = swelling, engorgement & bleeding of mucosa

Symptoms
- **Abdominal pain** – paroxysmal, severe, colicky
  → pallor, crying & draws up knees with each episode
- Abdominal distension / **'sausage-shaped' mass** (in RUQ)
- Anorexia & vomiting (may be bilious)
- Constipation
- **'Redcurrant jelly' stools** (blood/mucus) = **late sign**
→ **Dehydration & shock** = important complication

Investigations
- Hx & examination (**ABCDE**)
- FBC, U&Es – show blood loss / kidney injury
- Blood gas – raised lactate
- **AXR:** distended small bowel & no gas in rectum
- **Abdo USS:** 'target sign' → **First-line Ix**

Management[57]
- **ABCDE** → IV fluid resuscitation
- **First-line:** contrast enema reduction
- **Second-line:** laparoscopic resection

> **Causes of intestinal obstruction**
> - Idiopathic (majority)
> - Meckel's diverticulum
> - Polyps, tumours, inflamed appendix
> - Viral infection (Peyer's patch hypertrophy)
>
> **Associations**
> - Henoch–Schönlein purpura
> - Nephrotic syndrome
> - Obesity
> - CF

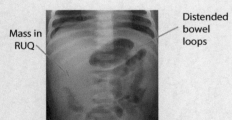
Mass in RUQ

Distended bowel loops

Fig. 5.49 Intussusception.

> **Usually <1m** but can be any time (especially within 1st y)

[57] BMJ (2021) Best Practice – *Intussusception*

VOLVULUS (MALROTATION) → *failed rotation of intestine during development causes volvulus after birth*

→ Presents as intestinal obstruction ± compromised blood supply

Symptoms
- **Bilious vomiting**
- Abdo pain & **distension**
- Constipation
- Bloody/dark red stools

Investigations
- Hx & examination
- FBC, U&Es
- **AXR**
- **Barium swallow** – corkscrew

Management: surgery to untwist intestine **(Ladd's procedure)**

→ **Signs of vascular compromise / shock = urgent laparotomy**

PYLORIC STENOSIS → *hypertrophied pyloric muscle obstructs gastric outlet*

Symptoms   Age of presentation = 2–7w
- **Projectile vomiting**
- Hunger & dehydration ± weight loss

Signs
- Palpable 'olive-like' mass in RUQ
- Peristaltic waves from LUQ → RUQ

Investigations
- Hx & examination
- Test feed
- AXR/USS – hypertrophied pylorus

Management
- Correct electrolyte imbalance – 0.45% saline + 0.5% dextrose + potassium
- **Pyloromyotomy** = division of hypertrophied muscle

The surgical scrotum

Embryology
→ Testes formed from **urogenital ridge** on **post. abdo wall** (near kidney)
→ Testes **migrate down through inguinal canal** into scrotum
  = preceded by **'processus vaginalis'** which normally obliterates after birth

INGUINAL HERNIA → Protrusion of abdominal viscera through inguinal rings
↳ In kids = almost always **indirect** due to **patent processus vaginalis**
↳ **Common:** 1 in 50 boys (much rarer in girls)

Signs/symptoms
- **Groin/scrotal swelling** – on crying/straining
  = reducible or irreducible firm, tender lump → **cannot get above it**
- ± vomiting
- ± irritability

Management: *prompt repair to avoid risk of strangulation → refer child*
- Analgesia & sustained gentle compression
- **Surgery** – ligation & division of processus vaginalis sac

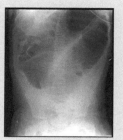

Fig. 5.50 Sigmoid volvulus.

DDx of pyloric stenosis: GORD, overfeeding, gastroenteritis, sepsis

hypochloraemic, hypokalaemic, metabolic alkalosis (↓ Cl⁻ & K⁺ from vomiting)

Risk factors for inguinal hernia
- Preterm
- DDH
- Undescended testes
- CF

HYDROCELE → Peritoneal fluid tracks down patent processus vaginalis & surrounds testes

Signs/symptoms
- **Scrotal swelling** – bluish colour
  - ▸ often bilateral
  - ▸ **transilluminable**
  - ▸ can get above it
→ *no other symptoms*

Management: most resolve spontaneously
Surgery if:
- persists >18–24m
- symptomatic / very large

VARICOCELE → Varicosities of testicular veins → **around puberty (>10y)**

Signs/symptoms
- **Scrotal swelling** – 'bag of worms'
- Dragging/aching
→ *associated infertility*

Management:
Surgery (obliteration/embolisation of testicular veins) **if acute pain/infertility/shrinking testes**

CRYPTORCHIDISM (UNDESCENDED TESTES) → Descent occurs in 3rd trimester (may continue to 3m of age)
↳ *PREMATURITY = RISK FACTOR*

Types
- **Retractile:** can manipulate testes into scrotum (eventually descends with age)
- **Palpable:** can palpate testes in groin but cannot manipulate into scrotum
- **Impalpable:** cannot palpate testes (may be in inguinal canal, intra-abdominal or absent)

Investigations
- **Examination** – palpate groin/scrotum → try to manipulate testes into scrotum
- **Laparoscopy** – 1st-line Ix if impalpable testes
- **USS** – if impalpable testes to confirm presence/absence
- **Hormonal** – if bilateral impalpable testes → HCG injection causes ↑ serum testosterone if testicular tissue present

Management: early referral to paediatric surgeon → need surgery if undescended by 6m
- **Orchidopexy** (surgical placement of testes into scrotum)

Acute scrotal problems

TESTICULAR TORSION = *twisting of testicular pedicle resulting in* **compromised blood supply** *& necrosis*

Signs/symptoms: easy to mistake for abdominal pathology!   EMERGENCY
- **Acute, severe pain** – in scrotum, groin or lower abdo
- Nausea ± vomiting ± fever
- Hot, swollen testes – lying higher than normal
- **Absent cremasteric reflex** – stroking inner thigh raises ipsilateral testicle

Management: within 6–12h to preserve testicular viability
- **Surgical correction**
- + bilateral suturing & fixation to tunica vaginalis – prevent recurrence

TORSION OF TESTICULAR APPENDAGE = *twisting of embryological remnant (hydatid of Morgagni) on upper pole*

Signs/symptoms
Similar to testicular torsion but:
- Pain less severe
- Longer Hx (pain ↑s over 1–2d)
- May be 'blue dot' seen/felt on scrotum

Management
Surgical excision of appendage

Complications of cryptorchidism
- Infertility
- ↑ risk malignancy
- Psychological

→ Scrotal examination needed in all acute abdomen presentations

---

Risk factors for torsion
- Ages 12–18y
- Congenital abnormality (e.g. Bell–Clapper testes)
- Trauma

Other differentials of scrotal swelling:
- Idiopathic scrotal oedema = painless, bilateral
- Incarcerated inguinal hernia
- Epididymal cyst = dragging/aching testicle

If cannot confidently r/o testicular torsion, then must have urgent surgical exploration

EPIDIDYMO-ORCHITIS = *inflammation of epididymis/testes usually due to **viral** or bacterial infection*

↳ *UTIs*
↳ *STIs*
↳ *Mumps*

Signs/symptoms
- **Testicular pain** – develops over days
- **Swollen, red, tender testicle**
- Fever & malaise
- ± dysuria – if UTI
- ± discharge – if STI
- **Positive Prehn's test** – scrotal elevation relieves pain

Management
1. Analgesia / scrotal support
2. ABX – if UTI/STI

Penile abnormalities

HYPOSPADIAS = *congenital abnormality where **urethral opening is on underside of penis***

↳ *Common:*
  1 in 200 boys

Features
- Ventral urethral meatus
- Hooded dorsal foreskin
- Chordee = ventral curvature of shaft

Symptoms: **may be none other than cosmetic**
- Difficulty weeing
- Erectile deformity
- ± other genitourinary abnormalities

Management
Surgery by 2y
→ Do not circumcise as need foreskin for later reconstructive surgery

Fig. 5.51

PHIMOSIS = inability to retract the foreskin

↳ **Physiological:** normal attachment of foreskin to glans at birth → by 4y 90% have retracted
↳ **Pathological:** due to localised skin disease: **balanitis xerotica obliterans** (BXO) → white scarring on the foreskin

Symptoms: **often asymptomatic**
- Difficulty weeing
- Dysuria/burning
- Swelling, erythema, soreness

Management
Circumcision if pathological/causing symptoms

> **Circumcision:** removal of the foreskin under GA
>
> **Indications**
> - Pathological phimosis
> - Recurrent UTIs
> - Recurrent balanoposthitis – inflammation of the penis & glans
>
> **Post-op complications**
> - Bleeding, infection, pain

> **Balanitis xerotica obliterans (BXO)**
>
> = skin disease of penis & glans
> → can result in urethral stenosis & phimosis due to scar tissue

> **Paraphimosis** = foreskin gets stuck in retracted position, resulting in swollen glans

Female genital disorders

LABIAL ADHESIONS = fusion of labia minora in the midline
Signs: translucent midline raphe
Symptoms: asymptomatic **OR** perineal soreness / urinary irritation & pooling
Management: topical oestrogen BD for 1–2w → surgery if unsuccessful

IMPERFORATE HYMEN = congenital abnormality where hymen has no opening
Symptoms: asymptomatic until menarche → abdo/pelvic pain, amenorrhoea, dysuria
Management: hymenotomy

Anorectal abnormalities

Types: imperforate anus, anorectal fistula, anal/rectal stenosis or atresia
Symptoms
- Fail to pass meconium/faeces
- **OR** faeces/urine exits in wrong place e.g. vagina/urethra
- Abdo distension
- Vomiting

Investigations
- Abdo X-ray
- Abdo USS
- Barium enema/swallow

Management: prompt referral to paediatric surgeon
- **Imperforate anus:** surgery
- **Stenosis:** may be able to stretch canal with metal dilator
- **Atresia/fistula:**
  - ► Temporary colostomy
  - ► Surgical reconnection of anus & rectum/fistula closure

Associations with anorectal abnormalities

- VACTERL syndrome
- Down syndrome
- Spinal problems
- GI tract problems
- Urinary tract

Community paediatrics

Normal child development

→ *steady progress in all fields with acquisition of skills before* limit ages

Limit age: 2SDs > mean

FEATURES OF NORMAL DEVELOPMENT
↳ Development of skills **follows a sequence**
↳ Rate of development **varies between children**
↳ Progress should be **similar in each skill area**
↳ Progress **relates to age** → *adjust for prematurity* by using age from EDD

> **Developmental screening:** overall developmental check of all children at set ages by trained professionals e.g. GPs → *includes newborn hearing screen & school entry vision test*
>
> **Developmental assessment:** detailed analysis of specific domain due to concerns from screening – specialist referral

Limit ages shown in red in table below → if milestone not achieved by this age then need to refer for further Ix (but most likely it is just normal for this child)

Median age	Gross motor	Fine motor / vision	Language	Social
Newborn **3m**	Flexed posture Holds up head (6m)	Fix & follow object (3m)	Startle to loud noise	Smile by 6 weeks (8w)
6m **9m**	Sit unsupported (9m) Crawl (12m)	Pass block between hands (9m)	Monosyllabic babble	Feed self
1y **12–15m**	Stand independently Walk steadily (18m)	Pincer grip	Respond to name 2 syllables 'mama'/'dada'	Drink from cup with 2 hands / finger feed
2y	Run	Scribble	2-word sentence 'want cat' (2.5y)	Remove an item of clothing / play alone
3y	Jump	Copy a line	3/4-word sentences	Put on item of clothing / use cutlery
4y	Stand on each foot for 3s	Copy a cross/square	Name 4 colours	Dress independently
5y	Walk heel-to-toe	Draw 6-part person/triangle	All speech understandable Count to 5	Play board games Brush teeth
Most rapid:	<1y	9–18m	18–30m	>2y

Fields of development
- Gross motor
- Fine motor & vision
- Speech, language & hearing
- Social, emotional, behavioural

Abnormal child development

→ *becomes more obvious with ↑ age (gap between child & 'normal' widens)*

Factors influencing development:

Prenatal	Perinatal	Postnatal
• Genetic disorders • Congenital infections • Maternal alcohol/drugs/ medications • Congenital malformations • Placental insufficiency	• Prematurity • VLBW • Hypoxia (difficulties during birth) • Maternal infection	• Nutrition • Accidents/injuries • Infection • Other illnesses e.g. metabolic • Environment / social situation

GLOBAL DEVELOPMENTAL DELAY (GDD)
= delayed acquisition of **all skill fields**, presenting in **first 2y** of life
→ likely associated cognitive difficulties (become apparent later)
→ needs Ix into causes

Causes of GDD
- Genetic/syndromic
- Infections, toxins, trauma
- Cerebral palsy
- Cerebral malformations
- Metabolic/endocrine

Investigating developmental delay
Physical: head circumf, weight, length/height
Cytogenic: karyotype, fragile X, FISH
Metabolic: TFT, LFT, U&Es, bone profile, CK
Infection screen: TORCH
Imaging: cranial USS/CT/MRI
Other: EEG, vision, hearing, physio, OT, SALT

late walking (>18m) may be normal if child was 'bottom-shuffler'/'commando-crawler'

Concurrent FTT / growth abnormalities / dysmorphic features suggest **chromosome abnormality** is the cause of delay

> **Delay:** slow acquisition of skills
> **Disorder:** maldevelopment of skill

↳ *delay may be a normal variant*

- *dysarthria: speech muscle weakness*
- *verbal dyspraxia: ↓ coord of speech muscles*

> **Asperger's syndrome:** social impairments of ASD but near-normal speech & language

> **Comorbidities**
> - General learning & attention difficulties
> - Seizures
> - Anxiety / sleep disturbance
> - ADHD
> - OCD

25–30h a week
= costly & time-consuming

MOTOR SKILLS DELAY: presents between 3m & 2y

Signs
- Slow to lift head, sit up, crawl, walk
- Floppy/stiff limbs
- Not weight-bearing by 1y
- Unbalanced/abnormal gait
- Hand dominance in first year – suggests hemiplegia

Causes
- Central motor deficit: cerebral palsy
- Congenital myopathy
- Spinal cord lesion: spina bifida
- Part of GDD: in many syndromes

Management
Ix: by neurodevelopmental paediatrician & physio
Ongoing support: from OT & physio

ABNORMAL SPEECH & LANGUAGE DEVELOPMENT: a delay or a disorder

Causes of delay
- Hearing loss
- Anatomical deficit e.g. cleft palate
- Environmental deprivation
- Multiple languages spoken at home
- GDD, autism, cerebral palsy

Investigations
- Hearing assessment
- SALT assessment

Management
- SALT
- Learning support at school
- Special schools – rarely

Types of disorder
- Language comprehension
- Language expression
- Speech production
- Pragmatics, sentence construction, grammar
- Social/communication skills e.g. autism spectrum disorder

AUTISTIC SPECTRUM DISORDER (ASD): Delayed development of social & communication skills

Affects 3–6 in 1000
Male > female

Triad of difficulties:

1. Impaired social interaction
- Poor eye contact
- Lack of social cues / inappropriate behaviour
- No interest in forming relationships
- No interest in playing with peers

2. Speech & language disorder *often have sensitivity to loud noise*
- Speech & language delay
- Limited gestures/facial expression
- Over-literal speech interpretation
- Echoes/repeats question/instructions

Diagnosis
- Behaviour observation
- Formal standardised tests

3. Ritualistic & repetitive behaviour
- Tantrums if routine is disrupted
- Repetitive movements e.g. hand-flapping

<10% will function independently as adults

Management[58]

1. **General:** personal space, quiet places, each day organised & explained / same routine
2. **Applied behavioural analysis:** behaviour modification approach to ↓ ritualism & develop language/social skills
3. **Appropriate schooling:** some special schools use above approach
4. **Educate parents:** reassure it is not the result of emotional trauma / poor parenting
5. **Consider & manage co-existing conditions** e.g. other mental health illness, insomnia, developmental delay

[58] SIGN (2016) Quick Reference Guide – *Assessment, diagnosis and interventions for autism spectrum disorders*

Learning difficulties

GENERAL LEARNING DIFFICULTIES
Significantly sub-average IQ (<70) apparent before 18y → **RF:** lower socioeconomic status

	Mild (85% cases)	**Moderate**	**Severe**	**Profound**
IQ	<70	<50	<35	<20
Presentation	At school/later	Delayed speech & language (2–4y)	Global developmental delay (apparent from infancy)	
Functioning	**Only need help if problems arise** • often not recognised as LD	**May need supervision** in some elements of daily living / work	**Need help with many ADLs** • often physical disability • limited communication	**Extensive/total help with ADLs** • minimal communication

Causes: 30% = unknown cause

- **Genetic/chromosomal:** Down's, fragile X, PKU, neurofibromatosis, tuberous sclerosis
- **Pre-natal:** hypothyroidism, fetal alcohol syndrome, pre-eclampsia, TORCH infections
- **Peri-natal:** birth hypoxia, hyperbilirubinaemia, intraventricular haemorrhage
- **Post-natal:** brain infection/tumour, head trauma, malnutrition, neglect/abuse

> **Comorbidities**
> - Poor sensory skills
> - ADHD
> - Depression
> - Bipolar/mania
> - Schizophrenia

SPECIFIC LEARNING DIFFICULTIES

1. **Dyspraxia / developmental coordination disorder (DCD)** = disorder of motor planning/execution

Signs
- messy, slow, irregular handwriting
- difficulties with buttons/laces/clothes
- difficulties cutting up food
- messy eating/drooling – cannot coordinate chewing/swallowing
- poorly established laterality e.g. handedness

Diagnosis
- features in history + OT assessment

Management → *should improve with ongoing therapy*
- OT – IT/educational support
- SALT
- vision & hearing assessment = useful

2. **Attention deficit hyperactivity disorder (ADHD)** = overactivity in most situations + impaired concentration

Cause: dysfunction of dopaminergic brain circuits
Diagnosis: assessed by paediatric & educational psychologists*

Features: → *short-tempered & difficulty making friends*
1. **Inattention** – ↓ concentration on work/play, distractible, don't listen
2. **Hyperactivity** – fidgety, excessive movement/noise, unorganised/lose things
3. **Impulsivity** – interrupt others, social disinhibition, difficulty sharing/taking turns

> **Risk factors for ADHD:** FHx, male, premature

> *based on clinical assessment and questionnaire filled out by parents & teachers*

> *NB Sx worse in unfamiliar environments → **must assess in >1 situation** e.g. home + school*

Management[59]   *need specialist community paediatrician/psychiatrist input*
1st-line: behavioural modification strategies – educate parents/teachers in clear rules, consistent rewards system
2nd-line: medication – stimulants (methylphenidate/Ritalin – see over) **or** non-stimulants (atomoxetine) → no meds if age <5y

> + additional lifestyle factors: diet, exercise, sleep hygiene

[59] NICE (2018, updated 2019) *Attention deficit hyperactivity disorder: diagnosis and management* [NG87]

DDx of ADHD
- Anxiety
- Personality disorders
- Autism spectrum disorder
- Hyperthyroidism

Causes of nocturnal enuresis

- **genetics** – $^2/_3$ have affected 1st-degree relative
- **emotional stress** = most common cause
- **UTI**
- **constipation**
- **osmotic diuresis** – diabetes mellitus
- **developmental disabilities/delays**

Side-effects of Ritalin: need specialist paediatric psychiatrist assessment
- Abdo pain, nausea, reduced appetite
- Insomnia, tics, anxiety/depression, palpitations
- Growth suppression

Requires monitoring → height & weight every 6m AND BP & HR every 3m

ENURESIS: *bedwetting*

Primary nocturnal enuresis: bedwetting >2 nights/week in child old enough to be continent (3–5y)

VERY COMMON:
→ 10% of 5 year-olds
→ 5% of 10 year-olds

Investigations
- **urinalysis:** if recent/sudden onset **or** Sx of UTI/DM
- diary of wet/dry nights
- drinking/urine volume charts

Management[60]
- **explanation:** common problem & no conscious control
- **advice:** fluid intake, diet, toileting before bed, etc.
- **reward systems / star charts:** avoid punishments
- **enuresis alarm:** sounds when becomes wet (must try before desmopressin if <7y)
- **desmopressin (ADH):** short-term relief e.g. sleepover

Primary daytime enuresis: lack of bladder control in day in child old enough to be continent (3–5y)

Causes
- **lack of attention to bladder sensation** – developmental problem or just preoccupied
- **neuropathic bladder** – associated with neuro conditions like spina bifida
- **detrusor instability**
- **bladder neck weakness / ectopic ureter**
- **UTI/constipation**

Management: treat underlying cause
→ star charts & alarms if no pathological cause

Investigations: r/o neuro cause
1. Examination: neuro, abdominal, rectal
2. Urinalysis – MCS
3. USS bladder
4. Urodynamic studies

Secondary enuresis: loss of previously achieved urinary continence

Causes
- emotional upset
- distraction (too busy playing)
- UTI **or** DM → urine dip & MCS

---

[60]NICE (2010) *Bedwetting in under 19s* [CG111]

Child & adolescent mental health

Sleep-related problems

Difficulty settling to sleep
What: won't go to sleep unless parent present – manifestation of separation anxiety in toddlers
Contributing factors: separation anxiety, napping in day, no bedtime routine, noisy environment, fear of the dark
Management: strict bedtime routine, **graded lengthening** of time between leaving room and checking on child

Waking at night
What: cannot settle back to sleep without parent present – often associated with difficulty settling to sleep
Management: treat difficulty settling to sleep first, **graded lengthening** approach

Nightmares
What: bad dreams that the child **can recall** = common
Management: REASSURE CHILD → professional input only if content indicates *morbid preoccupation* e.g. death

Night terrors
What: rapid emergence from period of deep sleep causes state of high arousal & confusion – 1.5h after settling
Features: child sitting up, eyes open, disorientated, confused, distressed, unresponsive – **no recollection** in morning
Management: reassure parents, improve bedtime routine, ensure **safe environment if concurrent sleepwalking**

Temper tantrums

→ *outbursts of anger & refusal to obey parents as an ordinary response to frustration*

MANAGEMENT
1. **Analyse tantrums**
   - **Antecedents** – what happened minutes before?
   - **Behaviour** – what exactly did the episode consist of?
   - **Consequences** – what was the result? – what parent did & outcome
2. **Examine child for medical/psychological factors**
   - e.g. global/language delay, hearing impairment, bronchodilators/anticonvulsants
3. **Interventions**
   - Avoid antecedents
   - **Distraction** techniques
   - **Ignore** until tantrum runs out
   - **Time-out** e.g. naughty step
   - Star chart to reward obedience

Aggressive behaviour

→ **usually learned** by copying parents, peers, siblings & **persistent if not actively managed**

RISK FACTORS: tired, stressed, communication impairment
MANAGEMENT: make clear rules & stick to them → 1–2–3 approach

School refusal

→ *inability to attend school due to overwhelming anxiety*

FEATURES: physical Sx of anxiety **confined to weekdays/term-time**
→ *nausea, headache, abdo pain, hyperventilation, general illness*
CAUSES
- Separation anxiety (<11y) – often provoked by life event e.g. death, moving house
- True school phobia (older kids) – anxiety provoked by an aspect of school e.g. bullying

---

Eating disorders covered in Chapter 6: Psychiatry

suggests psychiatric disorder e.g. PTSD

1. **Stop** doing that because…
2. **If you don't** you must go to your room…
3. **Go** to your room

Truancy: child leaves to go to school, but never arrives or leaves early
→ *associates with other behavioural difficulties*

Use **HEEADSS** assessment for adolescent consultations:
Home
Education & **E**mployment
Activities
Drugs/**D**rinking
Sex
Self-harm/**S**uicide
Safety (including **S**ocial media)

Symptoms of CFS

- Myalgia
- Migratory arthralgia
- Headache
- **Poor concentration**
- Irritability
- Stomach pains
- Scalp tenderness
- Eye pain/photophobia
- Cervical lymphadenopathy
- Depression
- **Disturbed sleep patterns**

↳ *Ix to r/o DDx: FBC, CRP, LFT, TFT, blood glucose, urinalysis*

MANAGEMENT: involve child, parents, teachers, psychologist

1. Separation anxiety: gently promote ↑ separation from parents & **graded return to school**
2. True school phobia: **address underlying cause** (e.g. bullying) **and** treat underlying emotional disorders

Chronic fatigue syndrome (CFS)

→ *persistent (>3m) high levels of **subjective fatigue** & rapid exhaustion **that limits daily activities***

CAUSES
- **Viral infection:** EBV, Coxsackie B → specifically known as myalgic encephalomyelitis
- **Psychological factors:** stress, trauma, mental health disorders
- **Genetics:** more common within some families

FEATURES: often worse 24h post physical/mental exertion

MANAGEMENT[61]: most remit spontaneously in months–years
- Energy management – educate on fluctuating energy limits
- Graded exercise therapy – slowly ↑ tolerance
- Diet & sleep optimisation
- ± CBT
- SSRIs if comorbid depression
- Consider analgesia if pain is a significant symptom: following neuropathic pain / headache guidelines

Depression, self-harm, suicide

Some differences to presentation in adults:
- Apathy/boredom & anhedonia more obvious than low mood
- Separation anxiety reappears
- Decline in school performance
- Hypochondrial ideas – complain of chest/abdo pain & headaches
- Irritable mood / antisocial behaviour

NB Poor sleep, lost appetites & slowed cognition = less common

MANAGEMENT[62]: RISK ASSESS!!!
Mild–moderate: low intensity psychotherapy (self-help) → high intensity psychotherapy (CBT)
Severe: high intensity psychotherapy (CBT) + SSRI (fluoxetine)

Drug misuse

SIGNS
- Intoxication / medical complications of use
- Unexplained absences from school/home
- Mixing with known users
- High spending / stealing money

MANAGEMENT: RISK ASSESS!!!
- Interview adolescent
- Urine sample for drug screen
- Referral to drug & alcohol services
- Medical Tx of any complications
- Tx of underlying psychological disorders e.g. depression

Psychosis

→ *breakdown in perception & understanding of reality* → *delusional ideas, hallucinations, odd behaviour*

CAUSES: schizophrenia, bipolar/mania, substance-induced (most common causes in adolescents)
INVESTIGATION: urine drug screen, medication review, exclusion of infection / metabolic disorders
MANAGEMENT: URGENT REFERRAL TO PSYCHIATRIST – antipsychotics, psychotherapy, family education

[61] NICE (2021) *Myalgic encephalomyelitis (or encephalopathy)/chronic fatigue syndrome* [NG206]
[62] NICE (2019) *Depression in children and young people* [NG134]

Safeguarding & abuse

Physical abuse

Suspicious features in history:
- Injury with no explanation / explanation doesn't fit injury
- Injuries to children not yet mobile
- Time delay in seeking medical support
- Varying explanations between carers/child
- Unconcerned/aggressive/vague parents
- Previous Hx of unusual/unexplained injuries

Suspicious features on examination:

Fractures
- In non-mobile child (<18m)
- Multiple fractures but no major trauma
- Rib & skull fractures
- 'Bucket-handle' fractures

Bruises
- In non-mobile child
- In shape of hand/bite/clusters
- Around neck, wrists, ankles, face (not on bony prominence)

Burns
- In shape of instrument e.g. iron
- Glove & stocking pattern – immersion

> **Investigations if abuse is suspected:**
> → Full skeletal X-ray
> → Bloods (r/o organic causes)

Sexual abuse

→ *forcing child to take part in sexual activities ranging from non-physical (watching porn) to rape*

Suspicious signs
- Vaginal/rectal bleeding, discharge, itching
- Soiling/secondary enuresis
- Unexplained STI – note this could be transmitted from mother
- Pregnant – if <13y this is legally sexual abuse
- Depression, self-harm, aggressive, poor school performance

Investigations
- **Examination** requires specialist doctor
- **Forensic testing** may be indicated
→ *often few physical signs*

Emotional abuse

→ *persistent emotional maltreatment that adversely affects child's emotional development*

e.g. telling them they are worthless/unloved, making fun of them, making them feel inadequate

Suspicious signs
- Negative interactions between child & carer
- Apathetic, fearful child
- Urinary & faecal incontinence
- Faltering growth / developmental delay
- Non-attendance at school
- Substance misuse / antisocial behaviour
- Depression, self-harm

> **Estimated prevalence of abuse in children <16y[63]**
> Physical abuse **7.6%**
> Sexual abuse **7.5%** (F:M = 3:1)
> Emotional abuse **9.3%**

> **DDx of physical abuse**
> **Bruises:** clotting/platelet disorder, HSP, Mongolian blue spots
> **Fractures:** osteogenesis imperfecta, osteoporosis (2° to steroids)
> **Burns:** bullous impetigo, scalded skin syndrome, healing skin infection

> **Risk factors for abuse/neglect**
> **The child**
> - Result of forced/commercial sex
> - Not meeting parental expectations
> - Disability / special needs
> - Known to social care
>
> **The carer**
> - Mental health problems
> - Alcohol/drug abuse
> - Young parental age
>
> **The family/environment**
> - Domestic violence
> - Social isolation
> - Poverty / poor housing

---

[63] ONS (2020) *Child abuse extent and nature, England and Wales: year ending March 2019*

Neglect

→ *persistent failure to meet basic physical & psychological needs which seriously impairs health & development*

e.g. inadequate food, clothing, shelter, access to medical care, education, emotional availability/support

deliberate or non-deliberate

Suspicious signs in child
- Consistently missed medical appointments
- Needs medical/dental care, immunisations/glasses
- Seems ravenously hungry
- Dirty, poor clothing
- Faltering growth / developmental delay

Suspicious signs in carer
- Alcohol/drug abuse
- Behaves irrationally/bizarrely/depressed
- Appears indifferent to child

Fabricated or induced illness (FII)

→ *exaggeration/fabrication of, OR deliberately caused symptoms of illness by carer* (>80% mother)

→ *leads to harm of child* e.g. through unnecessary investigations by healthcare staff

Types:
1. **Verbal fabrication:** parents invent signs/symptoms to healthcare staff, leading them to believe child is ill & resulting in unnecessary investigations & treatment e.g. special diets, restricted lifestyle, unneeded medications
2. **Induction of illness:** parents cause illness e.g. inhalation of noxious substances, suffocation, giving unneeded meds

Suspicious signs:
- Frequent unexplained illnesses / hospital admissions
- Symptoms only in presence of carer / not backed up by clinical findings

FII can be difficult to spot, as organic illness may be present concurrently

Managing child abuse: admit child to safety

1. **Thorough history** – be sensitive!
   - Ask to speak to child alone if possible
   - May wish to get background information from GP

2. **Thorough physical examination** – may want to measure height/weight/head circumference & plot on growth chart

3. **Carefully record any medical findings** – in notes / photograph injuries

4. **Observe & document interaction between carers and child**

5. **Treat injuries as necessary**

6. REPORT SUSPICIONS TO SENIOR
   - Assess if immediate protection from harm is needed
     → DO NOT DISCHARGE IF RISK
   - Consider risk to other siblings at home
   - Alert police & social services
   - **Follow local safeguarding policies**

Clinical investigations
1. Full skeletal survey
2. Bloods (r/o organic causes of injury)
3. CT brain (if head trauma)
4. Ophthalmological exam (if subconjunctival haemorrhage)

Emergency paediatrics

Assessment of the seriously ill child (ABCDE)

Airway & Breathing
- **Effort** – RR, WOB, accessory muscles, recessions, added sounds, resp. distress
- **Efficacy** – talking, air entry, SaO_2 (>92%)   *Look, listen, feel, measure*
- **Effects** – skin colour, conscious level

Circulation
- **Heart** – rate, rhythm, pulse
- **Blood pressure** – hypotension = **late sign**
- **Capillary refill** (<2s)
- **Peripheral temp., colour**

Disability (DEFG = Don't Ever Forget Glucose)
- **Level of consciousness** (AVPU)
- **Pupils** – size, reactivity
- **Posture & tone**
- **Blood glucose**

> **ALERT**
> **VOICE** responsive
> **PAIN** responsive
> **UNRESPONSIVE**

Exposure
- **Rash, injuries, bruises**
- **Pain** (GCS) – consider analgesia

Management of the seriously ill child

Airway & breathing
- **Open & maintain airway** – head tilt, chin lift, jaw thrust
- **5 initial rescue breaths if needed** – ideally via mask
- **100% high flow O_2** – non-rebreathe mask
- **Anaesthetist involvement** – if need intubation (ET tube)

Circulation
- **Chest compressions if needed** 100–120/min
- **Obtain IV access** – 2 wide-bore cannulas   **IO access after 3 IV attempts**
- **Take bloods** – FBC, U&E, glucose, X-match ± cultures
- **Fluid bolus** – 20ml/kg 0.9% saline over 10min
- **Catheterise** – guide fluid resuscitation
- **Consider inotropes** – guide fluid resuscitation

→ Continuous monitoring & reassessment

Shock

→ *inadequate circulation to meet metabolic demands of tissues*

CAUSES
→ **Hypovolaemic** (bleeds, burns, fever, D&V, urinary losses)
→ **Fluid maldistribution** (sepsis, intestinal obstruction)
→ **Obstructive** (cardiac tamponade, PE, tension pneumothorax)
→ **Cardiogenic** (RARE: myocarditis, congenital heart disease)

MANAGEMENT[64]
1. **Fluid resuscitation** = priority → 0.9% saline bolus (20ml/kg)
2. **If no improvement, involve PICU**
   - Tracheal intubation + mechanical ventilation
   - Invasive BP monitoring (arterial line)
   - Inotropic support
   - Correction of metabolic/biochemical/haem derangements
   - Support for liver/renal failure

[64] NICE (2015, updated 2020) *Intravenous fluid therapy in children and young people in hospital* [NG29]

Normal parameters

Age	RR/min	HR/min	SBP (mmHg)
Neonate: <28d	50–60	120–160	50–70
Infant: <1y	30–40	110–160	70–90
Child: <5y	25–35	95–140	80–100
Child: <12y	20–25	80–120	90–110

Clinical signs of shock

Early signs
- Tachypnoea, tachycardia
- Cap refill >2s
- ↓ skin turgor, sunken eyes/fontanelle
- Mottled, pale, cold skin
- Oliguria <0.5–1ml/kg/h

Late signs
- Hypotension, bradycardia
- Metabolic acidosis
- Depressed cerebral state

SEPTIC SHOCK

Causative organisms
Neonates: GBS, Gram −ve
Children: meningococcus

Clinical features
Features of shock plus:
- Fever, lethargy, misery
- Poor feeding
± purpuric rash (meningococcal)

Management
1. Fluid resuscitation
2. **IV ABX ASAP**
   - Ideally after cultures
3. Further support if need

Keep reassessing

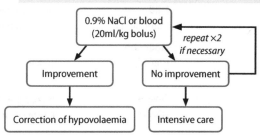

Fig. 5.52 Fluid resuscitation.

This accounts for the requirement of **1–2mmol/kg/d of potassium**

Deficit (ml) = % dehydration × body weight (kg) × 10

Example: 42kg child is clinically dehydrated (5%), but not shocked
Needs REPLACEMENT + MAINTENANCE
1. **Maintenance** = 1940ml/d (see above)
2. **Deficit** = 5% × weight × 10 = 5 × 42 × 10 = 2100ml/d
3. **Total replacement fluid over 24h** = 1940 + 2100 = 4040ml/d

If not shocked / clinical dehydration:
Deficit replacement = 50ml/kg (5% × weight × 10)

If shocked / severe dehydration:
Deficit replacement = 100ml/kg (10% × weight × 10)

Fluid therapy[65]

MAINTENANCE FLUIDS: if NBM / not drinking enough
Maintenance fluids for infants & children: 0.9% saline + 5% dextrose + 10mmol KCl

Estimate blood vol.: 80ml/kg
Estimate body weight:
<9y = 2(age+4)
>9y = 3 × age

	Fluid requirements over 24h	Fluid requirements per hour
1st 10kg	100ml/kg	4ml/kg
2nd 10kg	50ml/kg	2ml/kg
Subsequent kg	20ml/kg	1ml/kg

Examples of calculating maintenance fluids:
18kg child: 10×100 + 8×50 = **1400ml/d**
              10×4 + 8×2 = **56ml/h**
42kg child: 10×100 + 10×50 + 22×20 = **1940ml/d**
              10×4 + 10×2 + 22×1 = **82ml/h**

TYPES OF FLUID

	Na$^+$ (mmol/L)	Cl$^-$ (mmol/L)	Additives
Plasma	135–145	100–110	K$^+$, lactate, calcium, glucose
0.9% NaCl	154	154	–
Hartmann's	131	111	K$^+$, lactate, calcium
Plasmalyte	140	98	K$^+$, acetate, magnesium
5% dextrose	–	–	50g glucose
0.9% NaCl + 5% glucose	154	154	50g glucose

↳ *use a combination of fluids for replacement/maintenance to ensure it reaches all areas of the body*

Beware risk of hyperchloraemia with 0.9% NaCl
⅓ stays in vasculature
⅔ into extracellular space
Little enters cells = good for treating SHOCK
→ *Very little stays in circulation*

MANAGEMENT OF DEHYDRATION: if existing deficit

1. **Correct deficit** = % dehydration × body weight × 10
2. **Maintenance fluids** = see above
3. **Account for ongoing losses** (e.g. fever/GI)
   • **Gastric losses (vomiting)** = saline + K$^+$
   • **Diarrhoeal losses** = saline, K$^+$, glucose, HCO$_3^-$

Use oral route if possible!
weight loss = most accurate measure of dehydration

Degree of dehydration	Clinical signs	Fluid deficit	Management
Mild (sub-clinical)	Dry mucous membranes, ↑ thirst, ↓ urine output	**5% of body weight** = 50ml/kg	Maintenance fluids over 24h (oral intake / ORT if possible)
Moderate (clinical)	Tachycardia, CRT >2, ↓ turgor Tachypnoea	**5–10% of body weight** = 100ml/kg	Replace fluid deficit over 4h **PLUS** Maintenance fluids over 24h (oral/NG tube if possible)
Severe (shock)	Weak pulses, CRT >3, ↓ turgor Kussmaul breathing Hypotension, ↓ consciousness, very tachycardic	**>10–15% of body weight** = 150ml/kg	IV bolus: 20ml/kg 0.9% saline over 10min **Improvement:** replace deficit + maintenance **No improvement:** repeat bolus ×2 then PICU

[65]NICE (2015, updated 2020) *Intravenous fluid therapy in children and young people in hospital* [NG29]

Anaphylaxis

→ *life-threatening hypersensitivity reaction (IgE) with rapid onset airway & circulation problems*

ACUTE MANAGEMENT[66]

1. **IM adrenaline 1:1000** – repeat in 5min if no improvement
   - <6m = 100–150mcg (0.1–0.15ml)
   - <6y = 150mcg (0.15ml)
   - 6–12y = 300mcg (0.30ml)
   - >12y = 500mcg (0.50ml)

   1 in 1000 = fatal

2. **ABC** (AND CALL FOR HELP!)
   - **Airway:** secure airway
   - **Breathing:** high flow O_2 + SABA if wheezy
   - **Circulation:** lie supine with legs raised + IV fluids if shock (20ml/kg crystalloids)
3. **Non-sedating antihistamines**
4. **Monitor** – pulse oximetry, ECG, BP

LONG-TERM MANAGEMENT

- Prescribe EpiPen to keep at home/school – counsel on use
- Safety-net: allergen avoidance, signs of anaphylaxis
- Consider referral for allergy testing

> **Causes of anaphylaxis**
>
> - **Food allergy (85%)**   • Drugs
> - Insect stings   • Latex

> **Symptoms of anaphylaxis**
>
> - Difficulty breathing/swallowing
> - Stridor ± wheeze
> - Angioedema (swollen face/tongue)
> - Urticaria
> - Pale, clammy
>
> → **SHOCK may develop**

> **DDx:** asthma, panic attack, septic shock

Poisoning/overdose

→ *accidental* (young children), *deliberate self-harm* (adolescents), *abuse* (by carer)

Poison	Effects	Management
Alcohol	• Hypoglycaemia • Coma • Respiratory failure	• Check blood alcohol levels • **Monitor blood glucose** • Ventilatory support
Acids/alkalis	• Inflammation & ulceration of GI tract	• Early endoscopy
Ethylene glycol (antifreeze)	• Tachycardia • Metabolic acidosis • Renal failure	• **FOMEPIZOLE** • Haemodialysis
Paracetamol	24–48h: abdo pain, vomiting 3–5d: liver failure	• Measure plasma paracetamol conc. • **IV N-ACETYLCYSTEINE**
NSAIDs	Within 4h: • N&V, drowsiness, blurred vision, tinnitus • Hyperventilation • Acute renal failure	• Measure plasma salicylate conc. • Rapid BG, blood gases, Cr, FBC, ECG • **Supportive Tx:** fluids, dialysis etc. • **NO ANTIDOTE**
Iron	Initial: V&D, haematemesis, melaena, gastric ulcers **Latent period** 6h later: drowsy, coma, shock, convulse, liver fails	• Measure serum iron levels • **IV DEFEROXAMINE** (chelates iron)
Methadone	• Drowsiness, mitosis, vomiting • Tachypnoea/apnoea → resp. acidosis	• Activated charcoal within 1h • **IV NALOXONE**

TCAs	• Tachycardia, arrhythmias
	• Dry mouth, blurred vision
	• Agitation, confusion, convulsions
	• Respiratory depression
		• **IV SODIUM BICARB**
		  ▸ Correct metabolic acidosis
		  ▸ Ventilatory support
		  ▸ Sodium bicarbonate if arrhythmias
		  ▸ Diazepam if convulsions

GENERAL MANAGEMENT OF OVERDOSE/POISONING

1. **Identify agent & amount taken** (ask patient/parents, Sx, blood levels)
2. **Check if activated charcoal can be used to ↓ absorption**
3. **Investigations** – FBC, renal & liver function, ECG, ABG — ineffective for iron & pesticides
4. **Give antidote** – if available / toxicity high enough
5. **Supportive Tx:** ventilatory support, IV fluids etc.

Brief resolved unexplained events (BRUE)

→ *frightening combination of symptoms: most common in <10w*

- Apnoea
- Colour change
- Altered muscle tone
- Choking/gagging

POTENTIAL CAUSES

- **No cause identified = 50%**
- Upper airway obstruction
- Infections (URTI)
- Seizures
- Gastro-oesophageal reflux
- Cardiac arrhythmia

> **Further Ix to consider**
> - CXR – respiratory infection
> - EEG – seizure
> - Urinalysis (MCS) – infection
> - Oesophageal pH – reflux
> - Barium swallow – obstruction
> - Lumbar puncture – infection

MANAGEMENT[67]

1. **Detailed Hx & examination**
   → including social Hx to r/o abuse
2. **Admission to hospital**
   → basic investigations (FBC, U&E, LFT, glucose, lactate, blood gas, ECG)
   → usually need overnight monitoring (SaO$_2$, RR, HR, BP)
3. **Discharge if normal obs & no high risk features**
   → train parents in basic life support

> **High risk features**
> - <8w/o **or** was premature
> - multiple episodes **or** episodes >1min
> - suspect abuse
> - concerning Hx/examination features
>   *e.g. FHx cardiac death, infective Sx*

Sudden infant death syndrome (SIDS)

→ *sudden, unexpected death of an infant with no identifiable cause*

RISK FACTORS

The infant	The parents	The environment
Age: 1–6m (peak 2–4m)	Low income, poor/overcrowded housing	Co-sleeping
Preterm **or** LBW	Parental smoking	Overheated baby hot room, too many blankets
Male	• Single, unsupported mum • Maternal age <20y	Baby sleeping on tummy

> **DDx / underlying cause of SIDS**
> - Cardiac abnormalities
> - Metabolic abnormalities
> - Sepsis
> - NAI (shaken baby)

PREVENTION

- Put infants to sleep on back & 'feet to foot'
- Avoid heavy wrapping or hot room
- Do not co-sleep – esp. if tired/alcohol/drugs
- Sleep with baby in same room for 6m
- Do not smoke near infant
- Seek medical advice ASAP if baby becomes unwell

After sudden death of an infant

- Inform police & coroner
- Detailed Hx & examination of infant (post mortem)
- Allow parents to see baby
- Bereavement support & counselling

---

[67] Tate C, Sunley R Brief resolved unexplained events (formerly apparent life-threatening events) and evaluation of lower-risk infants—*Archives of Disease in Childhood—Education and Practice* 2018;103:95–98

Injuries & trauma

→ *major cause of death in those aged 1–14y*

ROAD TRAFFIC ACCIDENTS (passenger or pedestrian)
→ Most common cause of death / serious injury in childhood

HEAD INJURIES (most minor but 1 in 800 develop serious problems)
Assessment
- **ABCDE** (especially consciousness & pupils)
- **Monitor for 2° damage**

Management[68]
Mild: discharge with written advice
Potentially severe: monitor for signs of 2° damage
Severe: resuscitation, CT, neurosurgical referral

Complications
- **Hypoxia:** airway obstruction / ↓ ventilation
- **Hypo-/hyperglycaemia**
- **↓ Cerebral perfusion:** ↑ ICP, ↓ BP from bleed
- **Haematoma**
- **Infection:** open wound, CSF leak

BURNS & SCALDS (death usually due to smoke inhalation rather than burn)

Assessing the burn
A: early intubation if airway swelling
B: check for airway burns
  ▸ soot in nose, coughing black sputum
  ▸ stridor, hoarseness, cough
  ▸ breathing/swallowing difficulties
C: check BP & if low ensure no other cause for fluid loss e.g. bleed
D: assess pain with pain score
E: assess severity of burn: surface area, depth, involvement of delicate sites

Management
1. **Burns first aid:** cold water 20min + clingfilm
2. **Analgesia** e.g. IV morphine
3. **Fluid resuscitation** – if shock / >10% surface area
4. **Wound care**
   - **Superficial** = clean & dress
   - **Deeper, >5%, sensitive areas** = specialist review   *face, ears, eyes, perineum*

NEAR DROWNING → *BATHS* *(neonates),* ***POOLS/LAKES*** *(toddlers/children)*
1. Mouth-to-mouth resuscitation & CPR
2. Cover and keep warm
3. **Hospital admission:** monitor for respiratory distress, pulmonary oedema, development of pneumonia

CHOKING/ASPIRATION
→ **Unconscious:** paediatric BLS
→ **Conscious & ineffective cough:** 5 back blows, 5 abdo thrusts
(chest thrusts if aged <1y)

Red flags of head injuries

- LOC >5min
- Seizure
- GCS <15 2h post-injury
- Focal neurological deficit
- Amnesia >5min
- Signs of fracture
- High risk trauma
- ≥3× vomiting

Surface area
Patient's palm = 1% of body surface area
- Add 0.5% to each leg with every year >1y of age
- Subtract 2% from head with every year >1y of age

Specialist review of burn if:

- full thickness >5%
- partial thickness >10%
- sensitive area
- chemical/electrical burn

---

[68] NICE (2014, updated 2019) *Head injury* [CG176]

Status epilepticus

→ *seizure >30min OR successive seizures over 30min with no recovery between*

MANAGEMENT[69]
1. ABCDE
- Secure airway, high flow O$_2$, secure IV access
- **D**on't **E**ver **F**orget **G**lucose (r/o hypoglycaemia)
- Confirm it is an epileptic seizure (Hx, features, etc.)

2. Manage convulsion

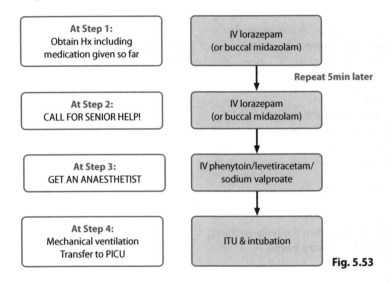

At Step 1: Obtain Hx including medication given so far	IV lorazepam (or buccal midazolam)
At Step 2: CALL FOR SENIOR HELP!	*Repeat 5min later* → IV lorazepam (or buccal midazolam)
At Step 3: GET AN ANAESTHETIST	IV phenytoin/levetiracetam/ sodium valproate
At Step 4: Mechanical ventilation Transfer to PICU	ITU & intubation

Fig. 5.53

Diabetic ketoacidosis

→ *see Chapter 2: Endocrinology in* General Medicine and Surgery, *the companion volume to this book*

PSYCHIATRY

06

ABBREVIATIONS

AD – Antidepressant
ADHD – Attention deficit hyperactivity disorder
ADLs – Activities of daily living
AMHP – Advanced mental health practitioner
AP – Antipsychotic
ASD – Autism spectrum disorder
BPAD – Bipolar affective disorder
BZD – Benzodiazepine
CAMHS – Child and Adolescent Mental Health Services
CBT – Cognitive behavioural therapy
CK – Creatine kinase
CNS – Central nervous system
CPN – Community psychiatric nurse
CTO – Community treatment order
DA – Dopamine
DBT – Dialectical behaviour therapy
DEXA – Dual-energy X-ray absorptiometry
ECT – Electroconvulsive therapy
EEG – Electroencephalogram
EMDR – Eye movement desensitisation & reprocessing
EPSE – Extra-pyramidal side-effects
EUPD – Emotionally unstable personality disorder
GABA – Gamma-aminobutyric acid
GAD – Generalised anxiety disorder
GGT – Gamma-glutamyl transferase
IAPT – Improving access to psychological therapies
ICD-10 – International Classification of Diseases 10th Revision
ID – Intellectual disability

LDL – Low density lipoproteins
LSD – Lysergic acid diethylamide
MAO(I) – Monoamine oxidase (inhibitor)
MBT – Mentalisation-based therapy
MCA – Mental Capacity Act
MCV – Mean corpuscular volume
MDMA – 3,4-methylenedioxymethamphetamine
MHA – Mental Health Act
MS – Multiple sclerosis
MSE – Mental state exam
MZ twins – Monozygotic twins
NA – Noradrenaline
NaSSA – Noradrenergic and specific serotonergic antidepressants
NMS – Neuroleptic malignant syndrome
OCD – Obsessive–compulsive disorder
OCP – Oral contraceptive pill
PD – Personality disorder
PPD – Postpartum depression
PPP – Postpartum psychosis
PTSD – Post-traumatic stress disorder
SLE – Systemic lupus erythematosus
SNRI – Serotonin-norepinephrine reuptake Inhibitor
SNS – Sympathetic nervous system
SSRI – Selective serotonin reuptake inhibitor
STI – Sexually transmitted infection
TCA – Tricyclic antidepressant
THC – Tetrahydrocannabinol

Mental Health Act (MHA 1983) & legislation

yellow highlight = **most important to know as junior doctor**

MENTAL HEALTH ACT 1983: legislation that allows people to be detained in hospital for assessment and/or treatment of their mental illness, providing certain criteria are met.

Only allows treatment of **mental illness**, not physical conditions. Treating physical illness against a person's wishes requires assessment under the **Mental Capacity Act** in patient's **best interests**.

See Chapter 2: Geriatrics for more information on MCA

Section	Type of order	Length	Staff involved	Explanation
2	Assessment	Up to 28d	2 doctors + AMHP • 1 'section 12' approved doctor (specific expertise in mental illness) • another doctor (who has ideally met patient before) • AMHP	**When diagnosis unclear / no treatment plan** • Allows detention **for period of assessment** (& Tx if needed) • After 28d must decide on **section 3 or informal Tx** *Cannot implement back-to-back Sections*
3	Treatment	Up to 6m		**When definitive diagnosis with treatment plan** • Allows detention and Tx against patient's will *Can be renewed after 6m & then after 12m* *Appropriate treatment **must be available at the** hospital named on the form*
4	Emergency	Up to 72h	1 doctor + AMHP	Allows emergency detention if only 1 qualified mental health doctor present & waiting for a second medical recommendation would involve undesirable delay *Can convert to Section 2/3 after 2nd doctor assessment*
5(2)	Emergency 'Doctor's holding power'	Up to 72h	1 registered medical practitioner **Not F1 as not fully registered** (ideally the responsible clinician OR nominated deputy – usually most senior team member)	• Allows detention by **any registered doctor** until formal assessment can be done • **Only inpatients** (excludes A&E) • **Cannot treat** • Tell an AMHP or psychiatrist that it has been implemented ASAP *Cannot implement back-to-back Sections*
5(4)	Emergency 'Nurse's holding power'	Up to 6h	1 registered mental health nurse / 1 learning disability nurse	• Allows detention until appropriate doctor can assess • Patient must be already receiving treatment for mental health as an inpatient *Cannot implement back-to-back Sections*
135	Power of entry	Up to 36h	Magistrate (AMHP applies to magistrates' court)	Allows police to enter home and remove person to place of safety *If they have a warrant*
136	Place of safety	Up to 36h	Police officer	• Allows police to remove person to a place of safety for formal assessment e.g. A&E, 136 suite, (police station in exceptional circumstances) • Applies to someone suffering from a mental disorder, is outside their home & is in immediate need of care or control for the safety of themselves or others
17A	Community treatment order (CTO)	As needed/ indefinitely	AMHP	• Allows Tx under MHA while living in community • Only relates to **psychiatric care** (not physical health) *Non-compliance can result in recall to hospital / revoking of CTO*

Alcohol & substance misuse

Definitions

Acute intoxication: transient physical & mental abnormalities shortly after administration e.g. altered cognition/behaviour

Harmful use: continued use despite evidence of damage to physical/mental health or social wellbeing but no dependence

Withdrawal: physical dependence causes physical symptoms on abrupt cessation e.g. seizures, delirium, psychosis

Tolerance: need to take more drug for same effect – often choose more rapidly acting administration route

Dependence syndrome: obtaining drug becomes priority in life (primacy), continued use despite negative consequences, loss of control of consumption, tend towards single preferred drug, tolerance & withdrawal

Alcohol misuse

↳ Costs NHS £3.5 billion per year

→ In UK **9% men & 4% women** are dependent

→ Younger people drink more heavily, older people drink more frequently

→ **Alcoholic liver disease** is greatest cause of alcohol-related deaths

↳ prevalence is increasing

RISK FACTORS:

- Genetics & gender – male > female
- Mental illness – depression, anxiety disorders, schizophrenia
- Stress, low self-esteem, social anxiety/isolation
- Significant life events – bereavement, trauma
- Lower socioeconomic status
- Occupation – bartenders, farmers, healthcare professionals

Complications of alcohol misuse

Medical consequences	Psychiatric consequences
CNS: cognitive/memory impairment, reduced brain volume, cerebellar degeneration, Wernicke–Korsakoff syndrome **PNS:** peripheral neuropathy, optic atrophy	**Alcoholic hallucinosis:** hallucinations while sober / after 12–24h of abstinence (usually visual) Respond well to antipsychotics & typically resolve in 24–48h DDx: acute psychotic episode, delirium tremens
Hepatic: fatty liver, hepatitis, cirrhosis*, hepatocellular carcinoma, hepatosplenomegaly, pancreatitis *risk in women	**Pathological jealousy** – primary delusion that partner is unfaithful → associated with violence towards partner
Gastric: gastritis/ulcer, carcinoma, oesophageal varices, Barrett's, Mallory–Weiss tears	**ARBD (alcohol-related brain damage):** cognitive/memory impairment & dementia
Renal: CKD, hepato-renal syndrome	Anxiety & depression
GI: malabsorption, diarrhoea, thiamine deficiency (Wernicke's) + niacin deficiency (pellagra), GI cancer	Suicide (10–15% risk)
CVS: cardiomyopathy, arrhythmias, HTN, cerebrovascular events ↳ esp. AF	Schizophrenia – increases risk of relapse & violence
Reproductive: sexual dysfunction, infertility, fetal alcohol syndrome	

Acute Wernicke–Korsakoff syndrome: due to thiamine (vitamin B1) deficiency**

Wernicke's encephalopathy: → progresses in 80%
- Acute confusion
- Ophthalmoplegia/nystagmus
- Ataxic gait

Treat promptly to prevent progression & death:
IV Pabrinex (vit B & C) + alcohol withdrawal Tx

Korsakoff syndrome:
- Antero-/retrograde amnesia
- Confabulation (false memories)
- Apathy (indifference/↓ interest)

ICD-10 diagnostic criteria: 5/6 in past year

Tolerance	Tremor (**withdrawal Sx**)
Control loss	Compulsion
Primacy	Persistence despite harm

One unit = 10ml ethanol
Guidelines = ≤14 units per week*

*spread over ≥3 days

Social consequences of alcohol misuse
- Relationship problems/domestic violence
- Risky sexual activity
- Missed work/poor performance
- Suicide/homicide
- Financial & legal problems (contact with criminal justice system)

****In alcoholics:** poor diet & ↓ absorption/hepatic storage

Wernicke's prognosis
15% mortality if untreated
20% complete recovery
25% significant recovery

Patients often non-compliant

Stages of change model describes how ready patients are to change behaviours

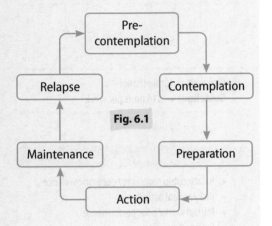

Fig. 6.1

Investigating alcohol misuse

→ *often missed (patient denial is a problem)*

HISTORY
Lifetime pattern of consumption
- When did they begin to drink regularly / first feel they had a problem?
- Reasons for periods of heavy drinking

Current pattern of consumption
- How often, what type of drink, how much?
- Where and when?
- Description of a typical day / heavy day of drinking

Signs of dependence
- Withdrawal symptoms in morning / if not had a drink
- Having to drink more for same effect (tolerance)
- Episodes of memory loss / blackouts (amnesia)

Social/occupational problems
- Missed days of work / lost job
- Relationship difficulties
- Financial impact, criminal charges

Previous treatment attempts
- Nature and effectiveness

Physical and mental health (often comorbid mental health Dx)
- Resulting from or exacerbated by drinking

INVESTIGATIONS
- **MCV** – stays raised 3–6m after abstinence
- **GGT** – alcohol-related liver inflammation
- **Liver USS** – if indicated

PHYSICAL EXAMINATION
- Of major systems (liver stigmata, cerebellar signs, peripheral neuropathy) & for symptoms of withdrawal

Withdrawal effects	Timeframe	Signs & Sx
Withdrawal symptoms	**>6h** after last drink. Resolve in 24–48h	Insomnia, tremor, anxiety, GI upset, headache, sweating, palpitations
Seizures	**12–48h** after last drink	Tonic–clonic seizures
Delirium tremens	**48–96h** after last drink. Last 1–5d	Hallucinations, disorientation, ↑HR, ↑BP, sweating, fever, agitation. **Emergency admission for Tx:** PO lorazepam, thiamine, hydration
Alcoholic hallucinosis	**12–24h** after last drink. Resolve in 24–48h	Vivid visual hallucinations (have insight)

Management of alcohol misuse[1]

→ *in the community unless severe/high risk delirium tremens / liver failure*

PSYCHOSOCIAL

RISK ASSESS

- Drug & alcohol services (e.g. Alcoholics Anonymous)
- Motivational interviewing, CBT, counselling, self-help resources
- Housing, financial, childcare support, avoid other users

BIOLOGICAL
1. **Detoxification/withdrawal management:** reducing regimen over 7–10d
   - Chlordiazepoxide – a BZD to treat withdrawal symptoms
   - Thiamine (B1) – to avoid/treat Wernicke–Korsakoff syndrome
2. **Maintaining abstinence:**
   - Disulfiram – irreversible inhibition of acetaldehyde dehydrogenase (ALDH) causing acetaldehyde build-up
     ↳ unpleasant symptoms of flushing, headache, nausea deter further alcohol consumption
   - Acamprosate – enhances GABA transmission to reduce alcohol cravings (contraindicated in renal failure)
   - Naltrexone – reduces euphoric effects (can raise liver enzymes)

Screening questions to detect misuse: CAGE

Cut down – ever felt you should cut down your drinking?
Annoyed – ever been annoyed by others criticising your drinking?
Guilty – ever felt bad/guilty about your drinking?
Eye opener – ever drunk first thing in the morning to steady nerves?

Poor prognostic factors

- Ambivalent about change
- Homeless / unstable accommodation
- Unemployed
- Lack family / social support
- Repeated treatment failures

[1] NICE (2011) *Alcohol-use disorders* [CG115]

Illicit substances

Class of substance	Mechanism	Effects
OPIATES • Heroin (diamorphine) • Morphine → smoked or IV • Methadone • Pethidine	μ opioid receptor agonist = GABA inhibition = reduced inhibition of dopamine release	**Effects:** euphoria, sedation, strong analgesia **SEs:** N & V, constipation, respiratory depression, ↓ consciousness, pinpoint pupils **Withdrawal:** irritable/anxious, **sweating**, shaking, restlessness, **insomnia**, fever/chills, **diarrhoea**, arthralgia/myalgia, **blown pupils** → very unpleasant but rarely serious
DEPRESSANTS • Alcohol • Cannabis – smoked • Barbiturates • BZDs – oral	**BZDs** Potentiate GABA at GABAa receptor	**Effects:** suppressed CNS activity, anxiolytic **SEs:** sedation, dizziness, impaired concentration/coordination, depression **Withdrawal from BZDs:** agitation, anxiety, insomnia, seizures, delirium, psychosis → may be fatal
STIMULANTS • Cocaine ('Charlie') – snorted • Crack cocaine – smoked • Amphetamines • MDMA (Ecstasy) – oral	**Cocaine** Monoamine reuptake inhibition (increased DA, NA, serotonin)	**Effects:** euphoria, feelings of extreme wellbeing, increased mental & motor activity, alertness, energy, confidence → risky/aggressive behaviour **SEs cocaine:** ↑HR, arrhythmias, septal necrosis, panic disorder / paranoia, psychosis **SEs MDMA:** nausea, blurred vision, dehydration, depression/anxiety **Withdrawal:** dysphoria/anxiety, fatigue, muscle aches/tremors, craving → unpleasant but rarely serious
HALLUCINOGENS • Cannabis ('dope') – smoked • LSD • PCP (phenylcyclidine) • Ketamine • Psilocybin (magic mushrooms)	**Cannabis** THC = active chemical → binds CB1 receptors to cause effects **LSD:** 5HT receptor agonist	**Effects:** altered sensory/perceptual experiences (delusions/hallucinations), detachment **SEs:** dizziness, dilated pupils, ↑HR, HTN, ↑appetite, anxiety/panic attacks Link between use of cannabis at young age and developing schizophrenia

New psychoactive substances (legal highs) → now illegal
→ plant-based/synthetic substances mimicking effects of illicit drugs

Management of illicit substance misuse

BIOLOGICAL

1. Detoxification/withdrawal management
→ α blocker for autonomic Sx

Symptom reduction: Lofexidine, loperamide, → diarrhoea
metoclopramide, Z-drugs, ibuprofen
→ nausea → insomnia → pain

2. Maintenance

Substitute medications: Methadone, buprenorphine
(opiate replacement) Long-acting opioid causes constant receptor occupation so taking illicit opioid on top has no effect

PSYCHOSOCIAL

• Drug & alcohol services (e.g. Narcotics Anonymous)
• Motivational interviewing, CBT, counselling, self-help resources
• Housing, financial, childcare support
• **Harm reduction:** promote use of sterile needles / don't reuse or share (if not willing to give up completely)

> **Complications of IV drug use:**
> • abscesses/cellulitis/osteomyelitis
> • bacterial endocarditis / septicaemia
> • transmission of viruses (HIV, Hep B/C)

Depression

Estimated 5% of global population (large increase since Covid pandemic); prevalence peaks in older adults >55y (but increasing numbers in younger population); F>M (including postpartum depression)[2,3]

ICD-10 criteria: symptoms for ≥2w

- **Mild:** 2 core + 2 other (total = 4)
- **Mod.:** 2/3 core + 3/4 other (total = 6)
- **Severe:** 3 core + 5 other (total = 8)

Somatic syndrome: physical Sx of depression

- ↓ appetite & weight loss (>5% in 1m)
- early morning waking
- psychomotor retardation/agitation
- ↓ energy & libido

Symptoms

Core symptoms	Other symptoms – 'GAPSSS'
1. Low mood worse in morning	**G**uilt/hopelessness
	Appetite changes (weight loss/gain)
2. Anhedonia loss of pleasure in activities	**P**oor memory, **P**essimism, **P**sychosis
	Sleep disturbance
3. Fatigue	**S**elf-harm / **S**uicidal thoughts
	Self-esteem = low

Hallucinations
= 2nd person, derogatory
→ Delusions
= persecutory, nihilistic
(e.g. rotting inside)
Big risk factor for suicide

Risk factors

MAO theory: ↓ noradrenaline, 5-HT, D2, GABA
- **Social:** life events, isolation, loss, childhood abuse
- **Biological:** FHx, hormonal changes, chronic/severe illness
- **Psychological:** negative thoughts, high expressed emotion, criticism, personality disorder
- **Medications:** steroids, antipsychotics, substance misuse

Prognosis for depression
- 50% recover in 1y (60% relapse)
- 25% = chronic depression (>2y)
- 5–15% die by suicide

Differentials

- **Psychiatric:** schizophrenia, anxiety disorder, SAD, BPAD, dysthymia
- **Neurological:** Parkinson's, MS, head injury, cerebral tumour, dementia
- **Endocrine:** hypothyroidism, hyperparathyroidism, Cushing's, Addison's
- **Infections:** HIV/AIDS, glandular fever, STIs
- **Systemic:** malignancies, SLE, RA, renal failure

Counselling newly diagnosed patients

- Be aware of stigma
- Explain different courses, outcomes, treatments
- **Remain positive** & highlight the benefits of treatment
- Stress importance of treatment adherence

Management[4]

All cases need assessment and active monitoring

BIOPSYCHOSOCIAL APPROACH

1. Biological interventions
   - **Antidepressants**
   - Atypical **antipsychotics** (if psychosis)
   - Augmentation with **lithium** (Tx-resistant)
   - Augmentation with **T₃** (Tx-resistant)

2. Psychological interventions
   - Psychoeducation   • Sleep hygiene
   - CBT   • Self-help e.g. apps
   - Mindfulness   • **IAPT services**

3. Social interventions
   - Support for education, training, employment
   - Support for housing/benefits
   - Carer support: info, support groups, assessment
   - CPN (monitor Sx, mood, mental state) if severe

Mild/moderate depression:
Primary care
Low intensity psychological interventions (IAPT)
Consider 1st-line medication (SSRI)

↓

Moderate/severe or Tx-resistant:
Primary care (may consider referral to 2°)
1st-line medication (SSRI) or alternative
High intensity psychological interventions

↓

Severe depression:
Inpatient or crisis resolution & home treatment
1st-line medication or alternatives/adjuncts (Li²⁺)
High intensity psychological interventions
ECT

NICE guidelines: not indicated if only **mild/subthreshold symptoms** for <2w & no Hx of depression

Inadequate response to Tx: Consider ↑ dose, combine or augment
No response to Tx: switch drug

[2] WHO (2021) *Factsheets: Depression*
[3] NICE CKS (2022) *Depression*
[4] NICE (2009) *Depression in adults* [CG90]

Antidepressants

Starting treatment
→ Rule out bipolar before starting antidepressant monotherapy!

1. Consider SEs, cautions, CIs
2. Start an effective but tolerated dose → trial for 3–4w before deciding if it is working
3. Review regularly
   ↳ 70% respond to 1st Tx

Withdrawal
DO NOT STOP ABRUPTLY: taper dose over 4w
- Withdrawal symptoms particularly noticeable with **paroxetine & venlafaxine**
- Continue **for at least 6m after resolution** of symptoms

St John's wort: unlicensed herbal remedy for treating depression
→ evidence of efficacy but difficult to guide on dosing

SJW = a cytochrome P450 inducer causing metabolism and therapy failure of:
- OCP
- Warfarin
- Digoxin
- Phenytoin, carbamazepine

Withdrawal symptoms
- Dizzy, numb/tingling
- Nausea/vomiting
- Headache
- Sweating
- Anxiety
- Sleep disturbance / strange dreams
- Shaking
- 'Shock' sensations

Types of antidepressant

Class	Drug	MOA & other notes	SEs, cautions & CIs
SSRI	**Sertraline** Fluoxetine Paroxetine Citalopram	Inhibit pre-synaptic 5-HT reuptake Take **up to 6w** for effect Symptoms may worsen before improving **1st line** (fewer SEs)	SEs: **nausea, insomnia**, fatigue, diarrhoea, dizziness, sexual dysfunction, restlessness Cautions: long QT, bleeding disorders (especially citalopram) BUT sertraline is indicated if post-MI CIs: poorly controlled epilepsy Paroxetine = teratogenic ⎡Advise against alcohol with antidepressants, as additive sedation effects⎤
SNRI	**Venlafaxine** Duloxetine	Inhibit 5-HT & NA reuptake 2nd/3rd line	SEs: more prominent **sedation & sexual dysfunction** & same as above Cautions: diabetes, uncontrolled HTN, bleeding disorders, epilepsy
TCA	Amitriptyline Imipramine Lofepramine Dosulepin	Inhibit 5-HT & NA reuptake 1st line in **pregnancy**	SEs: **sedation**, weight gain, dizziness, HTN, delirium, **antimuscarinic*** *dry mouth, blurred vision, constipation, urinary retention Cautions: bipolar, diabetes, epilepsy, high suicide risk CIs: arrhythmias, heart block, post-MI ↳ toxic in overdose
MAOI	Phenelzine Isocarboxazid Moclobemide	Irreversible MAO A & B inhibition Tx-resistant/atypical depression	SEs: nausea, diarrhoea, constipation, dry mouth, sleep disturbance, postural hypotension, headache Cautions: bleeding disorders, diabetes, elderly Interact with many drugs / tyramine-containing foods (hypertensive crisis) → rarely used
NaSSA	Mirtazapine	α2 receptor blockage = ↑ NA & 5-HT efflux Adjunct in Tx-resistant depression	SEs: **weight gain & sedation**, dizziness, headache Cautions: diabetes, seizures, urinary retention, elderly ⎡Especially good if sleep disturbance / lost appetite⎤

Anxiety disorders

Most common psych condition

Key feature for diagnosis

Pathological responses to **minimal environmental triggers**, resulting in **persistent symptoms** that **impair function** &/or cause **disabling behaviours** e.g. avoidance → discomfort too intense for patient to bear

Symptoms

Symptoms resulting from hyperventilation:
- Dizziness
- Tingling
- Numbness

Psychological symptoms	Physical symptoms
Worrying thoughts	Sleep disturbance
	Insomnia, night terrors
Sense of impending doom	
Sensitive to noise	Muscle tension
Fearful anticipation	Aches, tremors
Poor concentration	Autonomic arousal*

*Autonomic symptoms
- Dry mouth
- Sweaty
- Hot/cold
- Shortness of breath
- Chest pain, palpitations
- Diarrhoea, urgent micturition

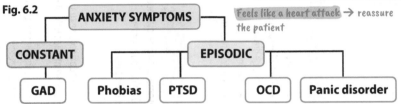

Fig. 6.2

Feels like a heart attack → *reassure the patient*

ANXIETY SYMPTOMS
- CONSTANT
  - GAD
- EPISODIC
  - Phobias
  - PTSD
  - OCD
  - Panic disorder

Generalised anxiety disorder (GAD)

ICD-10 criteria:
- **Generalised & persistent** somatic & psychological symptoms
- Present most days for **at least 6m**

- apprehension / fear of future
- insomnia
- motor tension
- autonomic overactivity & restlessness
- over-cautious behaviour

Panic disorder (episodic paroxysmal anxiety)

ICD-10 criteria:
- **Recurrent attacks of severe anxiety** (lasting <15min)
- In circumstances of **no objective danger**
  → not restricted to particular situations so **unpredictable**
- **Anticipatory anxiety** between episodes (fear of another attack)

→ *Difficult to get patients to face fear*

- sudden onset of **threatening body sensations**
  e.g. palpitations, choking, dizziness
- **loss of touch with reality / catastrophic thoughts**
  e.g. losing control, going mad, dying

Phobias

AGORAPHOBIA
Marked fear and avoidance of at least 2 of:
- Crowds / public places
- Travelling alone   } Lack immediate exit
- Travelling away from home

Symptoms experienced with phobias may progress to panic attacks

Unlike panic disorder:
Symptoms only occur *during* or *on contemplation* of *specific* (non-dangerous) situations, leading to *avoidance* of such situations.

SOCIAL PHOBIA
Marked fear and avoidance of being the **focus of attention/scrutiny/humiliation**
- Blushing/shaking
- Nausea/vomiting
- Urgency of micturition

SPECIFIC (ISOLATED) PHOBIA
Marked fear and avoidance of a **specific object/situation**
e.g. animals, birds, insects, heights, thunder, flying, small spaces, blood, injections, dentists, hospitals

Obsessive–compulsive disorder (OCD)

1. **Obsessions**: thoughts, impulses, images e.g. need for symmetry
2. AND/OR **compulsive acts/rituals**: physical behaviours e.g. washing hands
   - Present **most days** for at least **2w**
   - Cause **distress and interference with activities** → results in **functional impairment** (not seen in simple over-valued ideas)

Obsessions/compulsions often present in:
Schizophrenia, Tourette's, eating disorders, anankastic PD, **depression**, other anxiety disorders

OCD Sx in 20%

Originate in the mind of the patient
- Acknowledged as excessive/unreasonable
- Repetitive, intrusive, ego-dystonic

Give temporary relief

OCD is common in kids (average onset = 9y) & it is considered normal at this age

Differentials of anxiety symptoms

Endocrine
- Thyroid dysfunction
- Phaeochromocytoma

Metabolic
- Acidosis
- Hyper-/hypothermia

Neurological
- Seizures
- Vestibular dysfunction

Cardiac/hypoxia
- Arrhythmias
- CHF/angina
- COPD

Drug withdrawal/ intoxication
- Alcohol
- Opiates
- Amphetamine/cocaine

Psychiatric
- Depression
- Personality disorders
- ASD/Asperger's
- Delusional disorder
- Hoarding

DDx list guides investigations e.g. ECG, TFTs, FBC, U&Es, brain imaging

Management of anxiety disorders[5]

Step 1	Step 2	Step 3	Step 4
• Psychoeducation • Active monitoring **For all cases**	• Guided self-help • Low intensity psychological interventions	• High intensity psychological interventions e.g. CBT, psychodynamic psychotherapy • **AND** drug treatment	Refer to 2° care (MDT) • Complex therapies • Complex drug regimes

PSYCHOLOGICAL INTERVENTIONS: mild/moderate anxiety

1. **Psychoeducation:** improve patient and carer understanding of illness
   e.g. process, causes, treatment, prognosis
2. **Guided self-help/low intensity:** use few resources/less time-consuming
   e.g. books, computer, self-help apps
3. **CBT**
   - **Phobias:** systematic desensitisation/graded exposure
   - **OCD:** exposure & response prevention
   - **PTSD:** eye movement desensitisation & reprocessing (EMDR)

PHARMACOLOGICAL INTERVENTIONS: severe anxiety/psychological treatment failed

1. **Antidepressants (SSRIs)** – proven efficacy long-term (especially combined with psychological treatments)
2. **Beta-blockers** – symptom control (reduce HR & autonomic arousal)
   → **caution in asthmatics**
3. **BZDs** – acute management only (**max 4w** as addictive potential/sedative effect)

SOCIAL INTERVENTIONS: alongside other interventions
to promote long-term recovery by improving functioning e.g. help with work, access to benefits etc.

AIM: STOP AVOIDANCE (prolongs/reinforces problem)

Other Tx options: counselling, relaxation techniques, breathing exercises, social skills training

For SSRIs counsel patients:
- Cause short-term ↑ **anxiety**
- **Common SEs:** GI upset, insomnia, sexual dysfunction

CBT (cognitive behavioural therapy)

= **attempts to change thoughts which affect feelings, which in turn affect behaviour**

Pros: strong evidence base
Cons: patient must confront anxieties → can increase agitation

[5] NICE (2011, updated 2020) *Generalised anxiety disorder and panic disorder in adults* [CG113]

Reactions to stress and trauma

Acute stress reaction

A brief response (<1m) to a severely stressful event e.g. motor accident, violent crime

↳ *Many will develop PTSD*

SYMPTOMS: (overlap with anxiety/depression symptoms)
- Numbness, detachment, ↓ concentration, derealisation
- Insomnia, agitation, restlessness, anger
- Autonomic symptoms

MANAGEMENT
- Talking to friends/family/professionals to relieve anxiety
- Encouraging recall
- Learning effective coping strategies
- **Anxiolytics** (if severe anxiety)
- **Hypnotics** (if insomnia)

> **Coping strategies seen with acute stress reaction**
> - Avoid thinking/speaking of event
> - Denial / cannot remember event
> - Alcohol/substance misuse

Adjustment disorder

A psychological reaction to **a stressful life event / major change** e.g. new job/ home, divorce, bereavement
→ *starts within 3m (more gradual than acute stress reaction)*

SYMPTOMS: (overlap with anxiety/depression symptoms)
- Autonomic symptoms e.g. palpitations, shortness of breath
- Sleep disturbance
- Irritability / aggressive outbursts
- Social functioning impaired

MANAGEMENT
- Talking to friends/family/professionals: avoid denial/avoidance, encourage problem-solving behaviour
- Psychological interventions + medication (SSRIs) if severe

> **Coping strategies seen with adjustment disorder**
> Alcohol/drug abuse

Abnormal grief

Symptoms of normal grief persisting **>6m**

SYMPTOMS
- Low mood, guilt, worthlessness, disturbed sleep & appetite, suicidal thoughts
- Significant psychomotor retardation – very slow
- Prolonged, **serious functional impairment**
- **Hallucinatory experiences** other than those relating to the deceased person

Abnormal grief that is not severe enough to meet depression criteria = 'adjustment reaction'

> **Normal bereavement process: DABDA**
> **D**enial→ **A**nger → **B**argaining → **D**epression → **A**cceptance

Post-traumatic stress disorder (PTSD)

Delayed (often few months) response to a stressful event of an **exceptionally threatening/catastrophic** nature → symptoms persist **>6m** after event

SYMPTOMS: (overlap with depressive symptoms)
- **Hyperarousal** – persistent anxiety, irritability, insomnia, poor concentration, autonomic Sx
- **Re-experiencing** – 'flashbacks', recurrent dreams/nightmares, cannot recall event by will
- **Avoidance** – of reminders, detachment, numbness, anhedonia

MANAGEMENT[6]
1. **Psychological** – psychoeducation, CBT, EMDR
2. **Biological** – antidepressants (SSRIs = 1st line) ± antipsychotic
3. **Social** – educate family, social reintegration, alcohol & illicit substance avoidance

> **Coping strategies for PTSD**
> **Coping:** alcohol/drug abuse

> **Prognosis:** 50% recover in 1st year
> **Poor if:** comorbid mental illness, long duration, poor support & coping strategies

> **Complex PTSD:** overlaps PDs
> Added emotional element – often resulting from ongoing/multiple experiences of 'trauma' e.g. abuse

[6]NICE (2018) *Post-traumatic stress disorder* [NG116]

Health anxiety & somatisation

Definition

Health anxiety is an umbrella term encompassing:
- Excessive/unrealistic health-related concerns
- Somatic perceptions – preoccupied with bodily sensations e.g. pain
- Behaviours – reassurance seeking, repeated symptom checking, avoid medications/doctors

'Health anxiety' itself **is not a diagnosis**, but it is linked to other diagnosable disorders **(see below)**

HYPOCHONDRIACAL DISORDER
At least **6m** *of*:
- belief of 1 or 2 **serious physical diseases** (worried about a specific diagnosis e.g. cancer)
- OR preoccupation with **presumed deformity/disfigurement** (body dysmorphic disorder)

FACTITIOUS DISORDER (MUNCHAUSEN'S)
- **Feigns/exaggerates** symptoms for **no obvious reason** → *Internal motivation to adopt the sick role*
- May inflict self-harm to produce signs/symptoms

MALINGERING
- **Feigns/exaggerates** symptoms for **secondary gain** → *e.g. benefits / monetary gain or emotional gain / attention*

DISSOCIATIVE (CONVERSION) DISORDER
- Traumatic event disrupts consciousness, memory, identity or perception
- Patient **converts anxiety into more tolerable symptoms to attract benefits of sick role**
- Variable presentation: amnesia, stupor, trance, motor disorders, anaesthesia, convulsions

Somatisation
↳ also known as medically unexplained symptoms (MUS)
= expression of psychological distress through physical symptoms

SOMATISATION DISORDER F:M = 10:1
- Complaints for at least **2y of multiple & variable physical symptoms** from **at least 2 body systems** ↳ e.g. GI, cardio, genitourinary, skin ↳ complaint may change frequently
- **Symptoms are real to patient** but **cannot be explained** by a detectable physical disorder or investigations
- Causes **persistent distress, significant functional impairment** & **refusal to accept medical reassurance**
  - Assess impact on function/ADLs
  - Assess insight & explore their expectations

MANAGEMENT[7]: involves MDT*
- **General:** build rapport (acknowledge suffering, regular appointments), minimise investigations
- **Psychological therapy:** CBT, psychoeducation, self-help
- **Social:** encourage normal functioning, normal ADLs/hobbies, involve social network/support
- **Biological:** antidepressants → evidence of long-term efficacy is weak

IMPORTANT: Don't just assume all in patient's mind → ensure suitable investigations done

Possible predisposing factors/precipitants:
- Personal experience of a previous illness
- Significant illness of a loved one
- Early life trauma
- Family members with health anxiety

La belle indifférence: **Absence of distress despite symptoms of serious illness being relayed by the patient**

Differential diagnoses of health anxiety disorders / somatisation
- Depression/anxiety
- Personality disorder
- Over-valued ideas
- Schizophrenia/psychosis: hypochondriacal delusions
- Organic causes with vague symptoms: MS, lupus, porphyrias

especially with relationships

Explaining to patient is key!
Suggest link between physical symptoms and psychological factors

*GP, medical specialties (e.g. GI), psychology

May reinforce idea there is a physical problem

[7] NICE (2011, updated 2020) *Generalised anxiety disorder and panic disorder in adults* [CG113]

Personality disorders

Personality is thought to develop during childhood and adolescence

*PDs are enduring: unlike other mental health illnesses which may occur in discrete episodes

Aetiology of personality disorder is multifactorial

Attachment problems with PRIMARY CAREGIVER Patients find it difficult to trust people → intense unstable relationships

↪ *Screen for these in history*

Common comorbid conditions/DDx:
- Anxiety disorder
- Depression
- PTSD, OCD
- ASD/ADHD
- Adjustment disorder / stress reaction

↳ Comorbidities often missed as assumed to be due to difficult behaviours caused by the personality disorder **OR** comorbidities cause delayed diagnosis of the personality disorder itself

PDs (especially cluster B) are linked to **higher rate of suicide**

Definitions

Personality = combination of **consistent thoughts, feelings & behaviours** shown over time & in a variety of settings

Personality disorder = when unhelpful personality traits cause **functional difficulties/distress & interpersonal difficulties**

Problems caused by personality disorders are usually:
1. Pervasive – occur in all/most areas of life
2. Persistent* – evident from adolescence and into adulthood
3. Pathological – cause distress to self/others and **impair function** (occupation, relationships etc.)

Aetiology

- **Genetics / neurochemical imbalance:** e.g. impulsive behaviour / aggression & serotonin
- **Childhood temperament:** innate/biological disposition to an emotional response
- **Childhood experience:** neglect, trauma, abuse (upbringing & parenting style play a big role)

Classification

DSM-5 CLUSTERS: clusters overlap

Cluster A 'mad'	Cluster B 'bad'	Cluster C 'sad'
• Paranoid • Schizoid • Schizotypal	• Antisocial • Histrionic • Borderline • Narcissistic	• Obsessive–compulsive (anankastic) • Anxious/avoidant ↳ Different • Dependent to OCD

ICD-10 CLASSIFICATION

Paranoid	**S**uspicious, **U**nforgiving, **S**ensitive, **P**ossessive/jealous, **E**xcessive self-importance, **C**onspiracy theories, **T**enacious sense of self-rights **'SUSPECT'**
Schizoid	**A**nhedonic, **L**ack relationships, **O**nly small emotion range, **N**ormal conventions ignored, **E**xcess fantasy world **'ALONE'**
Dissocial	**S**ocial disregard, **I**rresponsible, **N**o concern for others, **G**uiltless, **L**oses temper easily, **E**gocentric **'SINGLE'**
Emotionally unstable	**Borderline**: **S**elf-image unclear, **C**hronic emptiness, **A**bandonment fear, **R**elationships unstable/intense, **S**elf-harm/suicide, **L**abile emotions, **I**mpulsive, **E**motions very intense **'SCARS LIE'**
	Impulsive: **N**o **P**lans, **L**acks impulse control, **A**ggressive outbursts, **N**o thought of consequences **'No PLAN'**
Histrionic	**A**ttention-seeking, **C**oncerned about self, **T**heatrical, **O**pen to suggestion, **R**acy/seductive, **S**hallow **'ACTORS'**
Anankastic	**P**erfectionist, **E**xcessive detail, **R**igid, **F**ull of doubt, **E**xcludes pleasure/people, **C**onscientious, **T**houghts are intrusive **'PERFECT'**
Anxious/ avoidant	**A**voids social contact, **F**ears rejection/criticism, **R**estricts lifestyle, **A**pprehensive, feels **I**nferior/Inadequate, **D**esires acceptance **'AFRAID'**
Dependent	**S**ubmissive/Subordinate, **U**nable to make decisions, **P**essimism, **P**oor confidence, **O**versensitive, **R**ely on others, **T**error of abandonment **'SUPPORT'**

Management[8,9]

Avoid admission where possible: fosters dependence & prevents adoption of coping strategies

→ RISK ASSESSMENT – consider admission if acute risk to self/others

→ CONSIDER COMORBIDITIES – admission may be needed to treat underlying mental illness

LONG-TERM MANAGEMENT

- **Psychoeducation:** especially for carers/family/friends
- **Self-help:** mood diary, coping behaviours, mindfulness, meditation, maintain physical health, sleep hygiene
- **Talking therapies:** CBT, DBT, MBT, CAT (cognitive analytical therapy)
- **Social support:** finance, housing, inclusion activities / activity scheduling, support with stigma   Most important

MEDICATION*

- **Antipsychotics:** for transient psychosis, reducing impulsivity/agitation
- **Antidepressants:** for comorbid anxiety/depression
- **Mood stabilisers**
- **Short-term sedative/anxiolytic** – in crisis situations
  ↳ Max 1w

GENERAL

Set clear boundaries, demonstrate you are reliable/consistent, beware of splitting/transference

---

Risks of personality disorder

- Impulsive behaviour
- Self-harm/suicide
- Substance abuse
- Self-neglect

Inclusion & involvement in their own care plan = key

Poor engagement/insight is a common cause of treatment failure

*Medication is only indicated for related symptoms/comorbidities (e.g. self-harm, unstable moods)

Transference: how patient feels about you
They subconsciously associate a feeling of the past in the present situation

(Don't take it personally!)

---

[8]NICE (2009) *Borderline personality disorder* [CG78]
[9]NICE (2009, updated 2013) *Antisocial personality disorder* [CG77]

Psychosis & schizophrenia

Persecutory: being stalked/spied on etc.
Grandiose: elevated self-importance, special power or ability
Somatic: think something physically wrong with themselves

PSYCHOSIS = a **syndrome** characterised by **a loss of contact with reality**

Key symptoms

- **Delusions** = fixed, false, unshakable beliefs, despite conflicting evidence
  – cannot be rationalised away
- **Hallucinations** = perception of something in the absence of external stimuli
  – auditory/visual/touch, smell, taste
- **Formal thought disorder** = pattern of **disordered language** reflecting disordered thoughts
  – tangential/circumstantial speech, derailment/thought disconnection (switch from one topic to another)

Differentials of psychosis

Organic:
- Delirium
- Medication-induced – DA agonists, corticosteroids, stimulants
- Endocrine disorders – Cushing's, hyperthyroidism
- Epilepsy

Psychiatric disorders:
- Schizophrenia
- Depression with psychotic features
- Schizotypal disorder – distorted thoughts but hallucinations/ delusions not prominent

- Schizoaffective disorder – 1st rank symptoms congruent to mood symptoms (mood & psychosis present **at same time**)
- Delusional disorder – delusions not so bizarre and no hallucinations

Other:
- Substance-induced – cannabis, hallucinogens, alcohol, cocaine
- Systemic – MS, SLE, HIV, syphilis, hypoglycaemia, Wilson's

Acute transient psychosis: *sudden onset* psychotic symptoms lasting **<28d** with no identifiable organic cause → linked to stress

---

SCHIZOPHRENIA = a **psychotic disorder** diagnosed if ≥**28d** of ≥2 of the following symptoms, with **no organic cause found**

Symptoms

SCHNEIDER'S FIRST RANK SYMPTOMS

Hallucinations (auditory)	Delusions
3rd person ('he' or 'she') Being talked about	Delusional perception Attribute false meaning to a true perception ↳ *e.g. red traffic light means aliens are landing*
Thought echo / thoughts spoken aloud	Delusion of control Believe thoughts/feelings/actions are being controlled by external force
Running commentary	Delusions of thought interference Insertion, withdrawal, broadcasting

OTHER SYMPTOMS

Positive: delusions, hallucinations, thought disorder
Negative: blunted/flat affect, social withdrawal, poverty of speech, anhedonia, avolition
Cognitive: poor attention, learning & problem solving (autism), disorganised behaviour
Motor: catatonic movements, waxy flexibility, stupor, posturing, negativism

---

Epidemiology of schizophrenia

Annual incidence: 1 in 500, M=F
Peak age males: 23–29y + 55–64y
Peak age females: 15–24y

Summary of 1st rank Sx

Auditory hallucinations
Broadcasting of thought
Control delusions (passivity)
Delusional perception

PANSS (Positive & Negative Severity Scale) can be used to assess severity of symptoms

↓ motivation

lack of response to stimuli

Aetiology & risk factors

→ *mixture of genetics (80%) and environment*

Genetic	Developmental	Psychosocial
• Family history (likely polygenic) 50% chance in MZ twins 10% chance in 1st° relative	• Low birth weight • Obstetric complications • Maternal illness in pregnancy e.g. influenza, malnutrition	• Urban living, migration (Afro-Caribbean minority) • Adverse life event (childhood abuse / parental death) • Poor premorbid personality • Abnormal family processes (e.g. overprotective/intrusive, arguing parents)

Course & prognosis

1. **Prodrome:** period of more subtle changes prior to obvious psychosis
   (not everyone experiences prodromal period)
   - non-specific negative symptoms
   - distress/agitation
   - transient psychotic symptoms

2. **Acute phase:** relapsing & remitting positive and negative symptoms

Good prognostic factors	Poor prognostic factors
Female	Male & unmarried
Married	FHx of schizophrenia
Acute onset	Early/insidious onset
Prominent mood symptoms	Prominent negative symptoms
Good premorbid personality	Substance abuse
Clear precipitating event	Long duration untreated
Early Tx with good response	Lack of insight / non-compliance

Key to ask in history

Investigations

To r/o organic cause & assess suitability for antipsychotics

- **History** (+ collateral) and MSE
- **Physical examination:** BMI, neurological
- **Bloods:** FBC, RFT, LFT, TFT, glucose, lipids, cholesterol
- **Urine:** drug screen
- **ECG**
- ± brain scan ± EEG if specifically indicated

Management[10]

BIOLOGICAL   BIOPSYCHOSOCIAL APPROACH
- Antipsychotics
- Annual physical health R/V: smoking, alcohol, BP, BMI, bloods, ECG
  FBC, RFT, LFT, glucose, lipids

PSYCHOLOGICAL
- CBT
- Psychoeducation: signs of relapse, prevent relapse, crisis plans
- Family Intervention Therapy (FIT): education and support for carers

SOCIAL
- OT assessment of functioning: ADLs, occupation, hobbies
- Social assessment for housing, benefits, finances, education/career
- Carer assessment: **carer stress**

ACUTE EPISODES: → *All patients need follow-up and monitoring*
- May need admission **OR**
- May prevent admission with community input from EIP (early intervention psychosis) team & CRHT (crisis resolution and home treatment team)

[10]NICE (2014) *Psychosis and schizophrenia in adults* [CG178]

Illicit substance use may ↓ age of onset & ↑ relapses

Outcomes
- 20% have only 1 episode
- 50% recover but relapse in future
- 30% develop chronic schizophrenia
- 10–15% die by suicide

Other risks: T2DM, CVD, ↓ life expectancy

Diagnosis consists of:
- Comprehensive psychiatric history
- Comprehensive medical history
- Risk assessment (to self & others)

Treatment-resistant schizophrenia
= no response to TWO different antipsychotics

Management:
1. Check Dx, compliance & substance misuse
2. CLOZAPINE: register with monitoring service for side-effects, including weekly FBC (SEs: agranulocytosis, neutropenia, cardiomyopathy)

Recovery isn't necessarily completely stopping symptoms BUT:
- Learning how to deal/cope with them
- Providing **social support** (financial, educational, housing etc.)
- Reducing stigma
- **Reducing risk** to self and others

Reasons for non-compliance with treatment:
- Side-effects
- Lack of insight
- Delusions about medication/prescriber
- Gains remission & thinks medication no longer needed
- Feels better when 'ill'

Treat acute episode then continue maintenance treatment for:

1y after 1st episode
2y if 2nd episode
5y if ≥3 episodes

Mania & bipolar affective disorder

Definitions

Acute mania: 1 episode of mania
Bipolar affective disorder: 2 episodes of mania **OR** ≥1 episode of mania + 1 episode of depression
Cyclothymia: persistent mood instability with numerous **subthreshold** manic & depressive periods
Dysthymia: chronically low mood but with no episode justifying a diagnosis of depression

Symptoms of mania

Mania = syndrome characterised by **abnormally elevated arousal, affect (incongruent) and energy levels**

➤ *FUNCTIONING IMPAIRED*

Hypomania = symptoms for 4d	Mania = symptoms for 1w
Mildly elevated or unstable mood	Elevated, expansive or irritable mood
Increased energy	Increased activity *(often goal-directed)*
Mild overspending and risk-taking	Reckless behaviour *(overspending, sexual)*
Increased sociability and overfamiliarity	Disinhibition
Distractibility	Marked distractibility
Increased sexual energy	Marked increased sexual energy
Decreased need for sleep	Sleep severely impaired / absent
hallucinations/delusions are mood-congruent {	**Flight of ideas & pressured speech**
	Grandiose/persecutory delusions
	Auditory hallucinations (2nd person)

> Overinflated self-esteem & grandiosity are common

Bipolar affective disorder (BPAD)

EPIDEMIOLOGY
→ 1–2% of population
→ peak onset = early 20s
→ F=M

4th most common mental health illness but often initially misdiagnosed as recurrent depression

RISK FACTORS: cause is unknown (mix of social & environmental factors)
Genetics: FHx of bipolar disorder (neurotransmitter imbalance – NA, DA, 5-HT)
Life events: prolonged stress, childbirth, physical illness, sleep disturbance
Substance misuse: amphetamines, cocaine, steroids, antidepressants

INVESTIGATIONS: to r/o organic cause
- Physical exam
- Bloods (FBC, TFTs, U&Es, glucose, Ca)
- Drug screen
- CT/MRI

REASONS FOR RELAPSES
- Non-compliance with medication
- Life events / stress
- Substance misuse
- Childbirth (puerperal)
- Disrupted circadian rhythm

> **Prognosis of BPAD**
> - Avg. episode: 6m
> - Recurrence = 90%
> - 10% die by suicide

> **Differential diagnosis**
> - Substance misuse
> - Hyperthyroidism, Cushing's
> - Space-occupying lesion
> - Metabolic disturbance
> - Epilepsy

MANAGEMENT[11]
1. Pharmacological Mx

Acute mania	Bipolar depression	Long-term Tx of bipolar disorder
1. Antipsychotic 2. ± 2nd antipsychotic 3. + Mood stabilisers → valproate (acute episode) → lithium (long-term/prophylaxis) 4. May consider BZDs **STOP routine antidepressants**	1. Antipsychotic (2nd generation) 2. + lamotrigine / other mood stabiliser **No evidence for routine antidepressants** → risk of rapid cycling – if prescribed, must be alongside anti-manic agents	1. Lithium OR continued treatment for mania 2. Valproate or olanzapine (if lithium intolerable)

haloperidol, risperidone, quetiapine, olanzapine

lorazepam

In acute manic phase consider use of MHA & inpatient admission
→ no serious decisions while unwell
→ psychotherapy not useful in the acute stage

2. Psychological Mx
- Psychoeducation: recognising relapses
- CBT
- CPN visits: monitor mood, mental state, symptoms

3. Social Mx
- Support for education, training, employment
- Support for carers and family

Physical health monitoring:
- Eating/exercise programme
- Weight and cardiovascular/metabolic parameters monitored annually
- Monitoring for medication effects e.g. lithium

Mood stabilisers

LITHIUM
Indications: Tx & prophylaxis of acute hypo-/mania & BPAD, Tx of refractory depression / aggressive self-harming

Side-effects

Common:
- GI upset
- Fine tremor
- Polyuria/polydipsia
- Metallic taste
- Weight gain
- Oedema
- Cognitive slowing
- Hyperparathyroidism

In lithium toxicity (>1.2mmol/L):
- Diarrhoea/vomiting/dehydration
- Coarse tremor
- Ataxia (fasciculations, jerks, stiff)
- Dysarthria
- Nystagmus / visual disturbance
- Confusion/convulsions/seizures
- Drowsiness/lethargy
- Renal failure
- Cardiac dysrhythmia

Cautions: cardiac disease, epilepsy, elderly
Contraindications: pregnancy, arrhythmias, long QT, Addison's disease, significant renal impairment, ↓Na

Lithium metabolised by kidneys:
- Check eGFR before prescribing
- Counsel patient to stay hydrated

Monitoring of lithium

Narrow therapeutic window: 0.4–1.2mmol/L
- Take sample 12h post-dose
- After dose change monitor levels weekly, then 3-monthly for 1y, then 6-monthly
- Monitor U&Es, LFTs & TFTs, calcium every 6m

Mx of lithium toxicity: STOP LITHIUM IMMEDIATELY
- Rehydration
- If severe: diuresis/haemodialysis

Lithium in pregnancy = risk of cardiac defects e.g. Ebstein anomaly
Must counsel women of child-bearing age on **contraception** & co-prescribe **folate** if pregnant

VALPROATE
Indications: acute hypo-/mania, BPAD, anti-epileptic
Contraindications: women of childbearing age / **pregnancy** (teratogenic) liver failure & cirrhosis

LAMOTRIGINE   → least teratogenic
Indications: BPAD, treatment-resistant depression, anti-epileptic
Side-effects: risk of Stevens–Johnson syndrome

CARBAMAZEPINE
Indications: prophylaxis of BPAD if unresponsive to lithium, trigeminal neuralgia, anti-epileptic
Contraindications: women of childbearing age / **pregnancy** (teratogenic)

Monitoring of valproate
- **LFTs** – hepatotoxic
- **Bone profile** – supplement vit D

painful rash, blisters on mucous membranes, flu-like symptoms

Antipsychotics

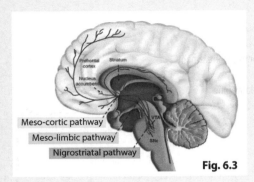

Meso-cortic pathway
Meso-limbic pathway
Nigrostriatal pathway

Fig. 6.3

General mechanism of action

Antipsychotics (APs) work by blocking postsynaptic receptors in dopaminergic pathways, therefore decreasing dopamine activity

Meso-cortic blockage ↓ psychotic symptoms
Meso-limbic blockage causes hyperprolactinaemia
Nigrostriatal blockage causes EPSEs

> **AIM** = reduce positive and negative symptoms with minimal SEs **(target mesolimbic pathway)**

Typicals / first generation antipsychotics

Examples: chlorpromazine, haloperidol, sulpiride, flupentixol, trifluoperazine

Mechanism: D2 receptor antagonists

Side-effects

Neurological	EPSEs, ↓ seizure threshold, sedation, neuroleptic malignant syndrome (NMS)
Psychiatric	Apathy, confusion, depression
Anti-muscarinic	Dry mouth, blurred vision, constipation, urine retention
Other	Arrhythmias, hyperprolactinaemia, hypotension, weight gain

EMERGENCY!
- hyperthermia
- muscle rigidity
- tremor
- acidosis
- tachycardia
- confusion

Extrapyramidal side-effects (EPSEs): due to dopamine blockage in nigrostriatal pathways

FROM START

>48 HOURS

DAYS—WEEKS
MONTHS—YEARS

Akathisia: uncontrollable urge to fidget e.g. pacing, crossing and uncrossing legs
Acute dystonia: involuntary muscle spasms causing abnormal movements/postures
Parkinsonism: tremor, rigidity, bradykinesia
Tardive dyskinesia: involuntary hyperkinetic movements e.g. lip-smacking, chewing

Respond to anticholinergics: PROCYCLIDINE

Atypicals / second generation antipsychotics

Examples: aripiprazole, olanzapine, risperidone, clozapine

Mechanism: D2 receptor antagonists ± 5-HT receptor antagonists (except aripiprazole, which is a partial D2 agonist)

Side-effects
- Nausea, constipation, dizziness (postural hypotension)
- Weight gain & metabolic syndrome*
- Sedation
- QTc prolongation (not aripiprazole)
- ± insomnia, ± prolactin

Generally, **atypicals are 1st line** as **SAME EFFICACY** but **FEWER EPSEs** than 1st generation medications

	AP with least effect	AP with most effect
Weight gain	Aripiprazole	Olanzapine & clozapine
Sedation	Aripiprazole	Clozapine
Metabolic complications	Aripiprazole	Olanzapine & clozapine

NB Risperidone is somewhere in the middle with causing the above side-effects, BUT causes the most EPSEs of 2nd generation APs

---

Prescribing antipsychotics:

- Start low & go slow
- Monitor for side-effects
- May take 2–3w for effects
- If **non-compliance,** consider **long-acting DEPOT INJECTION**

Stepwise progression of AP Tx

Initially: atypical AP
↓
No response 4–6w:
switch to another atypical AP
↓
Still no response: clozapine
(consider compliance first)

Clozapine = for Tx-resistant schizophrenia
(no response to 2 antipsychotics)
Side-effects: agranulocytosis, neutropenia, cardiomyopathies

*Metabolic syndrome

- Central obesity
- Insulin resistance
- Impaired glucose regulation (T2DM)
- HTN
- ↑ LDL and triglycerides

Psychiatric emergencies

Major	Minor	Medical
• Suicidal patients (30%) • Agitated/violent patients	• Grief reaction • Rape • Panic attacks	• Neuroleptic malignant syndrome • Serotonin syndrome • Delirium • Overdose/withdrawal

40% of psychiatric emergencies need admission to hospital

Acute behavioural disturbance

1. ASSESSMENT
History: need to rule out organic cause *e.g. infection*
- Establish any diagnoses & medication
- Any previous similar episodes & cause/Tx
- Consider medication compliance or SEs
- Use of alcohol / illicit drugs
- Recent changes in social life e.g. employment/relationships
- History of self-harm/suicide attempt/violence – risk assess

Behavioural disturbance may be due to psychiatric symptoms, non-psychiatric symptoms or substance misuse

Factors to consider when deciding need for treatment/admission
- Severity of illness
- Level of insight
- Risk of harm to self or others
- Other support available

2. NON-PHARMACOLOGICAL MANAGEMENT
- Encourage patient to move to area away from others
- Speak confidently, slowly, clearly
- Non-threatening body language, give space
- **Explore & acknowledge concerns with patient** – try to build rapport

3. PHARMACOLOGICAL MANAGEMENT / PHYSICAL RESTRAINT
Rapid tranquilisation → calm the patient without full sedation
- BZDs, antipsychotics, promethazine – minimum dose, **PO if possible**

LAST LINE! → Will need close medical monitoring afterwards

Neuroleptic malignant syndrome (NMS)

AETIOLOGY: RARE (<1%), adverse reaction to antipsychotics (DA blockade causes hyperactivity of SNS)
→ *Hard to predict*

SYMPTOMS:
- Fever, diaphoresis (sweating)
- Rigidity
- Confusion, fluctuating consciousness
- Autonomic instability (fluctuating BP, HR, salivation, incontinence)

INVESTIGATIONS
- Raised CK – may be >1000
- Raised leucocytes
- Deranged LFTs

MANAGEMENT: withdraw antipsychotic medication
- Rehydration
- Monitor temperature, BP, pulse
- Consider BZDs to ↓muscle activity & temperature (lorazepam, diazepam)

Risk factors for NMS:
Hx: previous NMS, brain damage, alcoholism
Mental state: agitation, hyperactivity, catatonia
Physical: dehydration
Treatment: recent ↑ or ↓ dose, high dose, IM injections
more likely with 1st generation APs

If severe:
- **Bromocriptine**
- **Dantrolene** (↓ rigidity)
- ICU, intubation + ventilation

Serotonin syndrome

AETIOLOGY: increased serotonin due to ↑ synthesis, ↓ uptake/metabolism or direct receptor activation → *more predictable*

SYMPTOMS
Psychiatric: restlessness, confusion, agitation
Autonomic: hyperthermia, diarrhoea, ↑ HR, hypo-/hypertension, mydriasis
Neuromuscular: myoclonus, rigidity, tremors, hyperreflexia, ataxia, convulsions

MANAGEMENT: stop precipitating medicine → restart **cautiously** after 48h
- Rehydration
- May need cyproheptadine (anti-serotonergic)
- BZDs if agitated (lorazepam, diazepam)

Common causes of serotonin syndrome:
- Switching antidepressant
- Combining antidepressants
(with other ADs or supplements)

May need ICU, intubation + ventilation if severe

Differentiating between neuroleptic malignant syndrome and serotonin syndrome

	Neuroleptic malignant syndrome	Serotonin syndrome
Associated treatment	Antipsychotics Idiosyncratic/normal dose	Serotonergic medications Overdose/combinations
Onset	Slow (days–weeks)	Rapid
Progression	Slow (24–72h)	Rapid
Muscle rigidity	Severe (lead pipe)	Less severe rigidity, clonus present (involuntary rhythmic muscle contractions)
Activity	Bradykinesia	Hyperkinesia
Blood results	↑↑ CK & WCC	↑ or normal CK

Self-harm

EPIDEMIOLOGY: F>M, ⅔ are aged <35y

> Overdose & cutting are the most common forms

RISK FACTORS

Biological	Psychological	Social
• Genetics • Age (teens/young adults) • Personality disorder (particularly EUPD)	• Abuse: sexual, physical, emotional • Bullying • Bereavement • Relationship breakdown • Endings/changes	• Substance misuse • Friends who self-harm • Financial/living concerns • Work/school pressures • Isolation/loneliness

> Risk of suicide is 66× greater if self-harmed

MANAGEMENT:

> Divorced > Single > Widowed > Married

1. **Assessment**
   - Physical & mental health
   - Safeguarding concerns
   - Further self-harm and suicide risk
2. **Treatment**
   - Of physical injuries
   - Specialist psychosocial assessment
   - Monitor in a healthcare setting to reduce risk of recurrence
   - Consider need for admission to mental health ward

Factors predicting repetition of self-harm

- Number of previous episodes
- Personality disorder
- History of violence
- Alcohol misuse
- Unmarried

Suicide

EPIDEMIOLOGY: second leading cause of death in those aged 15–29y

Factors indicating suicidal intent

- Trying to avoid intervention
- Feelings of hopelessness about the future
- Planning suicide
- Leaving a note
- Anticipatory acts (leaving a will, settling debts)
- Use of violent methods

RISK FACTORS

> Hanging/strangulation is most common method

- History of self-harm or suicide attempt
- Severe depression
- Occupation (farmers, doctors)
- Social isolation
- Anorexia
- Unemployed
- Alcohol
- Male

Risk assessment

- Impulsive or planned?
- Ongoing or resolved trigger?
- Precautions to avoid discovery
- Preparations (note/will written)
- Do they regret it? want to try again?
- Use of alcohol/drugs?
- Any protective factors?
- Social support network?
- Willing to engage in Tx?

Safety plan: identify support, recognise early warning signs, avoid alcohol/drugs, identify emergency contacts

Child & adolescent psychiatry

↳ Mental illness affects 10% children
↳ 50% present to GPs

↳ Impacts development, education, relationships

> **Child** <16y
> **Young person** 16–17y
> **Adult** ≥18y

Epidemiology

Children: neurodevelopmental disorders
Adolescents: mood/anxiety disorders*, eating disorders, substance misuse
*self-harm is common

Assessment

- History, MSE, risk assessment → SAFEGUARDING ISSUES?
- Consider impact on family/carers

Abuse may underlie PCx

Consent

Legally presumed that those ≥16y have capacity to make decisions regarding their care BUT encourage discussion with family.

- However, must **assess capacity on an INDIVIDUAL BASIS** (some <16y may have competence)
- If deemed to have competence, a child can consent to treatment BUT **parents can still override refusal** of treatment if it is in child's best interests (avoid if possible)
- If a child lacks competence, **a parent can consent to treatment on their behalf** if it is within scope of parental responsibility
- If a parent refuses treatment that is in child's best interests, further advice should be sought from courts.

There is no age restriction for Mental Health Act.

Summary of consent

	Capacity/competence	No capacity/competence
16–17y	Can consent/refuse admission or treatment	Parental consent may be adequate, may need MHA
<16y	Can consent, but if refuse can use MHA	Parental consent may be adequate, may need MHA

If ≥16y, capacity is presumed. If concerns regarding capacity to make a decision, this can be assessed under the MCA.

If <16y, capacity is not presumed & MCA does not apply. Instead 'Gillick competence' must be assessed to decide whether child understands enough to make the decision.

> Capacity depends on the decision – a child may be competent to consent/refuse a simple, low risk procedure, but not more complex, riskier ones

May lack competence/capacity due to age or a mental health disorder

Confidentiality

If child has competence, should respect their decisions regarding confidentiality/disclosure of information unless:
- There is **overriding public interest** in the disclosure
- Disclosure is **required by law**

If child lacks competence and refuses disclosure of information to parents you should:
- Firstly try to **persuade them** to involve parents/carers
- Disclose information to parents/authorities if you deem it **necessary in child's best interests**

> Should encourage child to involve family/carers in their care if possible

Management of mental health conditions in children

Biological: usually **less common/limited evidence** as 1st-line treatment
→ consider in ADHD and depression

Psychological: most commonly used are **CBT and family therapy**

Social: very important – especially regarding education and social services
→ need good intra-agency working

Use of antidepressants in children/adolescents

- Concerns of suicidal behaviour in teens taking SSRI
- **Only prescribed by specialist (child psychiatrist)**
- **FLUOXETINE = ONLY ANTIDEPRESSANT LICENSED FOR PAEDIATRIC USE** (although others sometimes used)

Eating disorders

Prevalence = 0.6% → most common in adolescent girls.
Peak onset = adolescence. F:M = 10.1

Anorexia nervosa

FEATURES

- **BMI <17.5**
- **Persistent restriction of energy intake**
- Fear of gaining weight / becoming fat
- Often excessive exercise (to compensate for food)
- **Lack of insight** into seriousness of low BMI
- Menstrual abnormalities

SYMPTOMS

Psychiatric: brain atrophy	**Reproductive:** hypothalamic changes	**Hair/skin**
• Inflexible thinking	• Reduced libido	• Broken skin, dry & brittle hair
• Obsessions/habits	• Amenorrhoea (females)	• Hair over face/body (lanugo)
• Poor concentration	• Low testosterone (males)	**Other**
• Irritable / flattened mood	• Reproductive dysfunction	• Cold extremities / hypothermia
• Interests centre around food	**Muscles**	• Infections
Heart	• Wasting/cramp	• Iron-deficiency anaemia
• Low BP & pulse	**Bones:** irreversible	• Leucopenia, thrombocytopenia
• Risk of arrhythmias & heart failure	• Osteopenia/osteoporosis	• Metabolic disturbances

Metabolic disturbances: hypokalaemia, ↑ cortisol, GH & cholesterol, ↓ hormone levels

MANAGEMENT[12]

BIOPSYCHOSOCIAL APPROACH

Biological   ↪ dietitian input
- **Weight restoration** – risk **refeeding syndrome**
- Regular monitoring – weight, FBC, U&Es, LFT, glucose, bone profile, Mg^{2+}, CK, B12
- ± DEXA scan
- ± ECG – prolonged QTc, HR <50, arrhythmias

Treat coexisting mental health illness e.g. SSRI for depression

Psychological*
- Psychotherapies: CBT, motivational interviewing, compassion-focused, interpersonal, family therapy
- Family therapy if <18y

*Psychological Tx has limited effect if BMI <13, **so restore weight first**

Social
- Education: dietary advice / multivitamins
- Involve family/friends for support
- Carer support

General risk factors

- Perfectionism
- Body image disturbances
- Weight stigma / teasing / bullying
- Low self-esteem
- Early sexual development
- History of abuse
- Personality disorder
- FHx of eating disorders
- Exposure to 'diet culture'
- Higher socioeconomic status
- Comorbid mental illness (e.g. anxiety disorders)

DDx anorexia nervosa

- Hyperthyroidism
- Depression, anxiety, OCD
- Psychosis, substance misuse
- Body dysmorphic disorder

Poor prognostic factors

- Low body weight
- **Late onset**
- Bulimic features
- Family difficulties
- Personality disorder
- **Longer illness duration**
- **Poor support/relationships**
- **Comorbid mental illness**

10-year prognosis

50% recovered
40% chronic problem
10% mortality (1/3 suicide)

Indications for hospitalisation

- BMI <13.5
- Very deranged bloods
- Syncope/arrhythmias

---

[12]NICE (2017, updated 2020) *Eating disorders* [NG69]

Bulimia nervosa

Prevalence = 1% → often a
history / coexisting anorexia nervosa

FEATURES
- **Recurrent binge eating** (no prominent weight changes)
- **Recurrent compensatory behaviour** (vomiting, laxatives, diuretics, fasting, exercise)

} ≥once a week for 3m

SYMPTOMS

Psychiatric
- Poor concentration
- Irritable

Mouth
- Tooth decay/erosion
- Hoarse voice
- Bleeding
- Swollen parotid glands ('chipmunk face')

Hands
- Russell sign: calluses, scars, abrasions on backs of fingers due to self-induced vomiting

Electrolyte imbalance:
can be life-threatening
- Seizures
- Muscle paralysis
- Arrhythmias

Abdomen
- Swollen/painful stomach
- Constipation
- Delayed gastric emptying
- Reflux/oesophagitis
- Rectal prolapse
- Renal failure

↳ *most important*

MANAGEMENT[13]

Biological
- Antidepressant – SSRI (usually fluoxetine)
- Advise laxative and alcohol cessation
- Regular monitoring – weight, FBC, U&Es, LFT, glucose and electrolytes

BIOPSYCHOSOCIAL APPROACH

Psychological
- Psychoeducation: regarding coping mechanisms
- Psychotherapies: CBT, compassion-focused, interpersonal, family therapy

Social
- Involve family/friends for support
- Carer support

10-year prognosis
70% recovered
1% mortality

Poor prognostic factors
- Low body weight
- Comorbid depression

[13] NICE (2017, updated 2020) *Eating disorders* [NG69] & NICE BNF *Fluoxetine*

Intellectual disability

↳ Significantly sub-average intellectual functioning (IQ <70)
↳ Impaired adaptive behaviour
↳ Onset of intellectual impairment before 18y

Epidemiology

- ↑ prevalence in lower socioeconomic groups
- M>F
- Association with overcrowding, poverty, irregular/unskilled employment

Classification

IQ tests are subjective – performed by clinical psychologists

	Mild (85% cases)	Moderate	Severe	Profound
IQ	50–69	35–49	20–34	<20
Prevalence	1.5–3%	0.5%	0.5%	0.05%
Functioning	Only need help if problems arise • Often not recognised as ID	May need supervision in some elements of daily living / work	Need help with many ADLs • Often physical disability • Limited communication	Extensive/total help with ADLs • Minimal communication

Aetiology

30% have no identifiable cause

GENETIC/CHROMOSOMAL CAUSES

Down syndrome

= trisomy 21
- Most common chromosomal cause
- Characteristic physical abnormalities
- ↑ risk of deafness, cataracts, hyperthyroidism, Alzheimer's

Phenylketonuria

= autosomal recessive: 1 in 10,000 births
- High serum phenylalanine
- Epilepsy, hyperactivity, irritability
- Short stature, hypopigmented, eczema

Cri du chat syndrome

= deletion of short arm of chromosome 5

Fragile X syndrome

= abnormality on long arm of X chromosome
- Most common genetic cause
- More common in males
- Elongated face / protruding ears / microcephaly
- Delayed development of speech & language by age 2y

Neurofibromatosis

= mutation on chromosome 7
- Usually mild ID
- Café au lait spots
- Skin, bone, soft tissue, nervous system abnormalities

Tuberous sclerosis

= mutated tumour suppressor gene chr 9 or 16
- Results in autism & epilepsy with ID
- Skin changes, brain/other tumours

NB Intellectual disability (ID) is not same as autism spectrum disorders (ASD)
→ but often exist as comorbid conditions, along with epilepsy

PRENATAL, PERINATAL, POSTNATAL FACTORS

Prenatal	Perinatal	Postnatal
• Fetal alcohol syndrome (most prevalent) • Congenital hypothyroidism • Pre-eclampsia • Placental insufficiency • **TORCH** infections	• Birth trauma / hypoxia • Intraventricular haemorrhage • Hyperbilirubinaemia	• Brain infection/tumour • Head injury • Chronic lead poisoning • Malnutrition • Neglect/abuse

ID & mental illness

→ *may present differently / patient has difficulty describing symptoms*
  ↳ Psychological therapies may need to be adapted/simplified

>50% of patients with ID have coexisting mental health problems

DIFFERENCES IN PRESENTATION:

Mania/bipolar
- Challenging behaviour
- Giggling
- Delusions less elaborate

Depression
- Exaggerated need for routine
- Suicidal ideas rare & poorly planned
- **Less likely to complain of low mood**

Schizophrenia:
- Delusions/hallucinations less elaborate
- Persecutory delusions / thought disorder rare
- Earlier onset
- Presents as fear/withdrawal, challenging behaviour, sleep disturbance

Perinatal psychiatry

Screening

- **All women should be screened** at antenatal clinic for previous/current/FHx of psychiatric disorder
- **Refer necessary cases** for psychiatric assessment & referral
- **Regularly monitor mental state of all peri-/postnatal women**, regardless of whether they've been referred

WHO TO REFER?   Pregnant/postpartum women should have
1. PHx ± FHx of: priority in psychiatric service pathways
- Schizophrenia/psychosis
- Bipolar disorder
- Puerperal psychosis
- Severe depression i.e. required secondary care input (depression treated by GP doesn't need referral)

2. On mood stabilisers

Postpartum psychiatric presentations

NORMAL PSYCHIATRIC SYMPTOMS → Due to **hormonal changes** ± physical & emotional exhaustion

'The Pinks': within 48h postpartum
Excitement, euphoria, overtalkative, overactive, insomnia

→ **spontaneous resolution**

'The Blues': day 3–10 postpartum
Emotional lability, tearful, anxious, irritable
Does not affect functioning (most do not develop PPD)

→ **spontaneous resolution after 48h**

POSTPARTUM DEPRESSION (PPD) → bipeak onset at **2–4w** & **3m** postpartum

Symptoms:
Similar to normal depressive illness with more prominent anxiety
→ guilt & concerns over parental ability = common
→ anxious preoccupation with baby's health
→ reduced affection for baby / **impaired bonding**
→ **obsessional phenomena** (ego-dystonic in nature e.g. harming baby)

Edinburgh Postnatal Depression Scale: used to assess Sx during & after pregnancy

Management[14]   RISK ASSESS
- **Psychotherapy:** CBT
- **SSRIs** = 1st line (sertraline/paroxetine) – may give prophylactically after birth if high risk
- Admission to mother & baby unit / ECT – if very severe / high risk to self or baby

Prognosis
With Tx: 2/3 resolve within 2–3m
No Tx: can take >6m to recover
→ *children of treated mother experience fewer psychiatric symptoms/disorders*
→ *if untreated, can result in insecure attachments, ↑ psychiatric problems in child, child less compliant with their own health visits*

POSTPARTUM BIPOLAR DISORDER → highest risk **9–14d** postpartum
Often affects those with Hx of bipolar disorder
→ high risk of relapse in pregnancy due to discontinuation of teratogenic mood stabilisers
→ should consider continuing mood stabilisers that are safer to use in pregnancy

---

Puerperium: period of about 6w after childbirth

1 in 10 women suffer a mental disorder postnatally

Important to **identify at-risk women antenatally** so we can effectively manage risks

Assess risk to baby
- Obsessional/delusional Sx
- Determine baby's location & carer

Prevalence of PPD: 10%

PPD is difficult to diagnose as overlaps with 'normal' postpartum experiences (exhaustion, ↓ sleep, anxiety) BUT difference = it IMPACTS FUNCTION

Risk factors for postpartum depression
- Previous episode of PPD / FHx of PPD
- Depression during pregnancy
- Hx of major depressive disorder

Predictors of PPD
- Anxiety in pregnancy
- Stressful life events
- Marital discord
- Poverty

Small amounts transferred in breast milk but can still breastfeed

e.g. lamotrigine

Prevalence: 0.2%

PPP can be difficult to differentiate from OCD as have obsessional thoughts BUT thoughts not recognised as ego-dystonic

Risk factors for postpartum psychosis
- Previous PPP
- Hx of bipolar disorder

Other RFs: primiparity, unmarried, obstetric complications

PUERPERAL/POSTPARTUM PSYCHOSIS (PPP) → onset normally within
2–3w postpartum   ↳ *50% by day 7*

Symptoms:
- **sudden onset** behavioural disturbances
- hallucinations/delusions – often a religious context

Management[15]: treat as EMERGENCY   RISK ASSESS
- Admission to **mother & baby unit** – may need MHA
- **High intensity physical & psychological care including:**
  ▸ mood stabiliser ± antipsychotic
  ▸ treatment of anxiety & insomnia
- **Support services:** support groups, help with childcare/housework etc.

Prevention of PPP and BPAD
- If treatment for ongoing BPAD/psychosis stopped during pregnancy, restart immediately after delivery
- If history of BPAD, continue treatment during pregnancy and postpartum
- If history of PPP/BPAD in **postpartum only**, start treatment immediately after delivery prophylactically

Prognosis
Good short-term progress if treated early: most severe symptoms last 2–12w, most make full recovery within 12m
BUT associated with significant morbidity & mortality

Summary of psychiatric medications in pregnancy

Valproic acid	Avoid in pregnancy & breastfeeding
Lithium	Avoid in breastfeeding
Lamotrigine	Safe in pregnancy & breastfeeding
Atypical antipsychotics	Safe in pregnancy & breastfeeding
Sertraline/paroxetine	Safe in pregnancy & breastfeeding (low levels in breast milk)
Fluoxetine	Safe in pregnancy & breastfeeding (higher levels in breast milk)

[15] NICE (2014, updated 2020) *Antenatal and postnatal mental health* [CG192]

DERMATOLOGY

07

ABBREVIATIONS

ABPI – Ankle brachial pressure index
ACEi – Angiotensin-converting enzyme inhibitor
BCC – Basal cell carcinoma
DLQI – Dermatology Life Quality Index
EASI – Eczema Area & Severity Index
HHV – Human herpes virus
HPV – Human papillomavirus
HSV – Herpes simplex virus
IBD – Inflammatory bowel disease

ICU – Intensive care unit
LN – Lymph node
OCP – Oral contraceptive pill
PASI – Psoriasis Area & Severity Index
PCOS – Polycystic ovary syndrome
PDT – Photodynamic therapy
SA – Surface area
SCC – Squamous cell carcinoma
SJS – Stevens–Johnson syndrome

SSMDT – Specialised Skin Multidisciplinary Team
TEN – Toxic epidermal necrolysis
TNF – Tumour necrosis factor
UC – Ulcerative colitis
URTI – Upper respiratory tract infection
UVA – Ultraviolet A
UVB – Ultraviolet B
VZV – Varicella zoster virus

Definitions of terms

Term	Description
Eruption	Rash
Lesion	Any small area of skin disease
Macule	**Flat** (non-palpable) area of colour change **<0.5cm**
Patch	**Flat** (non-palpable) area of colour change **>0.5cm**
Papule	**Raised** (palpable) lesion **<0.5cm** – usually dome-shaped
Nodule	**Raised** (palpable) lesion **>0.5cm** – usually dome-shaped
Cyst	**Fluctuant** papule/nodule containing **fluid/pus/keratin**
Plaque	**Palpable, flat-topped** lesion
Vesicle	**Fluid-filled** lesion/papule **<0.5cm**
Bulla	**Fluid-filled** lesion/papule **>0.5cm**
Pustule	**Pus-filled** lesion
Wheal/weal	**Smooth, skin-coloured** superficial swelling **lasting <24h** (often surrounded by erythema)
Erosion	**Partial break** in skin: loss of epidermis only
Ulcer	**Complete break** in skin: dermis included
Fissure	Small, slit-like break in skin
Excoriation	Erosion or ulcer due to scratching
Lichenification	Thickening of skin and increased markings due to chronic scratching/rubbing
Scale	Visible white loosening of outermost skin layer
Crust	Golden deposit on skin due to dried plasma

Psoriasis

Bi-peak onset: early 20s & 50s
2% population (M=F)

Things that impact the patient:

- **Symptoms:** pain, itching, bleeding
- **Psychological:** self-esteem
- **Treatment:** time-consuming & messy
- **Complications:**
↑ risk CVD, metabolic syndrome, lymphoma

Linked with other inflammatory conditions:
cardiovascular disease, metabolic syndrome, NASH (non-alcoholic steatohepatitis)

Other diseases associated with HLA gene:
lymphoma, asymmetric anterior uveitis, IBD

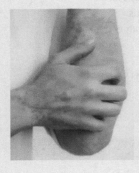

Fig. 7.1

Chronic, relapsing inflammatory skin disorder (↑ skin turnover & epidermal thickening)

Presentation

- Red, scaly plaques with sharp demarcation – extensor surfaces + scalp
- Psoriatic arthritis – in around 30%

Risk factors

1. **Genetics:** FHx, HLA-CW6, HLA-B27, HLA-B13, HLA-B17 genes
2. **Environmental:**
   - Strep throat infection, HIV
   - Medications – BBs, antimalarials, lithium, TNF-α inhibitors
   - Stress, alcohol, smoking, trauma (Koebner phenomenon)

Management[1]

→ *depends on severity & impact on patient**   *PASI/DLQI scores assess severity & impact*

1. **EDUCATION:** avoid lifestyle triggers e.g. smoking/alcohol/stress
2. **TOPICAL TREATMENTS**
   - Emollients e.g. E45   *Avoid vit D analogues in pregnancy or breastfeeding!*
   - Corticosteroids + vit D analogues (mild/moderate if sensitive area)
   - Keratolytics e.g. 5% salicylic acid → for thick plaques
   - Coal tar products (used on scalp)
3. **PHOTOTHERAPY** = needs 2° care referral
   - **Narrow band UVB** = superficial (good if pregnant)
   - **PUVA (psoralen tablets + UVA)** = deeper (not if pregnant)
4. **SYSTEMIC TREATMENTS**

Therapy	Side-effects	Monitoring
Methotrexate	Teratogenic, hepatotoxic, bone marrow suppression, GI upset/nausea	LFTs, FBC
Acitretin	Teratogenic, hepatotoxic, ↑ lipids	LFTs & fasting lipids
Ciclosporin	Nephrotoxic, ↑ BP, tingling peripheries	BP, U&Es

5. **BIOLOGICS** (monoclonal antibodies) for severe or recalcitrant disease

Topical steroid use

Mild	1% hydrocortisone	Any age	Anywhere
Moderate	Eumovate (clobetasone)		Caution on face
Potent	Betnovate (betamethasone)	Adults only	Not face/ genitals
V. potent	Dermovate (clobetasol)		

Side-effects
- Skin thinning
- Can trigger acne/rosacea
- Withdrawal can cause erythroderma

Phototherapy

- UV light exposure causes immunosuppression & ↓ skin inflammation → **UVB** or **PUVA**
- 2–3 × a week for 15–30 episodes
- Base starting dose on skin type & gradually ↑ time of exposure

Indications: acne, vitiligo, psoriasis, lichen planus

Side-effects
Of UV: erythema/pruritus, cold sores, skin cancer
Of tablets: nausea & headaches

Reassure
→ Only very short exposure (secs–minutes)
→ Dose is carefully calculated for skin type
→ Goggles protect eyes & genitalia covered

[1] NICE (2012, updated 2017) *Psoriasis* [CG153]

Acne vulgaris

Common inflammatory skin disorder commonly affecting ages **14–19y**

Pathophysiology

- **Abnormal keratinisation of follicle** = pore blockage
- **↑ Sebum production** = due to ↑ androgens at puberty
- **Overgrowth of *Cutibacterium acnes*** = Gram +ve commensal
  - ▸ releases pro-inflammatory mediators
  - ▸ follicles rupture & contents leak into surrounding dermis

Lesions of acne

1. Non-inflammatory
- Closed comedones (whiteheads) – small papules that may burst
- Open comedones (blackheads) – flat or raised with impacted keratin

2. Inflammatory
- Papules – burst comedones cause inflammation
- Pustules – papules containing pus
- Nodules – painful swellings lasting weeks–months

Sequelae of acne

1. Non-scarring
- Hyper-/hypopigmentation
- Erythematous macules

2. Scarring
- 'ICE-PICK' scars (atrophic) – collagen loss
- 'KELOID' scars (hypertrophic) – collagen formed

Management[2]

→ *depends on severity, psychological impact, response to previous Tx*

1. TOPICAL TX = 1st-line for mild/moderate acne
- **Retinoids** = affect keratin production
- **Antibacterials** e.g. benzyl peroxide
- **Antibiotics** e.g. erythromycin/clindamycin

2. SYSTEMIC ABX = 2nd-line OR 1st-line for severe acne
- Lymecycline/doxycycline (teratogenic / yellow teeth in kids)

3. ORAL ISOTRETINOIN (ROACCUTANE) = retinoid (↓s sebum made)
Indicated in:
- Nodulocystic acne
- Tx-resistant subtypes
- Visible scarring or risk of bad scarring
- Significant psychological distress

4. HORMONAL TX = Tx-resistant females / cyclical flares / hirsutism
- Combined oral contraceptive pill   CIs: pregnancy/lactation, PHx or FHx VTE

5. SCAR TREATMENT
- Microdermabrasion (removes dead skin) – superficial scars
- Laser resurfacing – atrophic scars
- Punch biopsy/excision – ice-pick scars
- Intralesional steroids – keloid scars

[2]NICE (2021) *Acne vulgaris* [NG198]

Risk factors for acne
- Male
- Cosmetic/hair products
- Excess washing
- OCP/steroids
- Endocrine disorders – PCOS

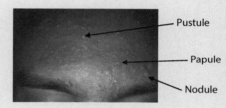

Fig. 7.2 — Pustule, Papule, Nodule

All Tx may cause irritation/erythema & photosensitivity

Side-effects of Roaccutane (key parameters to monitor in parentheses)
- **Teratogenic** – 2× contraception + monthly pregnancy test
- Hepatitis – avoid alcohol **(LFTs)**
- Photosensitivity & dry skin – protection
- Muscle aches
- Mood changes
- Anaemia & thrombocytopenia **(FBC)**
- ↑ Triglycerides & cholesterol **(fasting lipids)**

important monitoring requirements

Contraindications to Roaccutane
- Pregnancy
- Severe liver/renal disease
- Severe depression
- **Peanut allergy**

Eczema

Itchy skin condition characterised by **erythema, dry skin, scaling**

↳ { ± **vesicles & blisters** (acute)
  { ± **fissures & lichenification** (chronic)

Causes/risk factors:
- **Genetics**
  - ▶ mutated filaggrin gene
  - ▶ PHx/FHx atopies
- **Environmental**
  - ▶ irritants (chemicals, soap, nylon)
  - ▶ allergens (pets, dust, food)
  - ▶ illness/infection/stress
  - ▶ cold weather

Lotion → cream → gel → ointment
(become more oily from left to right = better moisture trapping BUT greasier)

EASI/DLQI scores: assess severity & impact

Atopic eczema

Prevalence: 20–30% schoolkids & 5–10% adults
Onset: usually <2y
Features: red, dry, scaly skin → affects flexures
Complications: susceptible to infection

↳ { **S. aureus / Strep:**
  - Weeping pustules / crusting
  - Fever/malaise

  HSV (eczema herpeticum)
  - Pain, fever, lethargy
  - Clustered blisters & punched-out erosions

Management of eczema[3]

→ *assess impact on life / psychological impact*

MILD ATOPIC ECZEMA
1. Emollients (e.g. Cetraben cream) – for dry skin: liberally as often as needed
2. Mild potency topical steroids – for **active** areas: 'finger-tip' portion 1/2 × daily

MODERATE ATOPIC ECZEMA
1. Emollients
2. Moderate potency topical steroids – for **active** areas
3. Topical calcineurin inhibitors e.g. tacrolimus, pimecrolimus (warn about stinging/burning sensation in first 2w of use)

MODERATE ATOPIC ECZEMA
1. Emollients
2. Potent topical steroids – for **active** areas
3. Topical calcineurin inhibitors
4. Phototherapy + emollients & topical steroids
5. Immunosuppressants: ciclosporin, methotrexate, azathioprine

GENERAL: avoid irritants/allergens/triggers

ADDITIONAL TREATMENTS
- Systemic ABX – if infection (flucloxacillin/ erythromycin or aciclovir)
- Antihistamines
- Dupilumab (monoclonal antibody)

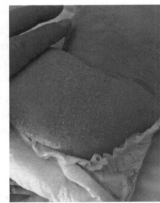

Fig. 7.3 Atopic eczema.

---

[3] NICE (2007, updated 2021) *Atopic eczema in under 12s* [CG57]

Skin infestations

Scabies

→ Sarcoptes *scabies mite*

FEATURES

- **ITCHY papules** (worse at night)
- Burrows / small tracts
- Usually symmetrical

Common sites:
- Finger webs
- Breasts
- Ankles
- Axillae
- Scalp
- Feet

Risk factors for scabies
1. Close contact – dorms, wards, care homes
2. Elderly, young, immunocompromised

→ *'crusted scabies' = severe form in elderly/immunocompromised*

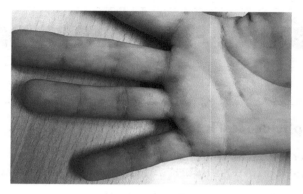

Fig. 7.4

Confirm Dx with microscopy

MANAGEMENT

1. **Permethrin/malathion creams**
   - Apply to whole body for 8–24h
   - Repeat in 1w
   - TREAT ALL CLOSE CONTACTS AT SAME TIME
→ For crusted scabies: ivermectin 200mcg/kg single dose
2. **Wash all bedding/clothing**

Head lice

→ *live on hair, feed on blood, spread via close contact*

FEATURES

- Persistent itching of scalp
- Redness & excoriated papules

MANAGEMENT[4]

1. Fine comb wet hair & conditioner REGULARLY = **most important**
2. Physical insecticide gels/sprays/lotions **OR** chemical insecticide (e.g. malathion 0.5% aqueous liquid) – apply from roots to tips of hair, leave on for 12h and then wash out using shampoo

---

[4] NICE (2016) Scenario: *Head lice management*

Bacterial skin infections

Normal skin commensals

- *Staph. epidermidis*
- Corynebacteria
- Micrococci
- Propionibacteria

Key to colours used in table

Primary infections
Secondary infections
Infections due to bacterial toxins
Hypersensitivity reactions (Group A Strep)

Staphylococcal infections can be 1° or 2° via toxins

Mx of Staph infections: take swab

- → **Topical ABX:** fusidic acid, mupirocin
- → **Oral ABX:** flucloxacillin, clindamycin

Impetigo = **contagious** – no school for 48h after starting ABX or until wounds crusted

Classification of skin infection

Staphylococcus	Streptococcus
Folliculitis	Erysipelas
Cellulitis	Necrotising fasciitis
Bullous impetigo	Scarlet fever
Staphylococcal scalded skin syndrome	Erythema nodosum
Toxic shock syndrome	Vasculitis
Both	
Impetigo, erysipelas	
Cellulitis	
Wound/ulcer/eczema infection	

Staphylococcal infections

→ Over 10 types of commensal staph on skin
→ *Staph. aureus* = **PATHOGENIC when associated with disease flares**

IMPETIGO

Sx: golden crust ± oozing blisters (affects young children)

Mx:
- Soak crust with soap + water
- Topical antiseptic/ABX
- Systemic ABX if widespread

BULLOUS IMPETIGO (specific strain of *Staph. aureus*)

Sx: 2–3cm blisters
Mx: oral flucloxacillin

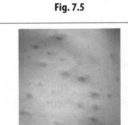

Fig. 7.5

FOLLICULITIS

Sx: erythematous pustules around hair follicles

Mx:
- Screen & treat nasal carriage (mupirocin cream)
- Topical or systemic ABX

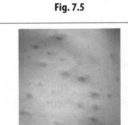

Fig. 7.6

STAPHYLOCOCCAL SCALDED SKIN SYNDROME

Sx: erythema & sheets of peeling skin, malaise & fever (affects children <5y, especially neonates)

Mx: ADMIT (emergency)
- Supportive (fluids & analgesia)
- IV flucloxacillin/erythromycin

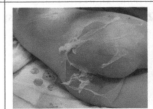

Fig. 7.7

TOXIC SHOCK SYNDROME

Sx: septic shock
Days 1–3: widespread macular erythema
Days 10–21: desquamation, mucosal oedema & ulceration

Mx:
- Supportive (fluids & analgesia)
- IV flucloxacillin/erythromycin

Associations:
- Tampons
- GIT infection

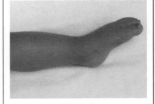

Fig. 7.8

Streptococcal infections

→ Usually **more acute onset** & **more severe** than staph infections
→ *Strep. pyogenes* (group A strep) = always PATHOGENIC

Streptococcal infections can be 1° or 2° via toxins or hypersensitivity

Mx of Strep infections: take swab

→ **Topical ABX:** clindamycin
→ **Oral ABX:** penicillin V

ERYSIPELAS (Infection **involving the dermis only** – not extending to the subcutaneous tissue) • unilateral 'beefy' red plaque = **painful** **Mx:** penicillin V	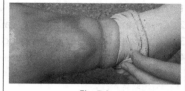 **Fig. 7.9**
NECROTISING FASCIITIS 1° or 2° infection **Sx:** • Rapidly spreading erythema & necrosis • Systemic sepsis: high fever, intense pain, vomiting **Cause:** group A strep ± *S. aureus* ± others **Mx:** 1. Surgical debridement 2. IV ABX (vancomycin ± gentamycin)	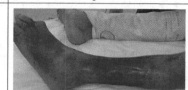 **Fig. 7.10**
CELLULITIS **Sx:** gross oedema, erythema, heat PLUS pain **Mx:** • Elevate • IV flucloxacillin • Bloods if systemically unwell	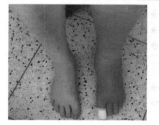 **Fig. 7.11**
SCARLET FEVER: toxin-mediated following STREP THROAT **Sx:** • Widespread pink/red papules • **Preceding sore throat, fever, lymphadenopathy** • **Strawberry tongue** **Mx:** systemic penicillin	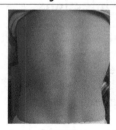 **Fig. 7.12**
ERYTHEMA NODOSUM = panniculitis **Sx:** red, tender nodules + fever, malaise, arthralgia 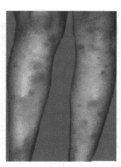 **Fig. 7.13**	**VASCULITIS** **Sx:** • Widespread purpura • Arthralgia, arthritis, haematuria • ± other organs 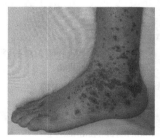 **Fig. 7.14**

Viral skin infections

Consider testing for HIV if widespread facial or perianal warts

→ 5min soak in warm water, apply Tx, nail file away dead skin

Viral warts (HPV)

→ **VERY COMMON** (*spread via direct or indirect contact* e.g. changing room floor)

MANAGEMENT: most warts disappear without treatment

1. **Topical paints** – salicylic acid + lactic acid
2. **Cryotherapy** – painful & may cause blisters
3. **Curettage & cautery** – need local anaesthetic
4. **Formalin soaks / podophyllin** – for **resistant** warts

FILIFORM WARTS → common on eyelids, face, neck, body folds **Recommended Tx:** • Most disappear without treatment • Keratolytic agents containing 10–26% salicylic acid • Curettage ↳ (warn patient about recurrence due to latent virus in the skin)	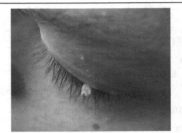 **Fig. 7.15** Filiform warts.
COMMON WARTS (HPV 2) → elevated papules → dorsum of hands → common in children	**PLANTAR WARTS** (HPV 1, 2, 4, 57) → may be uncomfortable to put pressure on → tend to be quite Tx-resistant
PLANE WARTS (HPV 3) → flat-topped → face & back of hands	**ANOGENITAL WARTS** (HPV 6 & 11) → risk factor for cervical neoplasia in women → refer patient for STI screen

VZV infections

CHICKENPOX → 10–14d **Sx:** • Widespread rash • Vesicles & crusted papules • Fever, headache, malaise **Mx[5]:** **Children:** symptomatic treatment with paracetamol, calamine lotion and chlorphenamine if ≥1y **Adults:** consider PO aciclovir in immunocompromised adult or adolescent if presenting within 24h of rash (800mg 5 times a day × 7d)	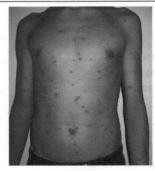 **Fig. 7.16**
SHINGLES → reactivated HSV in neural tissue **Sx:** • **Dermatomal** distribution of vesicles • Preceding pain/tingling **Mx with 7d PO aciclovir if:[6]** • >72h pain/tingling • Involves the eyes/perineum • Immunocompromised • Moderate/severe pain or rash	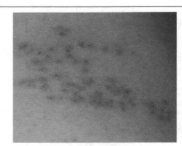 **Fig. 7.17**

consider PO valaciclovir as it has better bioavailability than PO aciclovir

Complications of shingles
• Persisting pain
• Ramsay Hunt
• Eye disease
• Deaf/dizzy
• Encephalitis

[5] NICE (2018) Scenario: *Chickenpox management*
[6] NICE (2021) Scenario: *Shingles management*

HSV infections

HERPES SIMPLEX VIRUS (HSV)
- **Cold sores (HSV 1)** *30–50% recur*
  - ▶ **Sx:** pain, tingling, vesicular eruption
  - ▶ **Mx:** topical aciclovir/valaciclovir
- **Genital herpes (HSV 2)** *95% recur*
  - ▶ **Sx:** pain, tingling, burning on urinating
  - ▶ **Mx:** oral aciclovir/valaciclovir

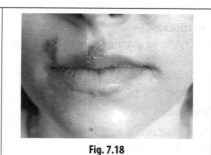

Fig. 7.18

Other infections

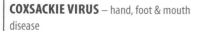

MOLLUSCUM CONTAGIOSUM –
Molluscipoxvirus (MCV)

Sx:
- Small, umbilicated papules (mainly trunk)
- Erythema, pus, crusting
→ *common in infants/children & is contagious*

Mx: self-limiting
(if not use cryotherapy or topical 1% hydrogen peroxide or 5% potassium hydroxide solution)

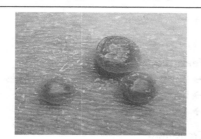

Fig. 7.19

COXSACKIE VIRUS – hand, foot & mouth disease

Sx: erythematous vesicles on hands, soles of feet, mouth
→ *common in infants / young children*
Mx: self-limiting (5–7d)

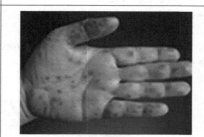

Fig. 7.20

PITYRIASIS ROSEA (thought to be caused by HHV6/7 virus)

Sx initially:
Herald patch (oval erythematous plaque + scaling)

Sx 5–15d later:
Generalised, smaller, well-defined erythematous macules
→ **'Christmas tree' distribution**

Mx: the rash usually clears in 8w
→ if symptomatic/itchy, topical steroid can be used

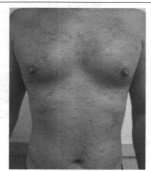

Fig. 7.21

Fungal skin infections

Levels of infection

Superficial: stratum corneum, hair, nails
Deep: subcutaneous tissue, dermis
Systemic: blood-borne

Risk factors for candida
→ Young/old
→ Immunocompromised e.g. steroids, ABX, DM

Candidiasis

→ *causes THRUSH* (genitalia, periungual, oral)

Features:
- Erythema extending from body folds
  → unclear border
- Small satellite lesions ± pustules at edges of eruption

Treatment

1. Topical azoles – clotrimazole
2. Systemic azoles – fluconazole
3. Nystatin / amphotericin B

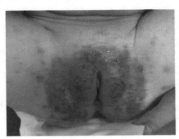

Fig. 7.22 Genital candida.

Malassezia/pityrosporum

→ *skin commensals*

PITYRIASIS VERSICOLOR
Features: on trunk
→ finely scaled, yellow/brown macules
→ hypo-/hyperpigmented
→ asymptomatic or slightly itchy

- Scaly in active phase
- Macular post-inflammatory hypopigmentation may persist for months, until melanocytes are stimulated by sun exposure

Treatment

1. **Topical treatment**
→ Ketoconazole shampoo – lather on affected areas for 10min before washing off – daily × 5d
2. **Systemic treatment:** widespread/resistant cases
→ Oral itraconazole – 200mg daily × 7d

Warn patients that it will take several months for skin colour to return to its original state

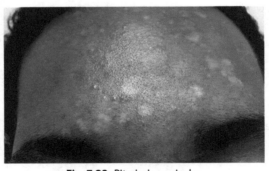

Fig. 7.23 Pityriasis versicolor.

SEBORRHOEIC DERMATITIS

Features: scalp, eyebrows, paranasal/periorbital
→ yellow/white flaking
→ ± erythematous, itchy, greasy skin
→ ± patchy hair loss

Treatment

→ Ketoconazole 2% shampoo – use 2–4 times a week then once every 2w as maintenance therapy
→ Low potency steroids e.g. Daktarin for a week
→ If more extensive and recalcitrant disease, use systemic itraconazole – 200mg OD × 7d

Consider HIV in patients with more severe symptoms

Dermatophytes

→ *cause TINEA/RINGWORM* *(most common fungal infections)*

Causes: *Microsporum, Trichophyton, Epidermophyton*

Investigations: skin scrapings, hair pluckings, nail clippings → microscopy & culture or under Wood's UV light

Treatment:

	Examples	Indications
Topical antifungals	Miconazole, ketoconazole, terbinafine, nystatin	Localised infection
Systemic antifungals	Terbinafine, itraconazole, griseofulvin for those aged <12y	Widespread **or** hair/scalp/nails **or** immunocompromised

TYPES OF DERMATOPHYTE INFECTION

TINEA CORPORIS = BODY
- Erythematous **annular scaly plaque**
- Central clearing
- **Very itchy**

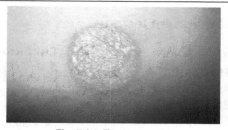

Fig. 7.24 Tinea corporis.

TINEA CRURIS = GENITALS • **Well-demarcated**, erythematous plaque • **Very itchy**	**TINEA MANUUM** = HAND • Scaling that spreads proximally • Asymmetrical involvement
TINEA UNGUIUM (ONYCHOMYCOSIS) = NAILS • Very common → often with athlete's foot **Hyperkeratosis:** • White discolouration • Loss of nail plate & lifting from bed (onycholysis)	**TINEA PEDIS** = FEET **Athlete's foot:** white maceration between toes *RFs: common floors, occlusive shoes, wet feet* **Moccasin foot:** more severe form (erythema, scaling, pustules, widespread)
TINEA CAPITIS = HEAD/SCALP • Patchy hair loss • Scales, erythema, pustules *More common in Afro-Caribbeans & children*	**KERION** = complication of tinea capitis **Boggy, painful swelling** (honey-coloured) + alopecia/lymphadenopathy (due to epidermal invasion & inflammatory response)

Melanocytic (pigmented) lesions

Benign lesions

1. **FRECKLES** – overproduction of melanin due to UV exposure
2. **CONGENITAL MELANOCYTIC NAEVI (MOLES)** – proliferations of melanocytes
3. **ACQUIRED MELANOCYTIC NAEVI (MOLES)** – proliferations of melanocytes
4. **ATYPICAL MELANOCYTIC NAEVI (MOLES)**

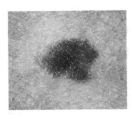

Fig. 7.25 Atypical naevus.

Causes: genetics, UV exposure, hormones (↑ with age to peak at 30y)

Features: similar to melanoma
- ≥5mm
- Irregular border
- Variable pigmentation
- Asymmetrical
- Flat or raised

Management
1. Monitor for changes
2. Sun protection advice
3. Excision if suspicious

Risk factors: FHx, UV, <30y

Malignant lesions

MELANOMA

FEATURES:
Asymmetrical
Border = IRREGULAR
Colour/pigmentation = VARIED
Diameter >6mm
Evolution (ABCD changes **or** bleeding/itching)

Risk factors

Genetic	Environmental
• PHx or FHx melanoma	• **Sun/UV exposure**
• Pale skin / red hair	• Phototherapy
• Many/large atypical naevi	• Tanning bed
• Increasing age	• **Immunosuppressed**

Differentials of melanoma
- Pigmented BCC
- Seborrhoeic wart
- Atypical naevus

INVESTIGATIONS: 2ww referral to dermatology
1. **History & skin examination**
2. **Excision** – if suspected melanoma (2mm margins)
3. **Histopathology** – Breslow thickness = depth of invasion → best prognostic factor

Stage of melanoma is determined by histopathologic features such as Breslow thickness

MANAGEMENT[7]: MDT (plastics, radiology, histopathology, oncology)

Breslow thickness <1mm
= WIDE LOCAL EXCISION (1cm margins)

Breslow thickness 1–4mm
= WIDE LOCAL EXCISION (1–3cm margins) ± SLNB

Breslow thickness >4mm
= WIDE LOCAL EXCISION (3cm margins) ± SLNB

POSITIVE SLNB
Discussion in SSMDT:
Total LN dissection + chemo-/radiotherapy

NEGATIVE SLNB
Discussion in SSMDT:
Monitoring as per SSMDT discussion

Patients are usually followed up for 2–5y depending on the MDT decision / Breslow thickness

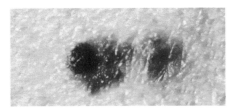

Fig. 7.26 Malignant melanoma.

[7]British Association of Dermatologists Guidelines (2010) *Revised UK guidelines for the management of cutaneous melanoma*

Non-melanocytic lesions

Malignant lesions

BASAL CELL CARCINOMA (BCC)
most common skin cancer (80%)
→ *from basal cells of epidermis*

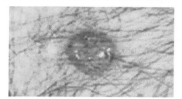

Fig. 7.27 BCC.

FEATURES
- **Slow growth** (months/years)
- Locally invasive but ↓ mets
- Asymptomatic or persistent bleeding/crusting

MANAGEMENT[8]: if elderly may not treat
1. **Simple surgical excision** – margins 4mm (5mm if high risk) (<2% recur)
2. **Moh's micrographic excision** – remove layer at a time & re-examine (<1% recur)
3. **Curettage & cautery** – scrape & cauterise to stop bleed (3–8% recur)
4. **Cryotherapy** – only if low risk tumour
5. **Photodynamic therapy (PDT)** – photosensitiser + UV → phototoxic reaction destroys lesion (only superficial BCC)

SQUAMOUS CELL CARCINOMA (SCC)
→ **2nd most common skin cancer (20%)**
→ *from keratinocytes*

FEATURES
- **Rapid growth** (weeks/months)
- Have metastatic potential ⟶
- Varied presentation (on hands/feet/head)

> **Risk factors for metastases**
> - >2cm or deep
> - Poorly differentiated
> - Lip/ear lesions
> - Previous Tx failure
> - Immunocompromised

MANAGEMENT[9]
1. **Simple surgical excision: margins depend on MDT risk stratification**
   - **Low risk:** ≥4mm margin
   - **High risk:** ≥6mm margin
   - **Very high risk:** ≥10mm margin
2. **Moh's micrographic excision**
3. **Radiotherapy** – if extensive surgery not an option

Premalignant lesions

BOWEN'S DISEASE (SCC *IN SITU*) = **epidermal dysplasia** (SCC if penetrate basement membrane)

Features: erythematous, scaly plaque/patch

Treatment
- 5-fluorouracil cream
- Curette & cautery
- Cryotherapy
- Photodynamic therapy

ACTINIC KERATOSIS = **10% risk of evolving to SCC in 10y**
Treatment: as for Bowen's

Benign

SEBORRHOEIC KERATOSIS = **benign proliferation of skin cells**

---

[8] British Association of Dermatologists (2021) *Guidelines for the management of adults with basal cell carcinoma*
[9] British Association of Dermatologists (2020) *Guidelines for the management of people with cutaneous squamous cell carcinoma*

Malignant lesions are the most common cancer in the UK

> **Risk factors for both BCC & SCC:**
> - **UV exposure**
> - Fair skin
> - Immunosuppression
> - Sites of inflammation/infection/wounds
>
> **Additional RFs for SCC only:**
> - **Smoking**
> - Actinic keratosis / Bowen's

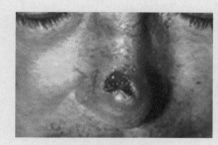

Fig. 7.28 SCC.

> **5-year survival of SCC**
> Non-metastatic: 75–90%
> Metastatic: 25%

↳ Follow-up is based on MDT discussion

> **DDx of Bowen's disease**
> - Psoriasis
> - Eczema
> - Actinic keratosis
> - Superficial BCC

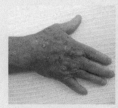

Fig. 7.29 Actinic keratosis.

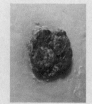

Fig. 7.30 Seborrhoeic keratosis.

Dermatological manifestations of systemic disease

ACANTHOSIS NIGRICANS

Symptoms:
- Velvety, thickened, hyperpigmented
- Affects skin folds (axilla, groin, neck)

Associations:
- Obesity, T2DM, Cushing's, Addison's, PCOS
- GI tract cancers

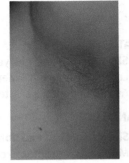

Fig. 7.31

PYODERMA GANGRENOSUM = chronic, recurrent ulceration   *DDx: venous or arterial ulcers*

Symptoms:
- Painful, ulcerated nodules
- **Gun-metal blue border**
- Heal to leave atrophic cribriform scar

± fever & systemic illness   *Mx: PO steroids*

Associations:
- UC, Crohn's, diverticulitis, vessel inflammation (Behçet's)
- Active hepatitis
- Haematological malignancy (leukaemia/myeloma)

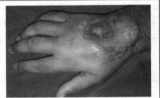

Fig. 7.32

DERMATOMYOSITIS = rare, acquired muscle disease + rash

Symptoms:
- **Violaceous rash** on photoexposed areas
- Heliotrope rash on eyelids   *(onset 50–70y)*
- Gottron's papules on knuckles

Associations:
- MALIGNANCY (breast, cervix, ovaries, lungs, pancreas, GI tract)
- Autoimmune conditions
- Drugs

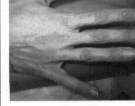

Fig. 7.33

ACQUIRED ICHTHYOSIS

Symptoms: 'fish-scale' skin (dry)

Associations:
- Hodgkin's lymphoma (and other malignancies)
- Drugs e.g. allopurinol

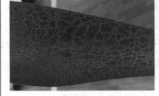

Fig. 7.34

ERYTHEMA MULTIFORME = inflammation of blood vessels

Symptoms:
- Red 'bull's-eye' lesions
- Usually on palms but target lesion could be anywhere on body

Associations:
- HSV infection (may follow cold sores)
- Drugs (penicillin, sulphonamides, allopurinol, phenytoin)

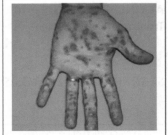

Fig. 7.35

ERYTHEMA NODOSUM = inflammation of subcutaneous fat

Symptoms:
- Tender, erythematous nodules (bruise-like)
- Usually lower legs
± fever, malaise, arthralgia

Associations:
- Infection: streptococcus, TB
- Inflammatory disease: sarcoid, IBD, Behçet's
- Drugs: sulphonamides, OCP

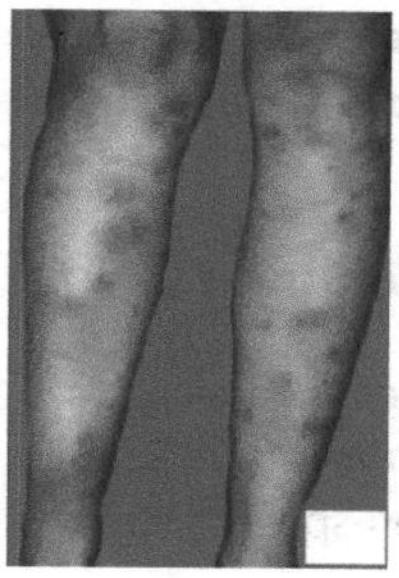

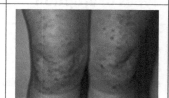

Fig. 7.36

DERMATITIS HERPETIFORMIS = chronic, recurrent, pruritic rash

Symptoms:
- Symmetrical vesicular rash
- On extensor surfaces

Associations: coeliac disease

Fig. 7.37

CUTANEOUS VASCULITIS = inflammation of skin blood vessels

Symptoms: non-blanching, erythematous, purpuric rash
± pustules, blister, wheals
± pain, itching, burning
± fever, arthralgia
→ legs, ankles, feet

Ix: Hx & exam
- Skin biopsy
- FBC & auto-antibodies
- U&Es & BP, urine dip

Triggers:
- Infection: meningococcus, strep, URTI, hepatitis C
- Autoimmune: RA, SLE, IBD
- Medications: ABX, NSAIDs, diuretics
- Haematological disorders/malignancies: myeloma

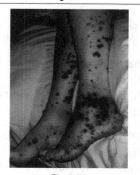

Fig. 7.38

PRETIBIAL MYXOEDEMA

Symptoms: mucin deposits = waxy plaques

Associations: Graves' disease

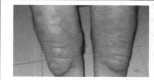

Fig. 7.39

SLE SKIN CHANGES

Acute: malar (butterfly) rash
Subacute: discrete ring lesions → red & scaly
Chronic: discrete discoid lesions → thick & scarring

± photosensitivity, arthritis, Raynaud's, renal disease

Diagnostic criteria:
- Malar skin rash
- Antiphospholipid/antinuclear/anti-DNA antibodies
- Persistent thrombocytopenia
- Persistent proteinuria

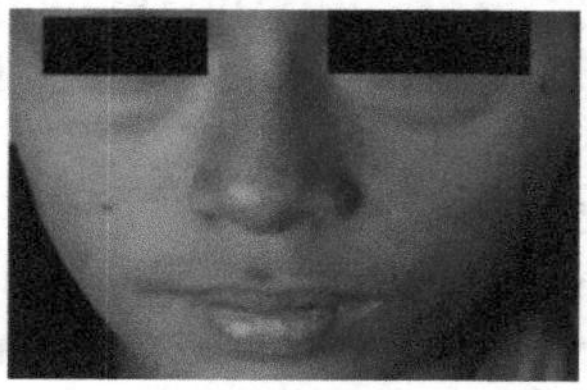

Fig. 7.40

DIABETIC SKIN CHANGES

Granuloma annulare: small papules in annular configuration → usually hands & feet

Necrobiosis lipoidica: symmetrical plaques with telangiectasia ± ulceration, red/brown colour
→ usually shins

Diabetic ulcer / gangrene / candidiasis

Acanthosis nigricans

Rubeosis & vitiligo

Drug eruptions

General management

1. **STOP DRUG**
2. Supportive care (burns etc.)
3. Wound care

Common rash-causing drugs

- Penicillins, sulphonamides
- Thiazide diuretics
- Gold, penicillamine
- NSAIDs
- Allopurinol
- Anticonvulsants

SCORETEN: measure of severity of SJS/TEN

Worse prognosis if any of:

- >40y
- Urea >10mmol/L
- HCO_3^- <20mol/L
- HR >120
- Glucose >14mmol/L
- **>10% SA**

Usually 8–21d post-exposure BUT can occur with drugs that have been used without issue for years

Mechanisms

1. **Allergy** e.g. ABX
2. **Intrinsic drug action** e.g. tetracycline & photosensitivity
3. **Non-specific** e.g. vasculitis

Types of eruption

TOXIC ERYTHEMA = 7–10d post exposure

Symptoms:

Morbilliform rash (measle-like)

- Symmetrical erythematous macules & papules
- May merge into larger plaques

± malaise, fever, pruritus

Complications:

Can progress to erythroderma/TEN

Management:

1. Stop drug (resolves in a week)
2. Consider emollients & antihistamines

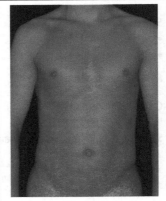

Fig. 7.41

URTICARIA (HIVES) = 24h post exposure

Symptoms:

Wheals = raised, pale red, itchy plaques

Causes:

- Drugs (salicylates, ACEis)
- Infection
- Sun, exercise, stress

Complications: angioedema

Management: antihistamines

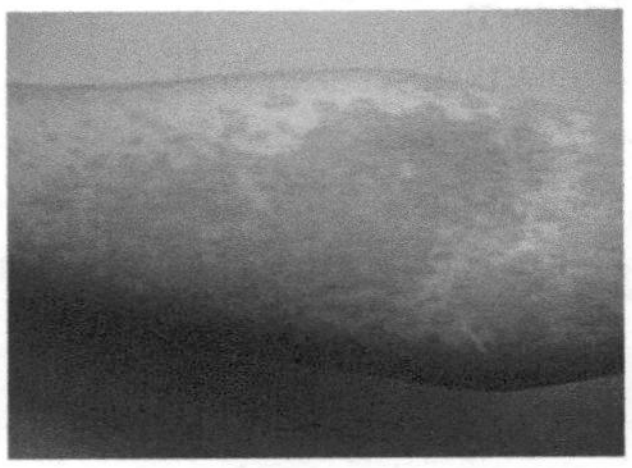

Fig. 7.42

STEVENS–JOHNSON SYNDROME (SJS) <10% SA

TOXIC EPIDERMAL NECROLYSIS (TEN) >30% SA

= **type 4 hypersensitivity**

Symptoms:

- Symmetrical red macules + central blistering
- ≥2 mucosal sites involved → **esp. mouth**
- Severe eye involvement
- **Dermal necrosis in TEN**

Causes:

- Drugs (penicillin, anticonvulsants, allopurinol)
- Infection (mycoplasma, HSV)

Complications:

→ sepsis, dehydration, electrolyte imbalance

Management:

1. STOP DRUG
2. ICU support (fluids, NG tube, analgesia)

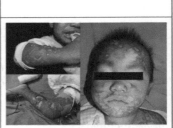

Fig. 7.43

ERYTHEMA MULTIFORME (see above)

Symptoms: red 'bull's-eye' lesions

Drug causes: penicillin, sulphonamides, allopurinol, phenytoin

EAR, NOSE AND THROAT 08

ABBREVIATIONS

AC – Air conduction

AOE – Acute otitis externa

AOM – Acute otitis media

AVM – Arteriovenous malformation

BC – Bone conduction

BCC – Basal cell carcinoma

BPPV – Benign paroxysmal positional vertigo

CHL – Conductive hearing loss

CPAP – Continuous positive airway pressure

CSOM – Chronic suppurative otitis media

dB – Decibel

EAM – External acoustic meatus

EBV – Epstein–Barr virus

ET tube – Endotracheal tube

FN – Facial nerve

FNAC – Fine needle aspiration cytology

FNE – Flexible nasal endoscopy

GA – General anaesthetic

GORD – Gastro-oesophageal reflux disease

HL – Hearing loss

HPV – Human papillomavirus

HSV – Herpes simplex virus

Hz – Hertz

HZV – Herpes zoster virus

LMN – Lower motor neurone

LN – Lymph node

LP reflux – Laryngopharyngeal reflux

MS – Multiple sclerosis

NICU – Neonatal intensive care unit

OME – Otitis media with effusion

OPG – Orthopantomogram

PPI – Proton pump inhibitor

PTA – Pure tone audiometry

RSV – Respiratory syncytial virus

SALT – Speech and language therapy

SAN – Spinal accessory nerve

SCC – Squamous cell carcinoma

SNHL – Sensorineural hearing loss

TB – Tuberculosis

TM – Tympanic membrane

UMN – Upper motor neurone

URTI – Upper respiratory tract infection

VC – Vocal cord

VZV – Varicella zoster virus

Head & neck malignancy = 6th most common cancer in world

Thyroid cancer

Symptoms:
- Neck lump moves when swallow / tongue out
- Hoarse voice / breathing difficulties

Management:
- Thyroidectomy, neck dissection ± radioactive iodine

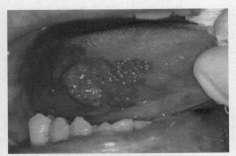

Fig. 8.1 Erythroplakia – red patches.

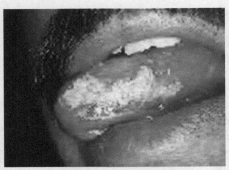

Fig. 8.2 Leukoplakia – white/grey patches.

---

*risk to structures e.g. SAN, brachial plexus, cranial nerves, phrenic nerve

MDT INVOLVEMENT: consultant, specialist nurse, surgeon, SALT, dietitian

---

Locations

- **Aerodigestive tract** (nasal/oral cavity, pharynx, larynx) = SCC most common
- **Salivary glands** = pleomorphic adenoma most common
- **Lymph nodes** = lymphomas, 2° tumours
- **Thyroid** = papillary, follicular, medullary, anaplastic
- **Skin** = SCCs, BCCs, melanomas

Risk factors

- Tobacco/alcohol – including chewing tobacco
- HPV 16 & 18
- Occupation – woodwork, textiles, nickel
- Erythroplakia – ½ become cancerous
- Leukoplakia – ⅓ become cancerous

Symptoms

→ *often unilateral*

- Unexplained dysphagia*
- Persistent, unexplained hoarseness*
- Trismus – oropharyngeal malignancy
- Referred otalgia
- Dyspnoea/stridor   *2ww referral

Signs

- Persistent, unexplained neck lump*
- Persistent mouth ulceration >3w*
- Leukoplakia/erythroplakia*
- Bleeding in mouth/throat

→ general B symptoms: weight loss, night sweats, fever

Diagnosis

- History & head/neck exam
- Flexible nasal endoscopy
- FNAC
- CT/MRI of neck – TNM staging
- CXR / CT chest – TNM staging
- Bloods – FBC, U&Es, LFT, TFT, glucose, albumin
- Assess nutritional status

→ **BIOPSY = DIAGNOSTIC** but avoid if possible, as need GA

Management[1]

→ *depends on **tumour location, TNM stage & patient health***

1. **Surgery**
   - Neck dissection* to remove LNs (LNs removed depends on site of primary)
   - Laryngectomy (for laryngeal tumour)
2. **Radiotherapy/chemotherapy**
3. **Transoral laser resection** (for early-stage disease)

Laryngectomy

→ Larynx is removed and the trachea opens onto the neck
→ no connection between oropharynx and trachea
→ unlike tracheostomy where still have proximal airway anatomically, although physically it may be obstructed

many may have mild lasting dietary impairment

Post-laryngectomy considerations:

(SALT) {
1. **Swallowing difficulties** – contrast swallow at 7–10d then rebuild oral intake over 3–6m
2. **Voice restoration** – often delayed until 6m → learn oesophageal speech / insert voice prosthesis
3. **Heat & moisture exchange** – air passes through device over stoma
}

---

[1] Head and Neck Cancer: United Kingdom National Multidisciplinary Guidelines (2016) *Journal of Laryngology & Otology*

Dysphagia

Causes

- Structural changes e.g. post-op/radiotherapy
- Obstructive e.g. malignancy, pharyngeal pouch
- Neurological e.g. CVA/stroke
- Muscular e.g. cerebral palsy, age-related weakness
- Gastro-oesophageal e.g. LP reflux/GORD

Signs/symptoms

- Difficulty initiating/coordinating swallow – e.g. dementia / stroke / neuro disease
- Food/fluid 'sticks' in throat – e.g. obstructing mass / narrowing
- Food regurgitation – pharyngeal pouch
- Aspiration – coughing, wheezing, recurrent chest infections
- Dehydration / weight loss

Investigations

- Video-fluoroscopy
- Barium swallow
- Endoscopy

Management

- Swallowing exercises
- Oral care – steam inhalations, artificial saliva
- Posture & positioning
- Adaptive equipment – cups/straws/spoons
- Modified diet – puréed, thickeners

Remember unexplained dysphagia = 2ww on upper GI cancer pathway

MDT involvement: SALT, dietitian, doctors, nurses, orthodontist, OTs

Differentials of neck lumps

Differential		Features	Associated Sx
Lymphadenopathy	Reactive (infection)	#1 cause of neck lump	• Hx of infective Sx • Fluctuate in size (<1cm reassuring)
	Neoplasm (lymphoma, metastatic, unknown origin)	Rubbery, painless lump	• B-cell Sx • Oropharyngeal/laryngeal Sx (depending on primary)
Thyroid	Cyst, neoplasm, multinodular goitre	Moves with swallowing	• Thyroid disease Sx
Congenital	Thyroglossal cyst	Moves up with tongue protrusion	• Common in those aged <20y
	Cystic hygroma (lymphatic lesion)	Soft, fluctuant, transilluminable Located in posterior triangle	• 90% present aged <2y
	Branchial cyst	Smooth, mobile, oval Located anterior edge of SCM	• Present in early adulthood
Salivary gland	Neoplasm	Depends on type	• Facial nerve palsy if malignant
	Sialadenitis	Swollen & painful	• Pain or swelling related to eating • Xerostomia & dry eyes
	Sialolithiasis		
Vascular	Carotid aneurysm	Pulsatile, lateral mass	• ± dysphagia, hoarseness
Skin	Sebaceous cyst, lipoma	Soft, mobile	• ± pain

Salivary glands

Anatomy

Minor glands: 600–1000 beneath mucosa

Major glands: 3 paired

1. Parotid – serous

→ fibrous capsule = painful if stretched

→ *Stensen duct* enters opposite 2nd upper molar

2. Submandibular – mixed

→ *Wharton duct* opens either side of frenulum under tongue

3. Sublingual – mucus

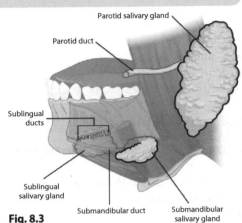

Fig. 8.3

Sjögren's syndrome: autoimmune disorder of ↓ saliva/mucus

Symptoms
- DRY MOUTH & EYES (+ vagina)
- Glossitis
- ± Parotid gland enlargement

Management
- Steroids
- Artificial saliva/tears
- Parotidectomy

Investigations:
- Genes: *HLA, B8, DR2*
- Specific antigens: SSA, SSB
- Labial biopsy = diagnostic

↑ risk of non-Hodgkin's lymphoma

---

* PAROTITIS = inflammation of **parotid gland**

Causes
- Infection – measles, mumps, HIV, TB, candidiasis
- Sarcoid
- Drugs

Xerostomia (dry mouth)

Causes:
- Depression/anxiety
- Drugs – antimuscarinics/sympathomimetics
- Radiotherapy to head/neck
- Sjögren's syndrome

Salivary gland disease

General symptoms
↳ SWELLING + PAIN ± xerostomia
↳ Dry, itchy eyes (lacrimal gland also involved)

SIALADENITIS (inflammation of gland)*

Causes: infection, stones, malignancy

Symptoms
- Swollen, tender gland
- ± pus from duct
- ± fever & systemic Sx

RF: dehydrated, poor oral hygiene, elderly

Management
- Hydration & analgesia
- High dose ABX ± pus drainage
- (Gland removal)

SIALOLITHIASIS (calculi in glands) → can cause **SIALECTASIS (dilated ducts)**

Symptoms
- **Post-prandial swelling & pain**
± palpable calculi in gland

Investigations
- CT/X-ray
- Sialogram = radio-opaque dye

Management
- Hydration & analgesia
- Duct massage
- Surgical stone removal (if necessary)

Salivary gland malignancy

→**RARE** (most commonly seen in **PAROTID** & are **BENIGN**)

SYMPTOMS

Benign	Malignant
• Well-defined	• Ill-defined border
• Discrete	• **PAINFUL**
• Mobile	• Fixed
• Slower growth	• Rapid growth ± nerve involvement

INVESTIGATIONS

- **Fine needle aspiration cytology (FNAC)** + core biopsy → for histology report
- USS – more information about tumour and lymph node status
- CT/MRI – to assess size, position and spread   **TNM STAGING IS USED**
  in malignant disease

MANAGEMENT[1]

Submandibular tumours
- **Benign:** simple excision
- **Malignant:**
  - ► wide excision (resection margins depend on grade of tumour)
  - ► + selective neck node dissection
  - ► + adjuvant radiotherapy unless small and low-grade

Parotid tumours
- **Benign:** complete excision
- **Malignant:**
  - ► parotidectomy (conserving any part of facial nerve that has not been infiltrated)
  - ► + selective neck node dissection if metastases
  - ► + adjuvant radiotherapy if tumour in close proximity to facial nerve or in high grade/large tumours

---

DDx of facial/neck swellings

Non-salivary swellings:
- Masseter hypertrophy
- Lymphadenopathy
- Dental infection/abscess
- Mastoiditis
- Cysts

Salivary swellings:
- Sialadenitis
- Sialolithiasis
- Sjögren's syndrome
- Neoplasm – benign/malignant

Most common types of salivary gland malignancy

Benign
- Pleomorphic adenoma
- Myoepithelioma
- Basal cell adenoma
- Warthin's tumour

Malignant
- Adenoid cystic carcinoma
- Mucoepidermoid carcinoma
- Acinic cell carcinoma
- Polymorphous adenocarcinoma

Throat infections

use CENTOR score to assess need for ABX

> **CENTOR SCORE:** 1 point each
> C: absence of Cough
> E: tonsillar Exudates
> N: tender cervical Nodes
> T: >38°C Temperature

↳ *score >3 = high chance strep A & need ABX*

> **Complications of tonsillectomy**
>
> - **Pain** (for 1–2w post-op)
> - **1° post-op haemorrhage** (needs surgery)
> - **2° post-op haemorrhage** (may be 2° to infection → conservative Tx or theatre depending on severity)

> Important DDx of unilateral throat swelling = TUMOUR

> **Glandular fever advice**
>
> - **Avoid intimate contact** = transmission
> - **No contact sport** = splenic rupture
> - **No alcohol** = liver damage

Tonsillitis[2]

→ *acute bacterial infection (Strep. pyogenes, staphs, M. catarrhalis)*

SYMPTOMS
- **Sore throat** + odynophagia ± pus on tonsils
- Pyrexia, malaise etc.
- Lymphadenopathy

MANAGEMENT: if **unilateral Sx** → ENT referral
- Analgesia, fluids, soft food
- **ABX:** PO phenoxymethylpenicillin (or clarithromycin) 5–10d
- Tonsillectomy if recurrent/complications (as per SIGN Guidelines[3])
  - ‣ 7× in 1y **OR** 5× in each of 2y **OR** 3× in each of 3y
  - ‣ **or** 2 episodes of quinsy

COMPLICATIONS
- Peritonsillar abscess (quinsy)
- Deep neck space infection

Peritonsillar abscess (quinsy)

→ *pus between tonsil capsule & lateral pharyngeal wall (Strep. pyogenes + others)*

SYMPTOMS
- Sore throat, odynophagia, dysphagia
- **Trismus** (limited mouth opening)
- **'Hot potato voice'** (muffled)
- Referred otalgia

SIGNS: usually unilateral
- Unilateral swelling **lateral to tonsil**
- Deviated tonsil & uvula **to opposite side**
- Limited mouth opening **(trismus)**

MANAGEMENT: ENT referral
- Needle aspiration / incision & drainage
- IV ABX ± steroids for swelling
- Analgesia, fluids, soft food

Glandular fever (infectious mononucleosis)[4]

→ *EBV infection affecting LNs, tonsils, liver*

SYMPTOMS
- **Prodromal illness:** fever, malaise, myalgia
- Sore throat, dysphagia
- Cervical lymphadenopathy
- Abdominal pain
- Hepatosplenomegaly (50%)

INVESTIGATIONS
- FBC, LFT, blood film
- Monospot test

MANAGEMENT: self-resolves in 2–4w
- **Supportive:** analgesia, fluids
- ABX **ONLY if tonsillitis** – not amoxicillin (causes skin rash)
- Monitor LFTs

---

[2] NICE (2018) *Sore throat (acute)* [NG84]
[3] SIGN (2010) National Clinical Guideline 117: *Management of sore throat and indications for tonsillectomy*
[4] NICE (2021) CKS Clinical Scenario: *Glandular fever*

Pharyngitis (sore throat)

ACUTE: sudden onset sore throat
- **Usually viral** (rhinovirus, coronavirus, influenza, HSV, VZV)
- **May be bacterial** (group A strep)

CHRONIC: long-standing sore throat
- **Specific** (syphilis, TB, toxoplasmosis)
- **Non-specific** (GORD, tobacco)

General Mx advice for sore throat: fluids, analgesia, gargle warm salty water

Supraglottitis (adults) / epiglottitis (children)

→ H. influenzae *B*

SYMPTOMS
- **Very sore throat + high fever**   Pharynx looks normal O/E
- Dysphagia, drooling
- **Stridor** – fast, noisy breathing, leans forward
- Altered/hoarse voice

MANAGEMENT: immediate admission
- **Airway protection** – intubation/tracheostomy
- IV ABX & steroids

→ *DO NOT try to examine throat/mouth in child, as upsetting them may compromise airway*

Deep neck space infection

→ *spread of throat infections (pus/abscess) via **para- or retropharyngeal space***

SYMPTOMS
- Sore throat + odynophagia
- Dysphagia, drooling
- Fever
- Trismus – if parapharyngeal
- 'Hot potato' (muffled) voice – if parapharyngeal

SIGNS
- **Poor head movement***
- **Neck mass***
- Septic

INVESTIGATIONS
- **CT** – shows deep neck spaces
- **OPG** – dental X-ray

MANAGEMENT: emergency (A→E)
- **Airway protection**
- IV ABX
- Surgical drainage

Complications of deep neck space infection
- Airway compromise
- Empyema
- Pneumonia
- Mediastinitis (50% mortality)
- Carotid artery erosion
- IJV thrombosis (Lemierre's syndrome)

*signs that differentiate it from quinsy

Other ENT symptoms

Symptom	Description	Causes
Catarrh	Build-up of **mucus** in the airway	infection, allergy, emotions, cold/heat, hormones
Cough	**Protective reflex** to clear irritants/ secretions. Dry or productive.	aspiration, reflux, infection
Referred otalgia	Ear pain caused by non-otologic source. Due to **shared nerve supply** between ear & facial structures/ oro-/ laryngopharynx (CNV, VII, IX, X)	dental pain, tonsillitis, thyroiditis, GORD
Globus pharyngeus	**Painless** sensation of 'sticking' / lump in throat **even when not swallowing**	LP reflux, stress/anxiety, minor inflammation → must exclude pathologies like cancer

Mx: *treat underlying cause, avoid caffeine/smoking, sip icy sparkling water, PPI, Gaviscon Advanced*

Airway obstruction

Signs of severe airway obstruction
• Tracheal tug/recession
• Accessory muscle use
• Tachycardia
• Hypoxia
• Confusion

Stertor: noisy breathing due to partial obstruction ABOVE the larynx → tonsils, adenoids, tongue, angioedema

Stridor: noisy breathing due to partial obstruction BELOW the larynx
→ needs ENT REFERRAL for laryngoscopy, or ANAESTHETICS REFERRAL for intubation (depends on severity)

Differentials of stridor

Congenital	Acquired	
	Acute	Chronic
• Laryngomalacia • VC web / VC palsy • Subglottic stenosis	• Laryngeal trauma • Foreign body • Croup • Epiglottitis • Allergic reaction • Deep neck space infection	• VC palsy • VC polyp/cyst • Tumour • Thyroid mass • Subglottic stenosis • Post radiotherapy

LARYNGEAL TRAUMA: usually the result of RTAs

Symptoms
→ stridor (may be delayed)
→ neck bruising
→ surgical emphysema (perforation)

Management: intubation ± tracheostomy

FOREIGN BODY

Symptoms
→ feel something 'stick' in throat
→ sharp pain
→ cannot eat/drink/swallow saliva

Investigations: lateral neck X-ray & CXR

Management: flexiscope ± theatre for removal

Management of stridor

1. **Basic history & assess severity** – cyanosis, RR, etc.

2. **A→E first aid** – ensure clear mouth

3. **Secure airway**
   - **Endotracheal tube:** first-line → need trained staff & equipment
   - **Cricothyroidotomy** → incision in midline of cricothyroid membrane & insert ET tube + bag valve mask
   - **Tracheostomy** → tube inserted between **2nd & 4th rings** of cartilage

Tracheostomy complications
• Tube blockage
• Wound infection
• Pneumothorax

Tracheostomy indications
• Bypass obstruction
• Aspiration prevention
• Secretion management
• Respiratory failure
• ICU weaning

Sleep apnoea

Repeated upper airway obstruction whilst sleeping, resulting in desaturation & awakening

↪ **Obstructive:** due to upper airway collapse ($\downarrow O_2$ causes reflex of waking slightly & taking deep breath)

↪ **Central:** fault with central respiratory drive *e.g. cerebral palsy, cognitive defect* → *diagnosed in childhood*

Symptoms

- Snoring/choking in sleep & witnessed apnoeas
- Restless/non-refreshing sleep
- Daytime sleepiness & $\downarrow$ concentration – **assess risk**, e.g. driving
- Irritability & $\downarrow$ libido

Investigations

- **History** – Epworth Sleepiness Scale[5]
- **Examination** – upper airway endoscopy
- **Sleep studies**
  - ▸ measure pulse, ECG, O_2 overnight
  - ▸ audio/video recording of sleep
  - ▸ **polysomnography** = gold standard version
    - → EEG, chest expansion, etc.

Apnoea Hypoxia Index (AHI)

	Adult AHI	Paediatric AHI
Mild OSA	≥5 to <15 events/h	≥1 to ≤5 events/h
Moderate OSA	≥15 to <30 events/h	>5 to ≤10 events/h
Severe OSA	≥30 events/h	>10 events/h

Management[6]

1. **Lifestyle** – weight loss, reduce smoking/alcohol
2. **Conservative** – nasal splints/tape & jaw advancers } 1 & 2 also for Mx of simple snoring
3. **Medical** – CPAP via mask = noisy & uncomfortable
4. **Surgery** – adenotonsillectomy, polypectomy, uvulopalatopharyngoplasty

Sleep apnoea in children

SYMPTOMS

- Snoring/choking in sleep & witnessed apnoeas
- Restless/non-refreshing sleep
- Daytime sleepiness or hyperactivity
- $\downarrow$ concentration – poor school performance
- Failure to thrive

INVESTIGATIONS

- **History** often all that is needed
- **Sleep studies** if complex/syndromic child/very young or small / multiple comorbidities

MANAGEMENT[3]

- **Clear clinical history** with no comorbidities = TONSILLECTOMY

If suspect more complex/central cause, further investigations and management may be required

Risk factors for sleep apnoea
- Older age
- **Obesity**
- Male
- Smoking/alcohol
- Sedatives
- Neuromuscular disease

Apnoea Hypoxia Index: measures no. of episodes to determine severity

Risk factors for childhood sleep apnoea
- Down syndrome
- Craniofacial abnormalities
- Neuromuscular disease
- **Obesity**

[5] Johns NW (1990–97) *Epworth Sleepiness Scale*
[6] NICE (2021) *Obstructive sleep apnoea/hypopnoea syndrome and obesity hypoventilation syndrome in over 16s* [NG202]

The larynx & voice disorders

VC = vocal cord

Fundamental frequency (F₀) = PITCH (Hz)
- determined by **density of vocal fold**
- density altered by **muscle contraction/relaxation**
- HIGHER DENSITY = LOWER FREQUENCY
  e.g. males, Reinke oedema

Intensity/pressure level = LOUDNESS (dB)
- Determined by **subglottic pressure**
- Pressure depends on **degree of VC closure / length of closure**
- LOWER PRESSURE = WEAKER VOICE
  e.g. recurrent laryngeal nerve palsy

Abnormal speech

Dysphonia: any voice impairment
Dysarthria: reduced voice muscle coordination
Dysphasia: receptive or comprehensive

Normal voice production

Due to VC vibration:
- Movement of air molecules in larynx causes oscillation of VC mucosa
- VCs drawn together, then apart
- Oscillation causes sound wave that resonates within vocal tract

Vowel production: vibration of OPEN VCs & mouth/tongue position

Consonant production: force air through NARROWED VCs

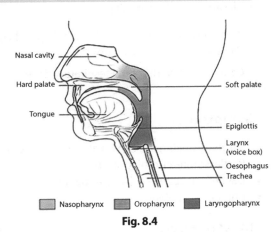

Labels: Nasal cavity, Hard palate, Tongue, Soft palate, Epiglottis, Larynx (voice box), Oesophagus, Trachea

Legend: Nasopharynx — Oropharynx — Laryngopharynx

Fig. 8.4

Voice disorders

STRUCTURAL/NEOPLASTIC

collection of fluid in Reinke's pouch

	Malignant	Benign	
	Laryngeal carcinoma	**Polyp**	**Reinke's oedema**
Causes	• Smoking • Genetics (FHx, male, black) • (+ alcohol >8units/d)	• Shouting • Voice abuse • Professional voice users	• Smoking • Voice overuse • LP reflux
Symptoms	**Progressive hoarseness** ± stridor, dysphagia ± referred otalgia ± cervical lymphadenopathy	**Husky (deeper) voice**	**Deep, gravelly voice**
Signs	• Irregular mass • Leukoplakia/erythroplakia	• Smooth, grey swelling → usually UNILATERAL	• Grey/red swelling → usually BILATERAL
Treatment	• Radiotherapy • Surgical excision	• Surgical excision ± medical Tx ± voice therapy	• Stop smoking / Tx reflux • Surgical reduction • Voice therapy

INFLAMMATORY

	Infectious	Non-infectious
	Laryngitis (bacterial, fungal, HPV)	**Laryngopharyngeal (silent) reflux**
Symptoms	• Hoarse/croaky/voice loss • Sore throat, odynophagia • URTI symptoms	• **Strained voice + ↓ pitch range** • Dysphagia & **globus sensation** • Cough & constant throat clearing • **NO HEARTBURN** unless concurrent GORD (often have both)
Signs	• Erythematous, sloughy VCs	• General erythema & oedema
Treatment	• Voice rest, analgesia, fluids • Steam inhalations → self-limiting	• Gaviscon + PPI • Vocal hygiene • **Dietary advice** – avoid fatty/fried food & caffeine

NEUROMUSCULAR – RECURRENT LARYNGEAL NERVE PALSY

Causes
- Miscellaneous
- **Surgical trauma** – e.g. thyroidectomy
- **Malignancy** – of bronchus, thyroid, oesophagus, larynx
- Idiopathic
- Neurological disorders

Symptoms
- **Weak, higher-pitched voice**
- Tires with prolonged use
- Choking on fluids
- Weak 'bovine' cough
- Diplophonia – 2-tone voice

Investigations

1. **Examination** – listen to voice, head & neck exam, cranial nerves, flexible nasendoscopy
2. **CXR** – exclude mediastinal mass
3. **CT (skull base to mid thorax)** – check for lesions along nerve
4. **Barium swallow** – if suspect oesophageal lesion

Management → may just wait for spontaneous recovery
- Voice therapy
- VC medialisation – inject collagen **or** surgery

MUSCLE TENSION IMBALANCE = excessive tension of laryngeal muscles

Causes
- Stress/anxiety
- Following URTI
- Long-term ineffective voice use
- Compensation for underlying VC problem e.g. cyst

Symptoms
- **Husky voice** – worse with use
- **Deeper or higher-pitched than expected**
- Unstable voice
- Sore throat

Management
- **Vocal hygiene** – steam inhalations
- **Lifestyle advice** – avoid irritants (smoke, caffeine, spicy food), drink plenty of water
- **Voice therapy** – practise projecting voice, relaxed posture, breathing control

> **Approximate incidence of VC palsy[7]:**
> **65%** = LEFT VC*
> **25%** = RIGHT VC
> **10%** = BOTH VCs
>
> ↳ *longer course of left recurrent laryngeal nerve leaves it more vulnerable to damage

Voice therapy

Aims: restore voice, eliminate benign nodules & avoid further vocal problems

Indications
- LP reflux
- Nodules, cysts, polyps
- Muscle tension imbalance
- Psychological voice problems

Components
- Semi-occluded airflow exercises – reduce muscle straining
- Efficient respiration
- Voice resonance & projection
- **Advice on vocal hygiene** – steam inhalations, avoid irritants etc.

[7] Yamada M, Hirano M, Ohkubo H (1983) Recurrent laryngeal nerve paralysis. A 10-year review of 564 patients. *Auris Nasus Larynx*, 10, S1–15.

Outer ear problems

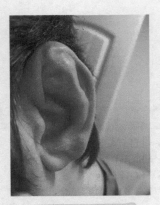

Fig. 8.5 Cauliflower ear.

Excess wax

→ Wax-softening drops e.g. sodium bicarbonate / olive oil
→ Ear syringing → **contraindicated if grommets, or perforation**

Foreign bodies

→ Wax hook/forceps/suction   *often in children*
→ GA if uncooperative / deep into canal

Pinna haematoma

→ *blood collects between cartilage & perichondrium*
→ **Cause:** trauma
→ **Complications:** avascular necrosis & infection → 'Cauliflower ear'
→ **Management:** IMMEDIATE DRAINAGE

Neoplasm

→ **Benign:** papilloma or adenoma   → **Malignant:** BCC or SCC

Acute otitis externa (AOE)

AETIOLOGY: inflammation of the ear canal

CAUSES
- Skin conditions e.g. eczema, psoriasis
- Generalised skin infections e.g. impetigo
- Localised skin infections e.g. ***Pseudomonas, S. aureus***, candida
- Trauma / foreign bodies (**cotton buds**)
- Water exposure

SYMPTOMS
- Pain & swelling
- Itching
- Hearing loss
- ± discharge (exudate build-up)

SIGNS
- **Tender pinna/tragus**
- Swollen/red canal
- TM not visible

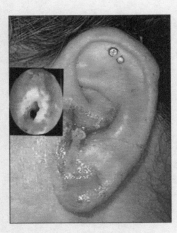

Fig. 8.6 Acute otitis externa.

Risk factors for AOE
- Immunocompromised/DM
- Atopies & skin conditions
- Swimmers

Differentials/complications of AOE
- Necrotising otitis externa
- Mastoiditis
- Pinna perichondritis
- Pinna cellulitis
- Middle ear infection (discharge but no canal swelling)

MANAGEMENT[8]
1. **Mild/simple** (TM visible)
   - Analgesia & keep dry
   - Topical ABX ± steroid
2. **Severe/complex** (TM not visible / Tx-resistant)   **Needs ENT referral**
   - Microsuction
   - Pope wick & topical antibiotic drops
   - PO ABX if pinna cellulitis

Necrotising/malignant otitis externa

AETIOLOGY: Complication of AOE → infection **spreads to skull base**

SYMPTOMS
- **Severe, often deep pain** – worse at night & when chewing
- **Nerve palsies** – CN VII, IX, X, XI
- **Canal granulations**   **Pathogen:** *Pseudomonas aeruginosa*

INVESTIGATIONS: CT/MRI

MANAGEMENT: → ENT referral
- High dose IV ABX (6w course)
- ± topical treatment
- Microsuction (twice weekly)
- Analgesia

[8]NICE (2021) CKS Management Scenario: *Acute otitis externa*

Middle ear problems

→ **Cause conductive hearing loss**

Acute otitis media with effusion (OME)

→ *'glue ear'*

AETIOLOGY: build-up of fluid within the middle ear

SYMPTOMS
- **Middle ear fluid** with **NO SX OF INFECTION** (painless)
- CHL 20–30dB = speech delay / school problems

CAUSES: Eustachian tube dysfunction
- Nasal/sinus infection
- Allergic response
- Ciliary dysfunction

MANAGEMENT[9]: 50% spontaneous resolution
- **If persists >3m:**
  - ▸ grommets – ventilate middle ear
    → pop out in 18m
  - ▸ hearing aids

Eustachian tube aerates middle ear & equalises pressure

Risk factors for OME
- Child
- Smoking
- Large adenoids
- Nasal abnormalities

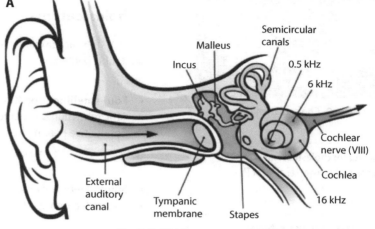

A

Semicircular canals

Malleus

Incus

0.5 kHz

6 kHz

Cochlear nerve (VIII)

Cochlea

16 kHz

External auditory canal

Tympanic membrane

Stapes

Fig. 8.7 Middle ear anatomy.

Acute suppurative otitis media (ASOM)

AETIOLOGY: acute infection of middle ear

- H. influenzae
- S. pneumoniae
- M. catarrhalis
- RSV/rhinovirus

SYMPTOMS
- **PAIN!** = crying/screaming child
- **Fever** / systemic upset
- Conductive hearing loss
- Otorrhoea (pus ± blood) if TM perforated → **relieves pain**

SIGNS
- Bulging TM **OR**
- TM perforation & pus/blood

MANAGEMENT[10]: by GP
1. Analgesia & wait for resolution in 3–7d
2. Antibiotic ear drops – **if TM perforation** & ongoing infection
3. PO amoxicillin **ONLY IF:**

- Aged <6m
- Risk of complications
- Otorrhoea
- Aged <2y with bilateral Sx
- Systemically very unwell
- Non-resolving infection (3d)

Complications of ASOM: refer to middle ear anatomy, *Fig. 8.7*
- Residual perforation/ effusion (CSOM)
- Ossicle necrosis
- Tympanosclerosis
- Intracranial sepsis/meningitis
- Facial palsy
- Labyrinthitis
- Mastoiditis

Mastoiditis: pus in air cells → bone necrosis & abscess

Symptoms
- Otalgia
- Hearing loss
- Malaise/pyrexia
- Post-auricular swelling
- Pinna down & forwards

Management: ABX ± surgery (ENT referral)

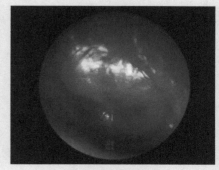

Fig. 8.8 Bulging TM.

[9] NICE (2008) *Otitis media with effusion in under 12s* [CG60]
[10] NICE (2018, updated 2022) *Otitis media (acute)* [NG91]

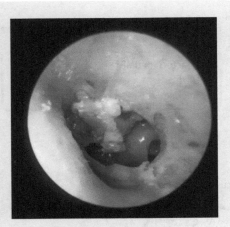

Fig. 8.9 Cholesteatoma.

Risk factor for cholesteatoma:
Retraction pockets (weaker areas of TM)
→ *dead cells accumulate in pockets*

Complications of cholesteatoma: due to erosion of bone & nearby structures
→ facial nerve palsy
→ vertigo
→ intracranial sepsis
→ CHL (ossicle erosion)

TEMPORAL BONE FRACTURE → Need CT
20% = transverse = SNHL
80% = longitudinal = CHL
Other complications: CSF leak, bleed, FN palsy

Chronic suppurative otitis media (CSOM)

AETIOLOGY: repeated ASOM (>6w) → non-healing TM perforation

SYMPTOMS
- Repeated otorrhoea
- CHL 10–20dB or more

MANAGEMENT: ENT referral to assess possible complications
- Regular aural toilet
- ABX + steroid ear drops

Cholesteatoma

AETIOLOGY: accumulation of keratinising squamous epithelium attracting anaerobic bacteria

Pseudomonas aeruginosa

SYMPTOMS
- **Foul-smelling otorrhoea**
- Attic retraction & squamous debris
- Conductive hearing loss

INVESTIGATION: Fine cut CT temporal bones / diffusion weighted MRI

MANAGEMENT[11]
- Surgical removal of sac
- Mastoidectomy if advanced disease

Foul otorrhoea + FN palsy needs ENT referral

Tympanic membrane perforation

SYMPTOMS
- **Conductive HL** (10–20dB)
± **pain, tinnitus, vertigo**

CAUSES
- AOM
- Foreign bodies
- Head injury – temporal bone fracture
- Barotrauma
- Sudden ↑ air pressure e.g. loud noise/slap

MANAGEMENT: heals in 6w
- Keep dry & wait
- GP follow-up in 6w → not healed = ENT

Tympanosclerosis

AETIOLOGY: calcification of scar tissue* on TM

*from previous infection, trauma or grommet insertion

SYMPTOMS: if large = conductive HL (50+dB)

Otosclerosis

AETIOLOGY: spongy bone forms around oval window = fusion with stapes → **familial condition**

SYMPTOMS: progressive, bilateral conductive HL ± tinnitus

MANAGEMENT: hearing aid / stapedectomy

Middle ear neoplasms

SQUAMOUS CELL CARCINOMAS = malignant
Sx: bloody otorrhoea & deep pain
→ may cause facial nerve palsy

GLOMUS TUMOURS (PARAGANGLIONIC CELLS) = slow growing & benign
Sx: pulsatile tinnitus & CHL + pulsatile red mass behind eardrum
→ may cause facial nerve palsy or CN IX/XII paralysis

---

[11] NICE (2020) CKS Management Scenario: *Cholesteatoma*

Inner ear problems

→ **Cause Sx of: tinnitus, SNHL, vertigo**

How we hear

1. Sound waves vibrate TM → transmits to ossicles
2. Ossicles **amplify** & transmit to oval window
3. Pressure waves through perilymph vibrate tectorial membrane
4. Hair cells are moved against **organ of Corti** & stimulate **cochlear nerve**
5. Signals carried to **cortex**

Tinnitus

DEFINITION: perception of noise with **no external stimuli**

CAUSES

Subjective/intrinsic = only heard by patient		Objective/extrinsic = heard by others as well
• Idiopathic • Drugs • Trauma • Presbycusis	• Labyrinthitis • Ménière's • Vestibular schwannoma • Otosclerosis	• Palatal myoclonus • Insect in EAM • Vascular

MANAGEMENT OF TINNITUS[12]

1. **Explain:**
   • Incorrect info reaching brain **OR**
   • Incorrect processing in brain

2. **Masking:**
   • Radio/television in background
   • 'Tinnitus maskers' – play noise into other ear

Treatment generally focuses on symptom control & acclimatisation rather than cure

3. **Counselling:**
   • CBT, mindfulness
   • Tinnitus therapy – techniques to avoid stress response
   • Support groups

4. **Hearing aids:** if associated SNHL

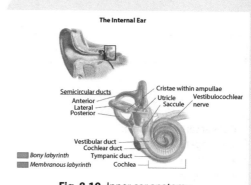

Fig. 8.10 Inner ear anatomy.

Vascular tinnitus = **PULSATILE**
→ AVM/glomus jugular tumour
→ Need CT/MR angiogram

Sensorineural hearing loss (SNHL)

→ **General Mx:** hearing aid, cochlear implant, hearing tactics

SUDDEN ONSET SNHL

Causes
• Ménière's
• Viral infection
• Ototoxic drugs
• Temporal bone fracture
• Tumour → exclude acoustic neuroma with CT/MRI

Unilateral SNHL	Bilateral SNHL
• Vestibular neuroma • Trauma • Vascular insult • Post-labyrinthitis • Otosclerosis • Congenital	• Presbycusis • Noise-induced • Metabolic • Otosclerosis • Congenital

Management: emergency → ENT referral
→ PO steroids **ASAP!** (prednisolone)

Prognosis: worse if severe vertigo as well

---

[12] NICE (2020) *Tinnitus* [NG155]

Must investigate ALL cases of UNILATERAL SNHL

Risks of surgical excision:
- damage to facial nerve
- intracranial sepsis
- hearing loss
- impaired balance

NON-ORGANIC HL = feigned loss to get compensation

VESTIBULAR SCHWANNOMA (ACOUSTIC NEUROMA)

Symptoms: caused by compression of CN VIII
UNILATERAL SNHL, tinnitus, vertigo ± **neuro symptoms**

Investigations
- Pure tone audiometry
- CT/MRI

Management[13]
→ 6-monthly monitoring + yearly MRI (most are small and slow-growing)
→ Surgical excision
→ Highly focused radiotherapy (gamma knife)

NOISE-INDUCED HEARING LOSS

Aetiology: chronic loud noise exposure (initially reversible but eventually = permanent)

Features
SYMMETRICAL SNHL & tinnitus
→ dip at 4kHz on tympanogram (Fig. 8.11)

Management: Prevention is key
- Tinnitus counselling
- Hearing aid

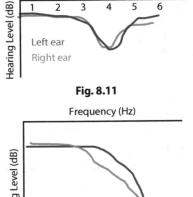

Fig. 8.11

PRESBYCUSIS

Aetiology: SNHL due to ageing (>50y) due to loss of outer hair cells of cochlea

Features
BILATERAL high frequency SNHL (Fig. 8.12)
± tinnitus → worse if background noise

Investigation
- Hx & otoscopy
- PTA / tympanogram

Fig. 8.12

Management
- **Reassure:** stress that low/mid frequency hearing is good & decline is gradual
- Hearing aid
- Hearing **tactics** e.g. facing speaker, ↓ background noise

OTOTOXICITY

Causes
- **Aminoglycosides:** gentamicin
- **Diuretics:** furosemide
- **Salicylates**
- **Chemotherapy agents**

Management

IRREVERSIBLE so prevention is crucial (careful monitoring of serum levels & PTA)

---

[13] NHS Clinical Commissioning Policy (2013) *Vestibular Schwannoma and Other Cranial Nerve Neuromas* – NHSCB/D5/P/a

Vertigo

DEFINITION
Abnormal sensation of movement / **'room spinning'** → usually with nausea &
vomiting

CAUSES

Central causes = brainstem	Peripheral causes = ears, eyes, somatosensors
• Space-occupying lesion • Head injury • Alcohol/drugs • Degenerative disease e.g. MS • Vascular ischaemia	• Labyrinthitis • Vestibular neuronitis • BPPV • Ménière's • Ototoxic drugs • Vestibular migraine

> **Non-vertigo causes of dizziness**
>
> • Postural hypotension/vasovagal
> • Arrhythmias
> • Presbystasis = age-related dysfunction of
>   vestibular system

DIFFERENTIALS OF VERTIGO SUMMARY

	Labyrinthitis	Vestibular neuronitis	BPPV	Ménière's disease	Acoustic neuroma
Pathophysiology	Inflammation of inner ear	Inflammation of vestibular nerve	Displaced semi-circular calculi	Excess endolymph	Compression of vestibular nerve
Aetiology	• URTI • AOM	Viral infection	• Spontaneous • Head injury	Unknown	Schwannoma of vestibular nerve
Onset	Sudden	Sudden	Sudden & episodic *(if head moved)*	Sudden, recurrent, progressive (stress may trigger)	Progressive
Duration	Hours – days	Hours – days	Secs – mins	30–40min	Constant
Symptoms	• N&V • Nystagmus ± SNHL	• N&V • Nystagmus • No ear Sx	• N&V • No ear Sx	• N&V • Nystagmus • Low freq SNHL • Aural fullness	• Facial palsies • Headache • Ataxia • SNHL • Tinnitus
Investigations	1. ENT exam 2. PTA	1. ENT exam 2. PTA	1. ENT exam 2. PTA 3. **Dix–Hallpike manoeuvre**	1. ENT exam 2. PTA 3. **Romberg test +ve** + CT/MRI: r/o *neuroma*	CT/ MRI head
Management	**Supportive:** • Vestibular sedatives* • Antiemetics • Bed rest	**Supportive:** • Vestibular sedatives* • Antiemetics • Bed rest *Vestibular sedative:* *Prochlorperazine*	• Eply manoeuvre • Cawthorne–Cooksey exercises **Reassure:** *spontaneously resolves in 12–18m*	**Supportive:** • Vestibular sedatives* • Antiemetics • Bed rest **Medical:** • Steroids • Intratympanic gentamycin **Prevention:** • Low salt/caffeine	**Medical:** Radiotherapy **Surgical excision** **Monitoring**

> **Advise patients NOT TO DRIVE while experiencing vertigo**

Hearing assessment

Assessment involves: history + otoscope + audiometric tests

CHL: outer/mid ear problem BC normal, AC ↓
SNHL: inner ear problem AC ↓ = BC ↓
Mixed: CHL + SNHL AC ↓ > BC ↓

Tuning fork tests

→ *use 512Hz tuning fork*

1. **Weber's test:** vibrating tuning fork placed in middle of forehead
2. **Rinne's test:** vibrating tuning fork placed on mastoid → when it can no longer be heard, it is moved next to the ear canal

Interpreting the results:

	Normal	**SNHL**	**CHL**
Weber's	Central/no lateralisation	Lateralises to opposite side to loss *Cochlear damage means no sound detection on that side*	Lateralises to same side as loss *Distracting external sounds not heard so fork seems louder*
Rinne's	AC>BC	**Positive:** AC>BC	**Negative:** BC>AC

Pure tone audiometry (PTA)

How is it performed?
→ Uses electrical equipment to control frequency & intensity of sound
→ Produces **audiograms**

Interpreting the results:
→ **Quantify HL** for diagnosis, monitoring & rehab

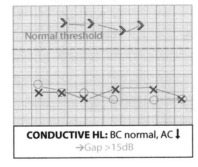

CONDUCTIVE HL: BC normal, AC ↓
→Gap >15dB

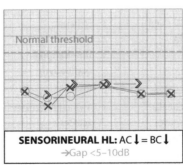

SENSORINEURAL HL: AC ↓ = BC ↓
→Gap <5–10dB

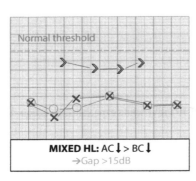

MIXED HL: AC ↓ > BC ↓
→Gap >15dB

Key to symbols most commonly used on audiograms[14]

	RIGHT	**LEFT**
AC	O	X
AC masked	△	□
BC	<	>
BC masked	[	]

Indications for masking other ear:

1. AC between ears >40dB different
2. BC >10dB more than AC in same ear

Fig. 8.13

---

[14] ASHA (1974) Guidelines for audiometric symbols. 16(5): 260–4

Tympanometry

How is it performed?
Measures 3 components:

1. canal volume
2. middle ear pressure
3. compliance

Interpreting the results:

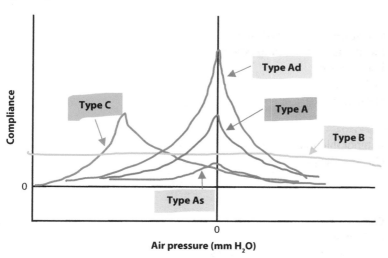

Fig. 8.14

TYPE A: normal

TYPE Ad: ↑ compliance
- healed TM perforation
- retraction pocket
- ossicle disarticulation

TYPE As: ↓ compliance
- TM scarring
- fluid in middle ear

TYPE B: no peak compliance
- middle ear effusion / tumour
- TM perforation
- grommet

TYPE C: peak compliance at low frequency
- Eustachian tube dysfunction

Paediatric hearing assessment

NEWBORN HEARING SCREENING PROGRAMME

Who for? All babies within 5w of birth

How is it done?

1. **Automated otoacoustic emission (AOE)** = play sound in ear & measure reflected vibrations – if fail AOE twice then:
2. **Automate auditory brainstem response (AABR)** = play sound in ear & measure brain waves – if high risk/fail both:
3. **AUDIOLOGY REFERRAL**

OLDER CHILDREN

Who for? Based on developmental age

How is it done?

1. **Visual reinforcement audiometry:** 6–36m
→ condition to look at toy when sound heard
2. **Play audiometry / performance test:** ≥30m
→ ask child to perform action when sound heard
3. **Pure tone audiometry:** >5y

High risk babies that automatically have AABR:

- Neonatal sepsis
- NICU stay
- FHx congenital deafness

Rhinosinusitis

Inflammation of nasal & sinus mucosa causing URTI Sx for >10d

↳ *Common cold usually <10d*

Acute rhinosinusitis

Risk factors for rhinosinusitis
- polyps
- deviated septum
- dental infections
- smoking

Acute: <4w
Subacute: 4–12w
Chronic: >12w

PATHOPHYSIOLOGY
→ Viral URTI causes **hyperaemia & oedema** of mucosa & ↑ **secretions**
→ **Stagnant secretions** become infected by bacteria (*H. influenza, Strep. pneumoniae*)

SYMPTOMS
- **Mucopurulent rhinorrhoea**
- **Nasal obstruction/congestion**
- ↓ Smell/taste
- Facial pain – over infected sinus, worse bending forward
- Malaise/pyrexia

INVESTIGATIONS
- Anterior rhinoscopy – inflamed mucosa
- FNE/endoscopy – mucopus in oropharynx
→ CT would show sinus opacification

Complications of acute rhinosinusitis
- Chronic sinusitis
- Osteomyelitis   *need CT
- Intracranial* (meningitis, brain abscess)
- Mucoceles
- Facial cellulitis
- Periorbital cellulitis

MANAGEMENT[15]
1. **Conservative**
   - Simple analgesia
   - Steam inhalations / nasal rinses
   - Nasal decongestants (pseudoephedrine)
2. **Medical**
   - Steroid nasal spray e.g. Beconase
   - Antibiotics (penicillin V or co-amoxiclav) – ONLY if severe pain/high fever/ persistent Sx
3. **Surgical (ENT referral)**
   - Maxillary sinus washout – ONLY if progressive pain/complications
   - Functional endoscopic sinus surgery (FESS) if complications

NB Facial pain without nasal symptoms = unlikely sinusitis

Facial cellulitis

Sources
- Orbital cellulitis
- Sinusitis
- Osteomyelitis

AETIOLOGY: infection spreads to skin
SYMPTOMS: red, warm, painful skin
MANAGEMENT: **high dose ABX** + sinus drainage

Periorbital cellulitis

MUCOCELE

= *collection of sterile mucus in obstructed sinus*
→ over years ↑ pressure causes sinus expansion

Symptoms:
- Eye displacement
- Visual problems
- Facial swelling

Management: surgical sinus drainage
- 2° infection of mucocele

AETIOLOGY: infection spreads into orbit (usually ethmoid sinus through thin ethmoid bone)

SYMPTOMS
- Unilateral eyelid swelling, pain, redness
- Proptosis/ophthalmoplegia
- Blurred vision / loss of colour vision
- Fever, headaches, meningism, septicaemia

CT indicated in periorbital cellulitis if:
bilateral; unable to assess eye; proptosis; reduced vision; failure to improve after 48h

MANAGEMENT: urgent ENT referral
- **High dose IV ABX**
- Nasal decongestant
- **Careful eye obs** (signs of abscess pressing on optic nerve)

- Colour vision
- Acuity
- Eye movements

[15] EPOS (2020) *European Position Paper on Rhinosinusitis and Nasal Polyps*

Chronic rhinosinusitis (>3m)

PATHOPHYSIOLOGY
→ **Infection:** viral/bacterial (anaerobes, *Staph. aureus*, Gram −ve)
→ **Allergens:** dust mites, pollen, animal hair

SYMPTOMS
- **Nasal obstruction/congestion**
- **POST-NASAL DRIP** – worse at night, morning cough to clear
- ↓ Smell/taste or unpleasant smell
- Intermittent facial pain – only with acute exacerbations
- Crusting/bleeding – **careful monitoring for vasculitis/septal perforation/neoplasm**

INVESTIGATIONS: diagnosis based on history
- Anterior rhinoscopy **and** FNE/endoscopy
→ *show inflammation, mucopus ± **polyps***

apply with head
upside down over
edge of bed
↓

MANAGEMENT[16]
- **Consider macrolide treatment for 3–6w**
- Topical nasal steroids (6–8w) e.g. betamethasone or fluticasone drops
- Steroid nasal spray (after finishing drops)
- Nasal douching

Nasal polyps

→ *grey/white, soft & mobile pedunculated swelling in nose/sinuses*

SYMPTOMS
- Nasal obstruction
- Anosmia
- Rhinorrhoea

> **Unilateral or bleeding** polyp = red flag
> **→ ENT referral**

ASSOCIATIONS/RISK FACTORS
- Cystic fibrosis
- Infective sinusitis
- **Samter's triad:** polyp + asthmas + aspirin sensitivity

INVESTIGATIONS
- Anterior rhinoscopy → biopsy if suspicious

MANAGEMENT
Medical: antihistamines, steroids (oral or drops/spray), decongestants → reduce size in 80%
Surgical: polypectomy → if significant blockage / red flag features

---

Nasopharyngeal carcinoma

→ *squamous cell carcinoma*

SYMPTOMS
- Cervical lymphadenopathy
- **Unilateral** otalgia (CN IX)
- **Unilateral** OME
- Nasal obstruction ± discharge ± epistaxis
- CN palsies (CN III–VI)

MANAGEMENT
- CT & MRI
- Radiotherapy
- Surgery

> **Specific form known as ALLERGIC RHINITIS:**
> → sneezing
> → itchy eyes
> → rhinorrhoea
>
> Mx: antihistamines, PO steroids, avoid allergens

> **If no improvement in 8w:**
> → ENT referral
> → Confirm Dx with nasal endoscopy
> → CT & surgery to clear drainage pathways

> **Nasal douching:** ½ tsp salt + ½ tsp sugar + ½ tsp bicarb dissolved in boiled water
> → draw up some with syringe
> → block one nostril with finger & sniff up mix with other nostril
> → let it run out after
>
> * should do before using nasal sprays/drops

> **Risk factors for carcinoma**
> - Southern Chinese origin
> - EBV

---

[16]ENT UK (2016) Commissioning Guide: *Chronic Rhinosinusitis*

Emergency presentations

Epistaxis

CAUSES
- Idiopathic ⎫
- Nose-picking ⎭ **most common**
- Trauma
- Infection
- Tumours

PREDISPOSING FACTORS
- Hypertension
- Anticoagulants, NSAIDs, aspirin
- Coagulopathies
- Hereditary haemorrhagic telangiectasia

MANAGEMENT[17] → **Examine with thudicum to find source of bleed**
1. **First aid**
   - Lean forward, pinch fleshy part → for 10min
   - Apply ice to bridge of nose
   - Avoid swallowing blood
2. **Resuscitation (if severe)**
   - Estimate blood loss, measure pulse/BP
   - FBC, coag screen, G&S
   - IV fluids if needed

   90% of bleeds are from 'Little's area'
3. **Cauterisation** – if bleeding from Little's area (anterior bleed)
   - Silver nitrate or bipolar diathermy
4. **Packing*** – if cannot visualise or cauterise bleed
   - **First-line:** anterior packing (RapidRhino/Merocel)
   - **Second-line:** posterior packing
6. **Surgery/theatre** – if cannot stop bleed
   - Sphenopalatine artery (SPA) ligation
   - Anterior ethmoid ligation (if trauma or SPA fails)

Nose fracture

→ *must rule out serious complications*

MANAGEMENT
1. **Manage epistaxis / acute problems**
2. **Rule out serious complications**
   - Zygomatic/facial fracture – diplopia, face numbness, trismus
   - Head injury – LOC, N&V, amnesia, pupils
   - CSF leak – unilateral clear nasal discharge
   - Obstructed airways
   - Chest/abdo injuries
   - Septal haematoma
3. **Clinic 7–10d later**
→ Assess bony nose injury once swelling has subsided
4. **Manipulation of bony deformity**
→ Must be done **within 14d of injury**

Unilateral epistaxis in adolescent boys consider juvenile angiofibroma

(nasopharyngeal vascular tumour) → needs CT & excision

*need prophylactic ABX if packing for >48h

Features suggesting posterior bleed:
- Profuse
- Bilateral
- Failed anterior packing

[17] NICE (2020) CKS Management Scenario: *Acute epistaxis*

Septal haematoma

AETIOLOGY: bleed between septum & perichondrium

ON EXAMINATION: bilateral red/purple bulge

COMPLICATIONS
→ Blocks nose & gets infected
→ Necrosis & septal perforation or saddle nose deformity

MANAGEMENT
→ Immediate ENT referral
→ Surgical drainage & IV ABX

Septal perforation

CAUSES
- **TRAUMA/SURGERY**
- Avascular necrosis – septal haematoma / cocaine
- Granulomatous infection – syphilis, TB, granulomatosis with polyangiitis

SYMPTOMS
- Sense of nasal obstruction
- Whistling
- Crusting/bleeding

MANAGEMENT
- Douching & Vaseline
- Surgery (septal button or flap repair)

Foreign body

SYMPTOMS   Be suspicious if child presents with these symptoms
- Unilateral offensive discharge
- ± epistaxis

COMPLICATIONS
- Inhaled foreign body
- Vestibulitis

MANAGEMENT
→ **Removal:** forceps/Johnson probe/suction

Facial palsies

> **Frontalis spared:** UMN problem
> **Entire facial palsy:** LMN problem

→ **ALL NEED THOROUGH ENT & NEURO EXAMINATION**

Investigations

- Hx, ENT exam, neuro exam
- PTA
- Electroneuronography = electrical stimulation of FN
- MRI/CT – if suspicious case

General management

Eye care: artificial tears, eye patch at night

Differentials of facial palsy

BELL'S PALSY (55%)

Aetiology: viral infection of FN
(↑ risk in diabetes & pregnancy)

Symptoms: sudden onset (hours)
- Ipsilateral facial palsy (inc. frontalis)
- ± Pain
→ No ear/CNS pathology

Management: 80% fully recover in 2m
- High dose PO steroids
- Eye care + analgesia

RAMSAY HUNT (7%)

Aetiology: HZV infection of facial nerve

Symptoms
- Ipsilateral facial palsy (inc. frontalis)
- Ear pain / vesicles
- Vesicular rash
± SNHL, vertigo, tinnitus

Management: palsy = irreversible
- **Aciclovir** + corticosteroids
- Eye care + analgesia

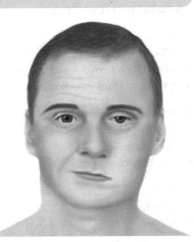

Fig. 8.15 Left facial palsy, frontalis not spared.

MIDDLE EAR DISEASE = AOM, cholesteatoma, mastoiditis

TRAUMA = temporal bone fracture, penetrating injury

TUMOUR = glomus jugular tumour, vestibular schwannoma, parotid gland

OTHER = CVA, multiple sclerosis, Guillain–Barré

> **Causes of facial palsy in kids**
>
> - Congenital
> - Forceps delivery
> - Chickenpox (VZV)
> - Acute OM

> **Red flags of facial palsy**
>
> - Associated ear infection / foul otorrhoea → cholesteatoma / complicated otitis media
> - Progressive palsy / parotid mass → neoplasm
> - Associated neuro symptoms → cerebrovascular accident

OPHTHALMOLOGY

09

ABBREVIATIONS

AION – Anterior ischaemic optic neuropathy
AMD – Age-related macular degeneration
AV – Arterio-venous
BB – Beta-blocker
CAI – Carbonic anhydrase inhibitors
CN – Cranial nerve
CPEO – Chronic progressive external ophthalmoplegia
CRA – Central retinal artery
CRAO – Central retinal artery occlusion
CRVO – Central retinal vein occlusion
CTD – Connective tissue disorder

EOM – Extraocular muscles
GCA – Giant cell arteritis
HSV – Herpes simplex virus
HZV – Herpes zoster virus
ICP – Intracranial pressure
IOL – Intraocular lens
IOP – Intraocular pressure
IRMA – Intraretinal microvascular abnormality
MS – Multiple sclerosis
NAAION – Non-arteritic anterior ischaemic optic neuropathy
NFT2 – Neurofibromatosis type 2

NPDR – Non-proliferative diabetic retinopathy
PCA – Posterior cerebral artery
PDR – Proliferative diabetic retinopathy
PG – Prostaglandin
RA – Rheumatoid arthritis
RAPD – Relative afferent pupillary defect
RPE – Retinal pigment epithelium
SLE – Systemic lupus erythematosus
VEGF – Vascular endothelial growth factor
VF – Visual field

Acute painless vision loss

Monocular causes	Binocular causes
• Vitreous haemorrhage • Ischaemic optic neuropathy (GCA) • Non-ischaemic optic neuropathy • Retinal vessel occlusion • Retinal detachment	• Pituitary tumour • Optic neuritis • Severe papilloedema • CVA • Dry eyes (± pain)

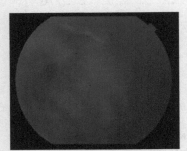

Fig. 9.1 Retinal tear.

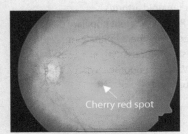

Fig. 9.2 CRAO.

Retinal detachment

CAUSES
- Age
- Post-op/trauma
- Diabetic retinopathy

RISK FACTORS
- Myopia
- Stickler's syndrome (in children)

TREATMENT: **refer for urgent surgery** = vitrectomy & reattachment

SYMPTOMS
Floaters
Flashes
Field loss
Fall in acuity

Floaters = small black dots in vision; patients may describe "blobs" or "ink splodge"

+ *absent red reflex*

Vitreous haemorrhage

CAUSES
- **Proliferative diabetic retinopathy**
- **Retinal vein occlusion with neovascularisation**
- Retinal tear
- Retinal detachment

INVESTIGATION: B-scan (USS of the eye used when blood blocks view of the retina)

SYMPTOMS
- **Floaters** – many small or one large
- Absent red reflex – if large bleed

TREATMENT
- **Proliferative/neovascular cause:** observation then pan-retinal laser once bleed settles
- **Tear/detachment:** vitrectomy

Retinal vessel occlusion

- **Retinal artery occlusions:** caused by CVD
  → cardiovascular assessment for cause & long-term Mx of diet/exercise/smoking
- **Retinal vein occlusion:** 2° to atherosclerotic thickening of CRA, compressing veins, or thick blood
  → HTN = major RF

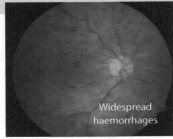

Fig. 9.3 CRVO.

	Symptoms	Signs	Investigations	Management[1]
CRAO	Sudden, profound, **entire** vision loss	• RAPD • Retinal oedema • Pale retina (ischaemic) • **Cherry red spot** ± carotid bruits	• BP • FBC, ESR, glucose • Carotid USS • Cardiac echo To r/o causes of: • HTN, DM • Heart problems • GCA (CRAO only)	**Refer to EYE CASUALTY & TIA CLINIC** • Rebreathe into paper bag = ↑ CO_2 dilates vessels • Ocular massage • Acetazolamide ↓ IOP • Paracentesis ↓ IOP *NB Little evidence for these, as once vision lost = often irreversible*
BRAO	Sudden central or **sectoral** vision loss	• Field defect • Signs of hypertensive retinopathy ± carotid bruits		**Refer to EYE CASUALTY & TIA CLINIC**
CRVO	Blurred, **widespread** vision loss	• RAPD • Flame haemorrhages (widespread) • Oedema • Disc swelling • Tortuous veins ± cotton wool spots	• BP • FBC, ESR, glucose • IOP To r/o causes of: • HTN, DM • Glaucoma • Blood problems	1. **Refer to EYE CASUALTY** 2. Manage cardiovascular risk factors 3. Manage complications of retinal vein occlusion (neovascularisation / macular oedema)
BRVO	Blurred, **central or sectoral** vision loss	Flame haemorrhages (focal)		

[1] RCOphth (2015) *Retinal Vein Occlusion (RVO) Guidelines*

Neuro-ophthalmology

Features on fundoscopy

→ *swollen optic disc*

- Blurred disc margin
- Haemorrhages around disc
- Smaller cup:disc ratio

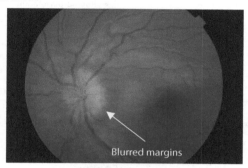

Blurred margins

Fig. 9.4 Swollen optic disc.

Causes of a swollen optic disc

Features of hypertensive retinopathy

Grade 1: subtle, arterial narrowing
Grade 2: AV nipping
Grade 3: cotton wool spots, haemorrhages, exudates
Grade 4 (malignant): + swollen optic disc

Optic nerve atrophy = death of nerve fibres

Causes: compression or ↓ blood supply
- after episodes of optic neuritis or ischaemia (arteritic or non-arteritic)
- compression by tumours e.g. pituitary chiasm tumours

Features on fundoscopy: pale neuroretinal rim

Ix: MRI/CT

	Cause	Symptoms	Management
Optic neuritis (consider if young/middle-aged)	Inflammation of optic nerve - **Demyelination (multiple sclerosis)** - Idiopathic - Infection – syphilis, HSV, mumps - SLE/sarcoid, diabetes mellitus - Ischaemia (GCA) **Most common cause**	**UNILATERAL** - Blurred vision & ↓ acuity - Central scotoma - **Red desaturation** - **RAPD** } Key Sx - **Pain on eye movement** ± neuro Sx e.g. numbness	**TYPICAL:** (unilateral & young) = likely MS cause **Mx:** observe **ATYPICAL:** (bilateral/older) = likely neuromyelitis optica **Mx:** PO/IV steroids (avoid PO prednisolone but can give PO methylprednisolone)
Papilloedema (BILATERAL disc swelling with **evidence of ↑ICP**)	Swollen disc due to ↑ICP - Brain tumour/abscess - Head injury / brain bleed - Meningitis/encephalitis - Idiopathic	**BILATERAL** **often asymptomatic** **(visual loss only if severe)** - Gradual progressive field loss - **Enlarged blind spot** - **Headache/vomiting**	1. **Neuroimaging** 2. Investigate for & treat underlying cause
Malignant HTN	Swollen disc due to rapid ↑ BP to >180/120 + fundoscopic features of hypertensive retinopathy	**BILATERAL** - ↓ acuity - Headache - Eye pain ± focal neuro signs	ANTIHYPERTENSIVES (hospital admission)
GCA / arteritic AION* Very unlikely if age <50y	Inflammation & occlusion of vessels supplying optic nerve = infarction **Pathognomonic for GCA**	**UNILATERAL** (may become bilateral) - **Headache**, tongue pain - Malaise, weight loss - **Jaw/temporal pain** - **SUDDEN DEVASTATING VISION LOSS**	**Ix:** ↑ CRP **Mx: emergency!** High dose steroids (for 2y) To prevent vision loss in other eye
Non-arteritic AION*	Occluded posterior ciliary artery = optic nerve infarction - **Atherosclerosis:** DM, HTN, ↑ lipids - Obstructive sleep apnoea - Viagra use	**UNILATERAL** - **SUDDEN VISION LOSS** - Crowded disc on fundoscopy of the contralateral eye - Altitudinal field defect (normal CRP and ESR)	**Ix:** cholesterol/TGs, glucose, BP **Mx:** control cardiovascular risk factors

*anterior ischaemic optic neuropathy

Acute red eye

Haemorrhages

Type of haemorrhage	Subconjunctival = blood pools behind conjunctiva		Retrobulbar = blood pools behind eyeball
Risk factors	• Post-surgery • Anticoagulants • Trauma	• Valsalva manoeuvres (coughing/vomiting) • Spontaneous (due to HTN)	• Anaesthetic injection • Trauma/perforation
Symptoms	Asymptomatic & harmless		• **Excruciating pain** • Significant ↓ vision • ↓ eye movement • Proptosis • ↑ IOP
Management	Reassure resolution in 2w		CT scan needed ± lateral cantholysis

Vascular congestion

LOCALISED CONGESTION → Episcleritis & scleritis

	Episcleritis = superficial inflammation of episclera	Scleritis = deeper inflammation of sclera ± episclera
Association	**Idiopathic** Sometimes with autoimmune disease e.g. SLE	Autoimmune, infectious, CTDs e.g. RA
Pain	Mild/achy	Very severe
Vision	Not affected	Blurring + photophobia
Blanches with phenylephrine	Yes	No (sclera may have **purple hue**)
Treatment	Observe / NSAIDs (steroid drops if severe) → self-limiting	Oral steroids ± immunosuppressants → needs referral

GENERALISED CONGESTION → Conjunctivitis, keratitis, uveitis
→ Ix: history & slit lamp

Keratitis usually presents with white patch(es) on the cornea

	Conjunctivitis inflamed conjunctiva	Keratitis inflamed cornea	Anterior uveitis inflamed iris	Acute angle-closure glaucoma sudden ↑ IOP
Redness	Diffuse, widespread	Ciliary	Ciliary	Ciliary
Vision	Normal	Blurry/impaired	Blurry/impaired	Poor
Pupil	Normal	Normal	Constricted	Mid-dilated
Discharge	✓	✓	✗	✗
Pain	Discomfort	Moderate/severe	Moderate/achy	Severe
Photophobia	+	+	++	−
Management	Observe / antibiotic eye drops	**Often infectious cause:** antibiotic eye drops	**Often inflammatory cause:** PO/topical steroids	Acetazolamide + pilocarpine + other glaucoma drops

Conjunctivitis

Cause	Viral adenovirus, HSV, molluscum	Bacterial *Staph. aureus, Strep. pneumoniae*	Allergic hay fever, pollen, dust
Uni-/bilateral	Unilateral or bilateral (often spreads from one eye to other)	Unilateral or bilateral (often spreads from one eye to other)	Usually bilateral
Eye Sx	Gritty & **crusting +++**	Gritty & crusting +	**Itchy**
Discharge	Watery	**Purulent**	Stringy
Lymphadenopathy	✓ (+ coryzal Sx)	±	✗
Treatment	Observation, lubricants, **hygiene**	**Topical ABX:** chloramphenicol/fusidic acid drops	Antihistamines

→ **Gonococcal conjunctivitis:** consider if prolonged in young adults → STI history → +++ crusting & hyperpurulent
→ **Neonatal conjunctivitis (<4w):** gonococcal/chlamydial infection → can cause permanent scarring & vision loss

Keratitis

CAUSES

→ **Infection:**
- Bacterial *(Staph., Strep., Pseudomonas)*
- Viral (HSV /HZV)
- Protozoan *(Acanthamoeba)*
- Fungal *(Candida, Aspergillus, Fusarium)*

Acanthamoeba = most serious → high risk of blindness

→ **Inflammation:** RA/SLE/Wegener's

COMPLICATION

Corneal ulcer → can perforate so needs **urgent ophthalmology referral**
↳ **Treatment: antimicrobial** or **steroids** depending on cause (must be initiated by ophthalmologist as wrong treatment can worsen ulcers)

Anterior uveitis

KEY SYMPTOMS: red, painful eye, photophobia, constricted pupil

CAUSES/RFs

→ **Idiopathic** = most common
→ **Inflammatory conditions:** Crohn's, ankylosing spondylitis, sarcoid, RA, TB

Acute angle-closure glaucoma → EMERGENCY

PATHOGENESIS: narrow anterior angle becomes suddenly blocked so no drainage (trigger = entering darkness & pupil dilating)

SYMPTOMS: sudden onset
- **Acute pain** + red eye
- Blurred & ↓ vision
- Headache, nausea, vomiting
± prodromal 'halos' around bright lights

SIGNS
- **Sudden ↑ IOP** >30mmHg
- Red eye
- Cloudy cornea (oedema)
- Fixed, mid-dilated pupil

MANAGEMENT: urgent hospital admission

Medical:
- Acetazolamide (CAI) ± timolol (BB) = ↓ aqueous humour production
- Pilocarpine* = constricts pupil to open drainage channel
- IV mannitol if other medical management fails

Surgical:
- Peripheral laser iridotomy** = burn hole in iris to allow drainage & angle to reopen
- Trabeculectomy if medical management fails

Risk factors for keratitis
Bacterial: contact lens use, poor contact lens hygiene, dry eyes
Viral: herpetic disease e.g. previous shingles, recurrent cold sores
Acanthamoeba – contact lens use, poor contact lens hygiene (contamination with soil, swim/showering with contacts in)

HSV keratitis = dendritic ulcers
DO NOT GIVE STEROIDS → Tx = PO/topical aciclovir

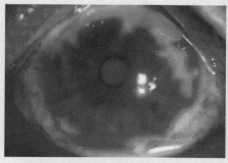

Fig. 9.5 Herpes keratitis dendritic ulcer.

RFs for closed angle glaucoma: 'CLOSE'
Chinese
Long-sighted (small eyeball)
Old age
Shallow anterior chamber
Ethnicity (East Asian)

*pilocarpine also given *prophylactically* in the other eye
**peripheral laser iridotomy also done *prophylactically* in other eye

---

BLEPHARITIS = inflammation of the eyelids & associated structures (lashes, skins, meibomian glands)

Aetiology: usually due to an inflammatory reaction due to the presence of bacteria **but it is not an infection**
↳ (usually *Staphylococcus, Demodex*)

Symptoms: usually bilateral
- Burning, itching, foreign body sensation, dry eyes
- Eyelid crusting, erythema, telangiectasias, skin flaking
- Blocked meibomian glands
- Associated with dry eyes

Management:
- Eyelid hygiene (eyelid scrubs)
- Warm compress twice daily
- Lid massage
- Lubricating drops if dry eyes

Topical ABX if unresponsive to hygiene measures

Investigations: slit lamp to r/o other pathologies
Commonly shows lash collarettes, blocked meibomian glands & chalazion (inflamed meibomian gland)
→ **Unilateral Sx (which persist or recur despite multiple treatments) may need investigation for malignancy**

Miscellaneous acute ocular problems

Assessment of ocular trauma

- Thorough Hx – has the object penetrated the globe i.e. intraocular foreign body? *(High speed? Sharp object?)*
- Visual acuity
- Ophthalmoscopy
- Slit lamp – check for abrasions
- Systemic examination – especially CNs
- CT – avoid MRI if could be foreign body

Blowout fracture

↑ Pressure in orbital cavity causes floor fracture into maxillary sinus

Symptoms
- Restricted eye movement
- Periorbital swelling

Investigations
- CT = GOLD STANDARD
- X-ray

Management
Conservative
↳ (unless muscle trapped or optic nerve affected – may need maxillary facial surgery but ALWAYS need maxillary facial opinion)

Causes of enophthalmitis

Post-cataract surgery: contaminated surgical equipment, blepharitis

Endogenous: other sources of infection in the body, IVDU, immunosuppression, diabetes, cancer, catheter, indwelling lines

Ocular trauma

→ *needs thorough assessment*

FOREIGN BODY (FB)
Symptoms: sudden onset irritation + photophobia
Management: eye casualty
- Extraocular: FB removal with needle/burr + ABX
- Intraocular: EMERGENCY – CT scan, ABX, urgent surgery

CHEMICAL INJURY
1. Immediate irrigation with water – continue until pH is 7
2. Determine if acid/alkali – alkali usually causes more damage
3. Careful eye inspection
4. **Ophthalmology referral:** topical ABX + steroids, topical dilating drops, analgesia, artificial tears

BLUNT TRAUMA
Presents in many ways:
- Hyphaemia
- Periorbital haematoma
- Retinal tear/haemorrhage/detachment
- Traumatic cataract
- Blowout fracture

Orbital disease

THYROID EYE DISEASE
Sx: periorbital oedema, eyelid retraction, exophthalmos, diplopia, restricted eye movement → *often bilateral but can be unilateral*

PERI-ORBITAL & ORBITAL CELLULITIS

	Peri-orbital	Orbital
Eyelid swelling	+	+++
Proptosis	×	✓
Acuity & colour vision	Normal (need to monitor)	May be reduced (need to monitor)
Extraocular movement	Normal	May be affected
RAPD	×	✓ or ×
Systemic symptoms	Systemically well	Systemically unwell
Management	PO ABX, no admission **unless child – then admit & treat as orbital cellulitis**	**Admit** + IV ABX + ENT referral (surgical drainage if ABX fail)

Complications of orbital cellulitis:
→ optic neuropathy, orbital abscess, brain abscess/meningitis, cavernous sinus thrombosis (most serious complication)

ENOPHTHALMITIS
Pathogenesis: inflammation of internal eye
Causes: trauma / post-op / endogenous
Mx: ABX (intravitreal), possibly vitrectomy

IDIOPATHIC ORBITAL INFLAMMATORY DISEASE
Pathogenesis: non-infectious/neoplastic inflammation = **Dx of exclusion**
Sx: rapid onset, painful, periorbital oedema & eye muscle paralysis, usually unilateral
Mx: steroids

Diabetic eye disease

Diabetic retinopathy

→ *most common cause of visual impairment in those aged 20–65y*

Pathophysiology

1. **Hypoperfusion of retinal vessels** – due to hyperglycaemia → ischaemia
2. **Pericyte death in vessels** – weakened walls → microaneurysms & oedema
3. **Macrophage accumulation** – to clear debris → exudates
4. **AV shunts open** – to overcome hypoxia → IRMAs (intraretinal microvascular abnormalities)
5. **Neovascularisation** – abnormal, weak vessels → haemorrhages

1. BACKGROUND / NON-PROLIFERATIVE (NPDR)

= after 8–10y → **asymptomatic**

Features

- Microaneurysms
- Exudates
- Haemorrhages (dot, blot, flame)
- Cotton wool spots (infarcted axons)

In severe pre-proliferative: 4-2-1 RULE

- **4 quadrants** with dot haemorrhages
- **2 quadrants** with venous beading
- **1 quadrant (anywhere)** with IRMAs

Management[2]

1. **Diabetes control** – most important!
2. Control of comorbidities (HTN, hyperlipidaemia etc.)
3. **Careful monitoring** – at least biannually

2. PROLIFERATIVE (PDR)

= 5% of DM cases → **asymptomatic until haemorrhage**

Features

- Irregular new vessels (over disc or elsewhere)
- Haemorrhage (vitreous or pre-retinal)
- Neovascularised iris (rubeosis iridis)

Management

1. **Diabetes control** – most important!
2. Pan-retinal laser photocoagulation

Diabetic maculopathy

→ *when retinopathy affects the macula* → ***GRADUAL LOSS OF VISION***

Features: focal or widespread retinal oedema, exudates within the macula

Treatment: mostly intravitreal anti-VEGF injections or macular laser (to treat macular fluid)

Diabetes control = still very important!

Risk factors for diabetic retinopathy

- **Duration & control of DM**
- HTN / renal disease
- Lifestyle – smoking/alcohol/diet
- Pregnancy
- Age

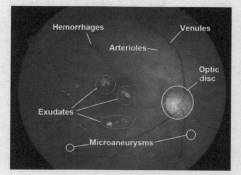

Fig. 9.6 Background retinopathy.

Pan-retinal photocoagulation

= burn away peripheral photoreceptors to ↓ O_2 demand & ↓ VEGF & new vessels

→ start far out, r/v in 4–6w, burn further in if needed

Diabetes increases risk of other eye disease:

- ↑ risk eyelid infections
- ↑ risk cataracts
- delayed healing abrasions/ulcers/wounds

[2]RCOphth (2012) *Diabetic Retinopathy Guidelines*

Age-related macular degeneration

AMD is the **most common cause of vision loss in UK**. Patients have progressive, irreversible **central vision loss**.

Risk factors for AMD
- Age (>50y)
- Smoking
- CVD – HTN, ↑ lipids

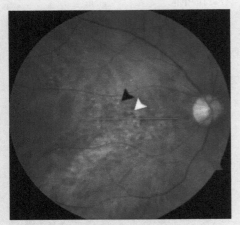

Fig. 9.7 Dry AMD with drusen.

AREDS2 formula = a combination of vitamins & nutrients that were shown to reduce progression of mild AMD to more advanced stages of the disease during clinical trials

Impact on life of AMD

- Struggle recognising faces
- Difficulty reading & driving
- Increased falls risk

General investigations
- Eye examination – fundoscopy, acuity, central visual field test (Amsler grid)
- Fundus photos

DRY AMD (90%) = *gradual vision loss (years)*

Pathophysiology
- Lipid debris thickens Bruch's membrane = **drusen** (discrete yellow spots)
- RPE atrophy = pale areas on retina
- RPE hypertrophy = black spots on retina

Management[3]: ophthalmology referral
- **Counsel patient:**
  - ▸ no real cure
  - ▸ smoking cessation
  - ▸ vitamin supplementation (AREDS2 formula) → just **slows** progression
- **Low level visual aids**
- **Regular eye checks**

WET AMD (10%) = *sudden*, **severe vision loss (months)** → starts with distorted images

Pathophysiology
- New, abnormal vessels pierce Bruch's membrane
- Leak fluid & blood = oedema, haemorrhage & RPE detachment
- Fibrotic tissue left once bleed settles = disciform scar

Management: as above + anti-VEGF

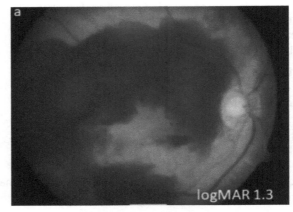

Fig. 9.8 Disciform scar.

[3]RCOphth (2021) *Commissioning Guidelines – AMD*

Cataracts

Clouded opacity on/within lens due to liquefaction of lens content. Cataracts are the most common cause of blindness worldwide.

Causes

- **Age** = leading cause
- Trauma – infrared/ultraviolet/X-ray or trauma
- Metabolic – **diabetes mellitus**
- Toxins – **steroids**, smoking
- Systemic disease – Marfan's, NFT2, atopic dermatitis
- Maternal infection
- Hereditary

General symptoms

- ↓ acuity & blurring (gradually)
- ↑ myopia (or sometimes hypermetropia)
- Faded colours
- Trouble with bright lights & night vision (glare)

Investigations/diagnosis

- Hx & slit lamp

Management[4]

→ *depends on impact on patient's life* (occupation/driving/ADLs)

1. **Patient assessment:** eye health (in both eyes), suitability for surgery, biometry results for each eye
2. **Phacoemulsification**
   - Ultrasound waves emulsify cataract & removed via incision
   - Corrective IOL inserted
     ↳ *the artificial lens can be designed to correct any vision impairment at the same time*

Complications of phacoemulsification
- Posterior capsule opacification (20%)
- Vitreous loss (7%)
- Retinal detachment (1%)
- Endophthalmitis (0.1%)

---

[4]NICE (2017) *Cataracts in adults* [NG77]

Glaucoma

Diseases causing characteristic damage to optic disc, **usually due to** ↑ **IOP** (>21mmHg)

Normal physiology

→ Ciliary bodies secrete aqueous humour into posterior chamber
→ Aqueous passes through iris into anterior chamber
→ From here it is drained via trabecular network

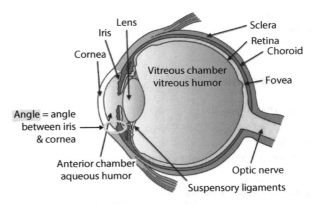

Fig. 9.9 Anatomy of the eye.

Open angle glaucoma

PATHOGENESIS
→ Wide anterior angle allows ↑ aqueous entry but ↓ drainage (ageing may cause sclerosis of meshwork)
→ ↑ IOP damages optic nerve fibres

SYMPTOMS
Asymptomatic until significant damage to optic nerve → **need screening**
• **Visual field loss**
  ‣ nasal step → superior arcuate scotoma
  ‣ progresses to tunnel vision → blindness

INVESTIGATIONS
• **Visual fields:** progressive ↓
• **Fundoscopy:** optic disc changes
• **IOP (tonometer):** >21mmHg

MANAGEMENT[5]

*Eye drops have many side-effects so compliance = poor

1. Medical eye drops (often combine)*

Eye drop	Mechanism of action	Side-effects
PG analogues (latanoprost)	↑ drainage	lash growth, dark iris
Beta-blockers (timolol)	↓ production	eye discomfort
Carbonic anhydrase inhibitors (acetazolamide)	↓ production	taste issues
Alpha agonist (brimonidine)	↑ drainage & ↓ production	dizziness

order of use

2. Laser trabeculoplasty
→ laser stimulates cells in trabecular network to increase drainage
3. Surgical trabeculectomy
→ make hole in sclera so aqueous humour can drain into reservoir under Tenon's capsule

[5]NICE (2017, updated 2022) *Glaucoma* [NG81]

Fig. 9.10 Increased cup:disc ratio.

Optic disc changes
• ↑ cup:disc ratio (>0.3/0.4, cut-off varies)
• Oval cup (no ISNT rule: **I>S>N>T**)

Management aims to prevent further loss, not reverse damage already present!

Normal tension glaucoma: normal IOP but damaged disc = due to ischaemia

Refractive errors

Measuring vision

DISTANCE VISION

A) Snellen chart* (need to read >½ of line for it to count)

Limitations:
- Letters more crowded further down
- May 'memorise' lines

B) Bailey–Lovie/logMAR* (need to read 4/5 letters for line to count)

Advantages over Snellen:
- Letters equally spaced / more uniform
- Illuminated & on wheels

C) Can also test with pinhole:
- No improvement / worsened vision suggests **pathological cause**
- Improvement suggests **refractive cause** (i.e. need updated pair of glasses)

> **DRIVING RULES for category 1 drivers**
> - Min. 6/12 with glasses & both eyes open
> - Read number plate from 20m
> - Sufficient VFs

NEAR VISION
→ Assess ability to accommodate using a hand-held card

Refractive errors

> Power of lens (D) $= \frac{1}{f(m)}$
> **Dioptre (D):** measurement of refraction
> **Focal distance (f):** distance from lens to point of focus
> *e.g. for a lens of 10D, focal distance will be 1/10 = 0.1m*

MYOPIA (SHORT-SIGHTED) → light focused **in front of** retina
- **Refractive:** eye refraction too strong
- **Axial:** eyeball too long

Risk factors: lots of close work / time indoors
Complication: ↑ risk retinal detachment

Correction: CONCAVE (negative) lens

HYPERMETROPIA (LONG-SIGHTED) → light focused **behind** retina
- **Refractive:** eye refraction too weak
- **Axial:** eyeball too short

Complication: acute angle-closure glaucoma

Correction: CONVEX (positive) lens
Hypermetropia = normal for infants (but corrects as eyeball grows)

ASTIGMATISM (UNEVENLY SHAPED EYEBALL) → asymmetry causes
different degrees of refraction & 2 focus points
Correction: CYLINDRICAL lens
→ has refractive power in only 1 meridian
→ can be used in conjunction with a spherical (convex/concave) lens
→ combination of spherical & cylindrical lens = **toric lens**

PRESBYOPIA = loss of accommodation due to thickening & sclerosis of lens with age (>40y)
Correction: 'add-on' positive lens for reading (aka reading glasses)
→ combined with distance prescription = **bi-/varifocals**

> **Visual acuity:** ability to resolve fine detail with *optimum optical correction*

Snellen	logMAR	
6/6	0.0	→ excellent vision
6/12	0.3	
6/24	0.6	
6/60	1.0	

*Major limitation of both methods = they are SUBJECTIVE (rely on patient being honest)

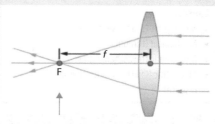

Fig. 9.11 Emmetropia if focal point directly on retina.

> **Emmetropia:** perfect focusing onto retina
> **Ametropia:** some form of refractive error
> **Hypermetropia:** long-sighted (can see far things)
> **Myopia:** short-sighted (can see near things)

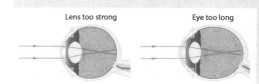

Lens too strong — Eye too long

Fig. 9.12 Myopia.

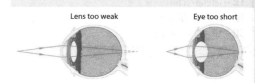

Lens too weak — Eye too short

Fig. 9.13 Hypermetropia.

Orthoptics

Diagnosis & management of binocular vision & eye motility disorders

Squint/strabismus

MANIFEST SQUINT (HETEROTROPIA) = visible deviation of one eye when eyes are open → **always pathological**

- **Sx:** diplopia
- **Dx:** cover test (bad eye fixates centrally when good eye covered) ↳
- **Ix:** to determine if serious cause

> The movement of the bad eye tells you what type of squint it is:
>
> **Inward movement:** divergent squint
> **Outward movement:** convergent squint

LATENT SQUINT (HETEROPHORIA)
= tendency for eye deviation **but normally compensated** → present in most people
→ **Sx:** headache, eye strain, intermittent diplopia (if decompensates after long period of focus)
→ **Dx:** cover–uncover test (bad eye deviates when covered – see it return to central when uncovered)
→ **Mx:** do not need treatment if controlled, sometimes need orthoptic exercises & prism (surgery if decompensated)

AMBLYOPIA ('LAZY EYE') = reduced vision in one eye → birth to 7/8y
Causes: lack of stimulation during critical period of visual development

- **Strabismic** – brain ignores image from squinting eye (suppression)

- **Stimulus deprivation** – something blocks image reaching retina e.g. ptosis/cataract
  ↳ Due to lack of stimulation in the affected eye, brain starts to ignore the affected eye.
  → worse eye becomes 'lazy'

- **Anisometropic** – difference in refractive errors of >1 dioptre
  ↳ Due to difference in uncorrected refractive error, there is a difference in uncorrected vision. The brain starts to ignore the visual input from the eye with worse vision.

Management: if treated in critical period, can reverse amblyopia
Occlusion of good eye with eye patch **OR** atropine drops in good eye to cause blurring (to make the bad eye "work harder")

Concomitant squint: squint is the same irrespective of gaze direction – less likely to be serious
Causes: accommodative esotropia, non-accommodative esotropia, constant/intermittent exotropia

Incomitant squint: degree of squint varies with gaze direction (↑ when look in direction of affected muscle)
Causes:
- Neurogenic (3rd nerve palsy)
- Mechanical (tumour)
- Myasthenic (myasthenia gravis)
- Myopathic (CPEO, myositis, thyroid eye disease)

Management of squints

1. **Correct refractive error ± orthoptic exercises**
   - 'BASE OUT' prism for CONVERGENT squints (accommodative esotropia)
   - 'BASE IN' prism for DIVERGENT squints (intermittent or near exotropia)
2. **Surgery to realign EOM** – if no refractive error / lenses don't help

Orthoptic exercises for convergency excess esotropias

Extraocular muscles:
SR – superior rectus
IR – inferior rectus
MR – medial rectus
LR – lateral rectus
IO – inferior oblique
SO – superior oblique

Ocular nerve palsies

3rd nerve palsy
- Ptosis – levator palpebrae
- Down & out – SR, IR, MR, IO
- Efferent pupil defect – dilated

Causes:
- **Microvascular disease** (age, HTN, DM, hyperlipidaemia)
- CVA
- Orbital trauma
- Demyelination
- PCA aneurysm ↓
- Tumour
NEEDS CT ANGIOGRAM

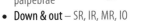

4th nerve palsy
- Up & in – SO
- Compensatory contralateral head tilt

Causes: trauma + same as 3rd nerve palsy (including microvascular)

6th nerve palsy
- Adducted – LR

Causes: same as others (including microvascular)

Pupil abnormalities

PUPILLARY LIGHT REFLEX

> **Afferent nerve:** optic nerve (CNII)
> **Efferent nerve:** oculomotor (CNIII)

Consensual reflex: light in 1 eye stimulates efferents to both
(2nd order neurones connect pretectal nucleus to BOTH Edinger–Westphal nuclei)

Afferent defect: pupil does not constrict

Relative afferent defect: affected eye dilates when performing swinging light test

ACCOMMODATION REFLEX: initiated by near fixation
(ciliary muscles contract, zonular fibres relax, lens more globular = ↑ refractive power)

Components:

1. **Accommodation** – constrict ciliary muscle = CNIII
2. **Constriction** – sphincter pupillae = parasympathetic fibres via CNIII
3. **Convergence** – medial & lateral rectus = CNIII activation & reciprocal CNVI inhibition

> **Pupil dilation (mydriasis):** SYMPATHETIC
> = **Dilator pupillae** (CNVI ophthalmic)
>
> **Pupil constriction (miosis):** PARASYMPATHETIC
> = **Sphincter pupillae** (CN3 oculomotor)

Maximum accommodation depends on lens rigidity
(↓ accommodation with age = PRESBYOPIA)

CAUSES OF PUPIL ABNORMALITIES

constriction in accommodation > in light

	3rd Nerve palsy	Horner's	Adie pupil	Argyll Robertson pupil	Marcus Gunn pupil
Signs	• Mydriasis (efferent defect) • Ptosis • Down & out	• Miosis (constricted pupil) • Partial ptosis • Anhidrosis	• Mydriasis (dilated pupil which then constricts with time) • Anisocoria increases in light **(pupil size difference more obvious in light)** • Sectoral iris sphincter palsy with **vermiform movements** of the pupillary margin • Absent light reflex ± ↓ tendon reflexes	• Small, irregular pupils • **Light-near dissociation** which disappears with time	RAPD
Causes	• **PCA aneurysm** • Tumour • CVA • Trauma • Demyelination	**Lesion of sympathetic chain** • Pancoast tumour • Cervical rib • Carotid artery aneurysm • Neck trauma • CNS disease (MS, syphilis)	**Ciliary ganglion lesion** (parasympathetic pathway) • Idiopathic • Viral infection • Trauma	Neurosyphilis	**Optic nerve pathology** **Young patients:** optic neuritis / MS **Older patients:** NAAION/GCA **Other:** tumour, orbital cellulitis, thyroid eye disease, trauma, CVA

Visual fields

Overlap between eyes allows depth perception (STEREOPSIS)

Anatomy

Blind spot: where optic nerve leaves retina (don't notice due to overlap in visual fields)
→ Behind retina, **optic nerve** becomes myelinated
→ Passes through **optic chiasm** & becomes **optic tract**
→ **Rotation of fibres 90° inwards**
  ▸ superior retinal fibres → medial (parietal lobe)
  ▸ inferior retinal fibres → lateral (temporal lobe)
→ Fibres reach **lateral geniculate nucleus (LGN) in thalamus**
→ Fibres rejoin to form **optic radiation** & rotate back to original position

> **Blood supply to occipital cortex:** posterior cerebral artery
> *NB Medial part also supplied by occipital branch of **middle cerebral artery***
> → *protects fibres coming from the macula*

Visual field defects

General rules
1. Any lesion in optic chiasm = bitemporal hemianopia
2. Any lesion posterior to optic chiasm = HOMONYMOUS defect on the CONTRALATERAL side to the lesion
3. Temporal or parietal lobe lesions = QUADRANTANOPIAS → ask about other symptoms

> **HOMONYMOUS:** field defects on same side in both eyes
>
> **HETERONYMOUS:** field defects on different sides in each eye

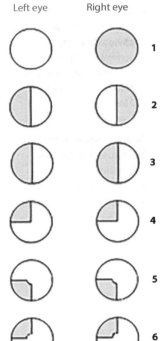

Fig. 9.14 Optic pathway.

Visual field defects

1. **Monocular blindness**
2. **Bitemporal hemianopia**
   = chiasm lesion
   Causes:
   (a) Pituitary tumour
   (b) Rathke's pouch meningioma
   (c) Craniopharyngioma (kids)
3. **Homonymous hemianopia**
   = optic tract or occipital lobe lesion
4. **Superior quadrantanopia**
   = temporal lobe lesion (inf. fibres)
   → Inferior fibres affected (superior VF captured by inferior retina)
5. **Inferior quadrantanopia**
   = parietal lobe lesion (sup. fibres)
   → Superior fibres affected (inferior VF captured by superior retina)
6. **Macular sparing**
   = lesion of PCA but spared MCA

In **elderly patients or patients with poor baseline vision**, it is important to **always assess visual fields** even when they complain of "monocular visual loss".
These patients **often cannot discern subtle visual loss in the other eye** and may therefore actually have binocular visual loss such as a homonymous hemianopia (which would be caused by a stroke/tumour and NOT ocular pathologies).

ANAESTHETICS

10

ABBREVIATIONS

AAA – Abdominal aortic aneurysm

ASA – American Society of Anesthesiologists

CNS – Central nervous system

CO – Cardiac output

COCP – Combined oral contraceptive pill

CPOC – Centre for Perioperative Care

CSF – Cerebrospinal fluid

DA – Dopamine

DOAC – Direct oral anticoagulant

Fe – Iron

GA – General anaesthetic

GIT – Gastrointestinal tract

HRT – Hormone replacement therapy

IBD – Inflammatory bowel disease

ICP – Intracranial pressure

LA – Local anaesthetic

LMA – Laryngeal mask airway

LMWH – Low molecular weight heparin

LVF – Left ventricular failure

MH – Malignant hyperthermia

MRSA – Methicillin-resistant *Staphylococcus aureus*

MSK – Musculoskeletal

N_2O – Nitrous oxide

NBM – Nil by mouth

NMBA – Neuromuscular blocking agent

PNS – Peripheral nervous system

PONV – Post-operative nausea & vomiting

POP – Progesterone-only pill

PPI – Proton pump inhibitor

SSRI – Selective serotonin reuptake inhibitor

SV – Stroke volume

TCA – Tricyclic antidepressant

TIVA – Total intravenous anaesthesia

Anaesthetics overview

Advantages of inhaled agents

- Children / needle phobia / tricky IV access
- Reduced incidence of awareness
- Rapid emergence with modern agents

Indications for TIVA

- Hx of malignant hyperthermia
- Hx of PONV

Advantages of TIVA:
- Reduced PONV
- Rapid emergence

Disadvantages of TIVA:
- Need secure IV access
- Increased incidence of awareness

Rapid sequence induction

In emergencies (patient not starved)
- Rapid production of optimal conditions for intubation
- Muscle relaxant immediately after inducing agent
- **Cricoid pressure protects against regurgitation & aspiration**

Malignant hyperthermia

= allergic reaction

Sx: very high temp, ↑ HR, ↑ RR, muscle rigidity

Signs: acidosis, rhabdomyolysis, ↑ K+

Tx: *stop causative drug*   CHECK FHX
- → 100% O_2 + dantrolene
- → Active cooling (ice/cool IV fluids)
- → **Monitor (ECG, temp, U&E, ABG)**

e.g. urinary retention

General anaesthesia (GA)

→ *drug-induced, controllable, reversible **loss of consciousness***

THREE COMPONENTS
- **Hypnosis:** IV, inhaled or IM agents (e.g. ketamine)
- **Analgesia:** opioids, NSAIDs, paracetamol   *no effect on consciousness/pain*
- **Muscle relaxation:** atracurium, rocuronium, suxamethonium

STAGES OF ANAESTHESIA:
1. **Premedication:**
   - Oral benzodiazepine if anxious
   - Ranitidine/PPI for gastric protection
   - Oral ondansetron as prophylactic antiemetic
2. **Pre-oxygenation**   *often causes PONV*
3. **Induction:** IV propofol / inhaled sevoflurane, isoflurane ± N_2O
4. **Airway control:** facemask ± oral airway **or** supraglottic airway (LMA, iGel) **or** ET tube
5. **Maintenance:** inhaled agents (above) **or** total IV anaesthesia (TIVA)
6. **Emergence:** time depends on drug distribution & lung exhalation of volatile agent

Physiological effects of general anaesthesia:
- → **Airway:** loss of tone & reflexes
- → **Breathing:** respiratory depression, atelectasis (collapsed alveoli)
- → **Cardiovascular:** hypotension, ↓ CO & contractility

RISKS OF GENERAL ANAESTHESIA

Minor	Major
PONV	Cognitive (delirium / worsen dementia)
Sore throat	Anaphylaxis
	Stroke, MI
	Chest infection
	Malignant hyperpyrexia (↑>1°C every 5–30min)
	Unintended awareness (1:1000 – 1:20,000)
	DEATH

Regional anaesthesia

→ *anaesthesia of a large region of the body, with **NO loss of consciousness***

INJECTION OF LOCAL ANAESTHETIC NEAR NERVES
- **Central/neuraxial:** into CSF e.g. spinal (into subarachnoid space), epidural (extradural)
- **Regional blocks / major nerves:** brachial plexus, femoral, sciatic

PHYSIOLOGICAL EFFECTS OF REGIONAL ANAESTHESIA
- → Reduction of sensory, motor, autonomic function of nerves
- → Some cardiorespiratory effects with central neuraxial blocks (↓ BP, bradycardia, ↓ intercostal muscle function)

RISKS OF REGIONAL ANAESTHESIA
1. **Wrong place:** total spinal block, respiratory paralysis, ↓ BP, intravascular injection (causing toxicity)
2. **Injury to structures:** nerves, blood vessels, adjacent structures
3. **Other:** spinal headaches, PONV (if opioids used), autonomic blockade

Local anaesthesia (LA)

→ *reversible blockade of nerve impulse conduction in small area*

↳ **Topical:** onset 15–20min → prior to injection, cannulation etc.

↳ **Local infiltration***: prior to minor procedures e.g. suturing   e.g. LIGNOCAINE

*often combined with vasoconstrictors (adrenaline) to ↑ duration of action (decreases local absorption)

Risks of anaesthesia

AIRWAY

- **Difficult airway** – difficulty or failure to intubate – important to assess airway pre-operatively
- **Structural damage** – oral irritation / bleeding / dental damage (1:4000)
- **Anaphylaxis** – most common with muscle relaxants, antibiotics, NSAIDs, latex – presents as CVS collapse if under GA
  - ▸ **Mx:** stop causative drug if possible, 100% O_2, **call for help**
    + **IV adrenaline 50mcg** or IM 500mcg + IV saline + lie flat & raise legs
    + chlorphenamine & hydrocortisone

BREATHING

- **Hypoxia** – airway obstruction, misplaced tube, aspiration, bronchospasm, pneumothorax, inadequate ventilation
- **Aspiration** – of gastric contents, blood (can result in obstruction/hypoxia ± bacterial infection) 1:3000
  - ▸ prevent by ensuring **NBM 6h pre-op** (clear fluids 2h pre-op)
  - ▸ if need emergency surgery / has severe reflux = **rapid sequence induction** (see above)

CIRCULATION

- **Hypotension** – common SE of many anaesthetic drugs, blood loss, vagal nerve stimulation (with bradycardia)
  - ▸ give IV fluids and metaraminol/ephedrine if BP drops significantly
  - ▸ **ketamine does not cause hypotension** – good in elderly / haemodynamically unstable patients

DISABILITY

- **Unintended awareness*** 1:15,000
  - ▸ due to equipment failure / under-administration of anaesthetic → more common with TIVA
  - ▸ less likely with volatile agents because of agent monitoring
  - ▸ will monitor during operation to ensure unawareness (e.g. BP, HR, pupils etc.)
- **PONV** – assess risk with Apfel score
  - ▸ warn patients
  - ▸ prescribe post-op anti-emetics prophylactically
  - ▸ avoid N_2O and minimise opiates

Apfel score for PONV	
Risk factors	**Points**
Female	1
Non-smoker	1
History of PONV	1
Post-op opioids	1
Total score	**0–4**

EXPOSURE

- **Hypothermia** – cold fluids, cold table, exposed skin, vasodilation, lack of shivering
  - ▸ regularly check temperature
  - ▸ warmed fluids / blood products
  - ▸ insulate patient, forced air warmer (Bair Hugger)

Common causes of anaphylaxis

- **Antimicrobials** (co-amoxiclav & teicoplanin)
- **Neuromuscular blocking agents (NMBAs)**
- **Chlorhexidine**
- **Colloids** (rarely used)
- **Patent blue injection** (a contrast dye for sentinel LN biopsy)
- **Miscellaneous** (ondansetron, propofol)

*this is a big worry for many patients, but can reassure that they will be monitored for signs of increased awareness throughout the procedure

Role of anaesthetists

In surgery:
- **Pre-op:** optimising, planning
- **Intra-op:** management
- **Post-op:** management, planning

Others:
- Chronic pain services
- Critical care
- Obstetrics
- Cardiac arrest calls

Pre-operative assessment

Estimate & reduce risk, educate patient, individualise care

Prehabilitation / optimisation

- Medical optimisation
- Exercise programmes
- Nutritional support
- Psychological/social support

Pre-operative starvation

- → Risk of aspiration of stomach contents under GA
  - **Food:** 6h (inc. milk)
  - **Fluids:** 2h (inc. tea/coffee)
  - **Breastfed infants:** 4h
  follow guidelines for T1DM & giving insulin

Also consider:

- Any bowel prep needed (enema)
- Prophylactic analgesia + antiemetic
- VTE assessment & prophylaxis

Precautions for MH

- Continuous temp. monitoring
- <5ppm volatile gases used & TIVA

History

BACKGROUND

- Identify patient
- Check understanding of need for surgery (check capacity)
- Check understanding of all options, benefits, risks

CURRENT HEALTH

- Recent/current illness (within 2w)
- Exercise tolerance / **functional capacity** (expressed as METs)
- Sleep apnoea
- Smoking, alcohol, weight
- Any chance of pregnancy?

PMHX

- DM, HTN
- Asthma/COPD
- CVD/IHD
- Liver disease
- Coagulopathies / bleeding Hx

DHX

- **Anticoagulants** – what, when last taken, why?
- Antihypertensives, diuretics, digoxin, steroids (affect renal function)
- **Allergies** – drugs, plasters, antiseptics

SURGICAL & ANAESTHETIC Hx

- Previous anaesthetics & reactions e.g. PONV

FHX: Malignant hyperthermia → negative FHx doesn't exclude MH

Examination

- **Multisystem:** cardiorespiratory, CNS, PNS, abdominal
- **Anaesthetic:** airway assessment: '**LEMON**'
  → **L**ook: neck size, jaw size, dentures, loose teeth
  → **E**valuate: adequate mouth opening (3 fingers between teeth)
  → **M**allampati score: grade IV = soft palate not visible
  → **O**bstruction: obesity, tumours
  → **N**eck mobility: trauma, ankylosing spondylitis

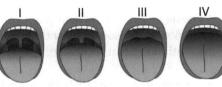

Fig. 10.1 Mallampati score.

ASA classification[1]

→ *describes health of patient before an operation*

Class	Definition	Example
1	A normal healthy patient	Non-smoking & min. alcohol
2	Mild systemic disease	Smoker, pregnancy, obesity Well-controlled DM or HTN
3	Severe systemic disease, with some functional limitations	Poorly controlled DM or HTN Distant Hx of CVA/MI Pacemaker
4	Severe systemic disease that is a constant threat to life	Recent Hx of MI/CVA/TIA Current cardiac ischaemia/HF
5	Moribund patient who is not expected to survive without the operation	Ruptured AAA Intracranial bleed Ischaemic bowel
6	Already declared brain dead (organs being removed for transplant)	

[1] American Society of Anesthesiologists (2020) *ASA Physical Status Classification System*

Investigations

→ *only undertake those necessary for that patient*

ALL PATIENTS FOR MAJOR SURGERY
- FBC (Hb & platelets), U&Es, clotting, G&S
- MRSA swabs – especially in **orthopaedic surgery** → decolonise

OTHERS
- **ECG:** if >65y or ASA >1
- **LFTs:** liver disease, metastatic disease, alcoholism
- **Blood glucose/HbA1c:** diabetics, long-term steroids
- **Clotting:** Hx of bleeding disorder, anticoagulated
- **CXR:** cardio-respiratory disease, malignancy
- **ABG/respiratory function tests:** COPD, asthma
- **ECHO:** LVF, IHD, valvular disease
- **Pregnancy test:** women of child-bearing age

Special cases for preoperative management

Condition	Pre-operative management considerations[2]
Anaemia (Hb <13g/dl)	• If non-urgent, delay surgery until Hb >13g/dl • Fe supplements PO (6–8w for effect) • IV Fe (<6w for effect)

Diabetes mellitus[3]	• Comprehensive pre-op assessment
	• **Optimise diabetes control** (HbA1c <69mmol/mol)
	• Plan admission & management of existing therapy
	  → only missing 1 meal = manipulate current treatment (*e.g. miss one dose*)
	  → missing >1 meal = variable rate IV insulin infusion
	• Place **first on operating list** (to minimise fasting times)
	• Close glucose monitoring throughout

Hypertension	BP controlled to <160/100mmHg before referral for surgery
Coagulopathies	• Stop anticoagulant drugs prior to surgery (see guidelines for timings before & after surgery to take medications) • If coagulation disorder, counsel patient on risks of anaesthesia/surgery • Ensure clotting screen is performed
Long-term steroids	May have insufficient adrenal response → consider extra corticosteroid cover i.e. hydrocortisone pre- and peri-operative

Medications that need stopping/changing pre-op: 'LICK SOAP'
- **L**ithium: stop day before
- **I**nsulin: start sliding scale
- **C**OCP/HRT: see box, right
- **K**+-sparing diuretics: day of surgery
- **S**teroids: switch to IV
- **O**ral hypoglycaemics: see guideline
- **A**nticoagulants/antiplatelets: see box, right
- **P**erindopril/ACEis: day of surgery

[2] NICE (2020) *Perioperative care in adults* [NG180]
[3] CPOC (2021) *Guideline for perioperative care for people with diabetes mellitus undergoing elective and emergency surgery*
[4] BSH (2016, updated 2022) *Peri-operative management of anticoagulation and antiplatelet therapy*

Investigations not usually indicated if only minor/intermediate surgery
unless patient is ASA ≥3

Medication management for diabetes mellitus

Depends on multiple factors:
- Type of diabetes
- Usual dosing regimen
- Type of insulin / oral hypoglycaemic
- Timing of surgery / whether NBM post-op
Always check CPOC guidelines for details

If high risk of thrombotic event without medication (e.g. recent VTE/CVA), use bridging therapy → switch to LMWH & stop this night before op

Drugs affecting coagulation[4]
- **Warfarin:** stop 5d before (& restart same/next day)
  → only start surgery if INR <1.5
- **DOACs:** stop 24–48h before (depending on DOAC, CrCl & bleed risk)
- **Clopidogrel:** stop 5–7d before (discuss with haematology/cardiology)
- **Aspirin:** usually safe to continue
- **COCP/HRT:** stop 4w before major ops & restart ≥2w after → **ensure alternative contraception** (e.g. switch to POP)

Post-operative care

See *General Medicine and Surgery* companion volume for more details

Appropriate rate for post-op fluids:
• 1000ml over first 4h
• 1000ml over following 6h
• 500ml over final 4h

Water requirements:
25–30ml/kg/d **or** 1.5ml/kg/h

Fluid need increases 10% for every degree of pyrexia

Post-operative fluids

- Providing patients drink after 1–2h post-op, no fluids are needed unless increased fluid loss (e.g. vomiting)
  - ▸ consider type of loss to help guide type of fluid given as replacement
- If surgery prolonged or patient fails to drink, then IV maintenance is required
  - ▸ **replacement = maintenance + deficit**
  - ▸ (1.5ml/kg/h) + (losses/time without fluids)
- e.g. 70kg patient fasted since 8am and unable to take fluids at 6pm requires
  - ▸ 1.5ml/kg/h to make up the deficit = $1.5 \times 70 \times 10 = 1000$ml
  - ▸ 1.5ml/kg/h from 6pm to 8am the following morning = $1.5 \times 70 \times 14 = 1400$ml
  - ▸ total = 2400ml
  - ▸ also needs 1mmol/kg of Na and K → use Hartmann's **or** saline + K + dextrose

Post-operative oxygen

Why?

→ **Reduced respiratory drive:** due to anaesthetic agents (& opioids)

→ **Reduced respiratory effort:** due to pain → *Some hospitals protocolise supplemental O_2 for ALL post-op patients, others just for high risk (e.g. COPD) or low O_2 sats (<92%)*

→ **Gas exchange failure:** if atelectasis

Oxygen delivery: nasal cannulae, Hudson, Venturi, non-rebreathe mask

Monitoring: vital signs, PaO_2 & ABG

Post-operative nausea & vomiting (PONV)

→ *20–30% patients*

RISK FACTORS

REMEMBER to consider other causes of nausea & vomiting (e.g. infection, ↑ICP, obstruction)

Patient	Surgical	Anaesthetic
Female	ENT / squint surgery	Opioid analgesics
Younger adults	Adenoids/tonsillectomy	Inhaled analgesics
Obese	Abdo-/gynae surgery	N_2O
Non-smoker	Longer operations	Spinal anaesthesia
Hx PONV / motion sickness	Intraoperative dehydration	
Gastric contents (emergency op)	Hypotension	

Vomiting centre = in medulla
It receives input from higher structures, Chemoreceptor trigger zone, GIT & vestibular system

Prevention is better than cure! (use TIVA)
• Minimise opiates, inhaled agents & spinal anaesthetics
• Prophylactic anti-emetics (dexamethasone/ondansetron)
• Ensure adequate hydration & post-op analgesia

ASSESSING THE PATIENT: ABCDE approach

→ What was the operation – was it likely to cause PONV?

→ Are there other factors contributing to nausea?

→ Which anaesthetic/post-op drugs have been used?

→ Which anti-emetic would suit them best?

MANAGEMENT[5]

Apfel score for PONV	
Risk factors	**Points**
Female	1
Non-smoker	1
History of PONV	1
Post-op opioids	1
Total score	0–4

Drug	MofA	Dose	Time given	Contraindication/caution
Ondansetron	5HT3 antagonist	4mg IV/IM **or** 8mg PO	End of op or prophylactic	Long QT syndrome
Droperidol/prochlorperazine	DA (D2) antagonist	0.625–1.25mg IV	End of op	Bradycardia, CVD, DM
Cyclizine	Antihistamine (H1 antag.)	50mg TDS PO/IV/IM	End of op	HF, IHD, elderly, glaucoma
Metoclopramide	D2 antagonist	10mg PO/IM/IV	GI cause of N&V	**Bowel obstruction**
Dexamethasone	Glucocorticoid	4–8mg IV	Intra-op or prophylactic	CHF, DM, glaucoma, HTN

often as an adjunct unless diabetic

[5] Gan TJ *et al.* (2014) Consensus guidelines for the management of postoperative nausea and vomiting. *Anesth Analg.* 118:85

Pain management

→ *fewer cardiorespiratory complications, earlier mobilisation (↓ risk VTE), faster recovery, ↓ mortality*

ADVERSE EFFECTS OF PAIN

- **Reduced respiratory effort:** ↓deep breathing / hypoventilation → atelectasis, pneumonia, respiratory failure
- **GI atony:** N&V, ileus
- **Bladder atony:** urinary retention
- **Psychological impact**

PRINCIPLES OF ANALGESIC USE[6]

- Take by mouth (where possible)
- Take by the clock (regularly)
- Guided by the ladder (step up)
- Ensure individualised treatment
- Use adjuvant drugs

1. **Evaluation**
   - Cause, type & severity of pain (**SOCRATES**)
     ▸ nociceptive vs. neuropathic
   - Start Universal Pain Assessment Tool: 0–10
     ▸ **assess pain during function:** deep breathing and coughing
2. **Explanation & reassurance** – of aetiology & Mx options to patient & family
3. **Management**
   - Correct the correctable e.g. radio-/chemotherapy, surgery
   - Consider non-drug treatments e.g. massage, heat, TENS, CBT, mobility aids
   - Prescribe **regular drugs** for **persistent pain**
4. **Monitor** – continuously review response to treatment & development of side-effects

Strong opioid → Morphine, fentanyl
± non-opioid
± adjunct

Weak opioid → Codeine, dihydrocodeine, tramadol
± non-opioid
± adjunct

Non-opioid → Paracetamol, NSAIDs, aspirin
± adjunct

→ SSRIs, amitriptyline (TCAs), gabapentin, muscle relaxants, magnesium

Fig. 10.2 WHO pain ladder.

Patient-controlled analgesia

Pro: immediate relief
Con: excess side-effects
Need patient education

ALWAYS COPRESCRIBE metoclopramide + laxative with opioids

Options for pre- & post-operative analgesia

Type of analgesia	Dose & route	Indications	Cautions/CIs	
Paracetamol	0.5–1.0g/4h PO (max 4g/d)	Mild–moderate pain	**Cautions:** • Hepatic impairment	
NSAIDs (ibuprofen, diclofenac)	**Ibuprofen:** 400mg/4h PO (max 2.4g/d) **Diclofenac:** 50mg TDS PO	Mild–moderate pain **Especially:** • Inflammation • MSK pain • Renal/biliary colic	**Contraindications:** • Peptic ulcer • Clotting disorders • Anticoagulants	**Cautions:** • Elderly • Asthma • Renal/hepatic impairment
Codeine (opiate)	30–60mg/4h PO or IV (max 240mg/d) *Can use nerve blocks for severe pain if cannot tolerate opiates*	• Mild–moderate pain • Diarrhoea • Cough suppression	**Contraindications:** • Respiratory depression • Acute abdo • Delayed gastric emptying	
Morphine (opiate) (Oromorph PRN = for breakthrough pain) Oxycodone if CKD	**Depends on condition/pain level:** **Diamorphine:** 5–10mg/4h PO **Morphine:** 10–15mg/4h PO/SC **Oxycodone:** 5mg/4h PO	• Moderate–severe pain • MI • Pulmonary oedema • Chronic pain	**Cautions:** • Impaired respiratory function • Acute asthma attack • Hypotension/shock • Elderly / liver disease • CKD • IBD **SEs:** N&V, constipation, sedation	

[6] Ventafridda V, Saita L, Ripamonti C, De Conno F (1985) WHO guidelines for the use of analgesics in cancer pain. *Int J Tissue React*, 7(1):93.

PALLIATIVE CARE

11

ABBREVIATIONS

CBT – Cognitive behavioural therapy
CSCI – Continuous subcutaneous infusion (syringe driver)
DNACPR – Do not attempt cardiopulmonary resuscitation

IR – Immediate release
MR – Modified release
PRN – Pro re nata (as required)
SC – Subcutaneous
SR – Sustained release

SSRI – Selective serotonin reuptake inhibitor
TCA – Tricyclic antidepressants
TENS – Transcutaneous electrical nerve stimulation

Key principles of palliative care

an approach which improves the **quality of life** of patients and their families facing life-threatening illness, through the **prevention, assessment and treatment** of pain and other **physical, psychosocial, and spiritual problems**.

- Provides **relief from pain & other distressing symptoms**
- Aims to **enhance quality of life** by setting clear goals of treatment, and regards dying as a normal process
- Intends **neither to hasten nor postpone death**
- Integrates **psychological & spiritual** aspects of patient care
- Offers support to help patients **live as actively as possible**
- Offers **support system** to those close to the patient e.g. family
- Early involvement of palliative care teams has shown **survival benefit in some settings**[2]
- **Uses a team approach:** all those involved in patient care with support of the palliative care team

Supportive care: 'umbrella term' for services helping patients & family to cope with life-limiting illness & its treatment (from pre-diagnosis to cure/continuing illness/death).
- Self-help & support
- Psychological & social support
- Information giving
- Symptom control
- Rehabilitation
- Palliative care
- Bereavement care

Assessment in palliative care

Holistically assess individual, family & carer requirements to determine a care plan
- Ask the patient what is **important to them**
- Consider **physical & psychological** symptoms – may use scoring tool e.g. Edmonton Symptom Assessment System[3]
- Consider **consent & mental capacity**
- Consider **social & practical** needs e.g. financial, family, residential circumstances
- Consider **spiritual needs**
- Ensure **confidentiality** (share info only with consent)

End-of-life decision-making

- Identify important individuals to share information with & get contact details e.g. family
- Discuss patient's priorities for end-of-life care (e.g. where they want to die, DNACPR)
  - ▶ put in place advanced directives / care plans / LPAs / organ donation
  - ▶ if lacking capacity, for best interest decisions with involvement of family

---

End of life care: usually refers to last 6–12m of life.

Consultant, nurse specialist, physio, OT, dietitian, pharmacist, social worker, psychologist, chaplain

Services available
- Inpatient units
- Outpatient hospices
- Specialist outpatient clinic
- Inpatient palliative care team
- Care at home

---

[1] WHO (2002) *National cancer control programmes. Policies and managerial guidelines*. World Health Organization
[2] Hoerger M, Wayser GR, Schwing G, Suzuki A, Perry LM (2018) Impact of interdisciplinary outpatient specialty palliative care on survival and quality of life in adults with advanced cancer: a meta-analysis of randomized controlled trials. *Ann Behav Med*, 53:674
[3] Bruera E, Kuehn N, Miller MJ, Selmser P, Macmillan K (1991) The Edmonton Symptom Assessment System (ESAS): a simple method for the assessment of palliative care patients. *J Palliat Care*; 7:6

Symptom management

KEY PRINCIPLES OF SYMPTOM CONTROL
→ **Treat underlying/reversible causes**
→ Consider non-drug treatment
→ Stop any unnecessary medications & **prescribe anticipatory medications**

Symptom	Pharmacological management[4]
Pain	WHO pain ladder[5]
Nausea & vomiting	Cyclizine, metoclopramide, haloperidol
Shortness of breath	Morphine, midazolam
Agitation	Levomepromazine, midazolam
Airway secretions	Hyoscine hydrobromide/butylbromide
Constipation	Laxative e.g. senna, lactulose
Cough	Saline nebs, glycerol syrup, opioid (codeine)
Hiccup	Metoclopramide, PPI, baclofen
Pruritus	Topical antipruritic, antihistamine (chlorphenamine)

Anticipatory medications to control symptoms in final days of life

Consider stopping these when coming to end of life

Pain management in palliative care

1. Evaluation
- Determine the cause, type & severity of pain (**SOCRATES / pain charts**)
  - ▸ **nociceptive** → usually responds to opioids
  - ▸ **neuropathic (nerve)** – 'burning/tingling' → less responsive to opioids
  - → **remember psychological factors can influence pain**

2. Explanation – explain aetiology & management options to patient & family

3. Management: individualised
- **Correct the correctable** e.g. radio-/chemotherapy, surgery
- **Consider non-drug treatments** e.g. massage, heat, TENS, CBT, mobility aids
- **Prescribe analgesia regularly for persistent pain**

4. Monitor – continuously review response to treatment & any side-effects

WHO PAIN LADDER[4]
Principles of analgesic use
- Take by mouth (where possible)
- Take by the clock (regularly)
- Guided by the ladder (step up)
- Ensure individualised treatment
- Use adjuvant drugs

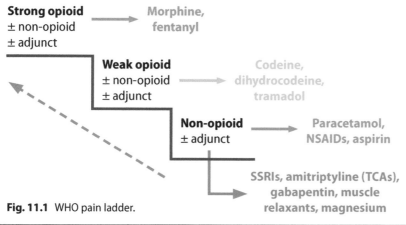

Fig. 11.1 WHO pain ladder.

Factors influencing pain

Physical: symptoms, treatment side-effects, insomnia
Psychological: anger, fear, depression
Spiritual: personal beliefs
Social: worry about family, finances, loss of role/job, isolation

Bone pain due to mets

- Radiotherapy
- NSAIDs/opioid
- Steroids (e.g. dexamethasone)
- Bisphosphonates
- Neuropathic agents / nerve blocks

---

[4] Twycross R, Wilcock A (2018) *Introducing Palliative Care*, 5th edition. Pharmaceutical Press
[5] Ventafridda V, Saita L, Ripamonti C, De Conno F (1985) WHO guidelines for the use of analgesics in cancer pain. *Int J Tissue React*, 7:93

Side-effects of opioids:
- N&V
- Constipation
- Delirium
- Drowsiness

Conversion of opioids

Oxycodone (Shortec IR or Longtec MR) = alternative if morphine not well tolerated
20mg PO morphine = 10mg PO oxycodone

Codeine
60mg PO codeine = 6mg PO morphine

Worked example
Patient taking Zomorph 30mg BD
24h dose = 2 × 30 = 60mg
PRN dose = 60/6 = 10mg
24h SC morphine dose = 60/2 = 30mg
24h SC diamorphine dose = 60/3 = 20mg

Using strong opioids

1. **Start by calculating 24h need**
   - **Use immediate release morphine (Oramorph)** → 4h duration of action
   - Start with: 2.5–5mg 4-hourly
2. **Convert 24h need to modified release / sustained release (MR/SR)**
   - **Use modified release morphine (Zomorph: tablets/capsules)** → 12 or 24h duration of action
   - Direct conversion of 24h oral dose to 12h capsule (take total 24h immediate release (IR) need and divide by 2 to get 12h MR dose)
3. **Calculate breakthrough (PRN) dose**
   - 1/6th to 1/10th of 24h morphine dose
   → If PRN frequently needed ≥2 per day, a **prompt review is needed**
4. **If oral route no longer an option**
   Convert to SC route (syringe driver = CSCI: continuous SC infusion)
   - **For CSCI morphine:** divide 24h oral morphine dose by 2
   - **For CSCI diamorphine:** divide 24h oral morphine dose by 3
   - **Ensure patient has PRN SC option:** 1/6th to 1/10th of 24h SC dose

Caution with morphine & oxycodone in eGFR <30 = drowsy, jerks, hyperalgesia. Seek specialist advice for opioid in poor renal function. Commonly used are fentanyl, alfentanil or buprenorphine

Get specialist advice if prescribing fentanyl patches

Figure acknowledgements

Where no acknowledgement is given, the figure was created by the author

CHAPTER 1

Fig. 1.5 Reproduced from a-fib.com/2-overview-of-atrial-fibrillation-2 with permission

CHAPTER 2

Fig. 2.3 OpenStax College, Biology (2013). Provided by: OpenStax CNX. Figure 3. Located at: http://cnx.org/content/m44749/latest/?collection=col11448/latest

Fig. 2.4 Created by the author based on figures from Alzheimer's Society UK (2022)

Fig. 2.7 Adapted from Azam, M. (2021) *Mind Maps for Medicine*. Scion Publishing Ltd

CHAPTER 3

Fig. 3.1 Reproduced from https://commons.wikimedia.org/wiki/File:Extragenital_endometriosis.jpg – Author: Hic et nunc under CC 3.0

Fig. 3.2 Reproduced from Blausen.com staff (2014). "Medical gallery of Blausen Medical 2014". WikiJournal of Medicine 1 (2). DOI:10.15347/wjm/2014.010. ISSN 2002-4436. – Endometriosis

Fig. 3.3 Reproduced from https://openstax.org/books/anatomy-and-physiology/pages/27-2-anatomy-and-physiology-of-the-female-reproductive-system – Figure 27.10 The Vulva – under CC 3.0

Fig. 3.5 Reproduced from Yuan, C., Yao, Y., Cheng, B. *et al.* (2020) The application of deep learning based diagnostic system to cervical squamous intraepithelial lesions recognition in colposcopy images. *Sci Rep* 10, 11639. https://doi.org/10.1038/s41598-020-68252-3 Open Access under CC 4.0

Fig. 3.6 Reproduced from https://commons.wikimedia.org/wiki/File:MenstrualCycle.png – Author: Chris 73 | Talk – under CC 3.0

Fig. 3.9 Reproduced from "Medical gallery of Blausen Medical 2014". WikiJournal of Medicine 1 (2). DOI:10.15347/wjm/2014.010. ISSN 2002-4436. – The Female Reproductive System

CHAPTER 4

Fig. 4.1 Adapted from: https://commons.wikimedia.org/wiki/File:Ectopic_Pregnancy.png –Author: Bruce Blaus Blausen.com staff (2014) – under CC 4.0

Fig. 4.2 Dufendach, K. (Artist). (2008). Placentation. [Web]. Reproduced from http://commons.wikimedia.org/wiki/File:Placentation.svg – under CC 3.0

Fig. 4.3 Reproduced from Gray, H. (1918) *Anatomy of the Human Body* – Figure 448. The diameters of the inlet of the true pelvis (female)

Fig. 4.4 Reproduced from https://commons.wikimedia.org/wiki/File:Bumm_352_lg.jpg - Bumm, E. (1902). Grundriss zum Studium der Geburtshülfe. Wiesbaden: J.F. Bergmann – now under Public Domain

Fig. 4.5 Adapted from: https://commons.wikimedia.org/w/index.php?curid=19780765 – Author: PhantomSteve/talk – Own work, CC BY-SA 3.0

CHAPTER 5

Fig. 5.1a, b, e and f Reproduced from Haveri FTTS & Inamadar, AC (2014) A cross-sectional prospective study of cutaneous lesions in newborn. *International Scholarly Research Notices*, vol. 2014, Article ID 360590. https://doi.org/10.1155/2014/360590 under CC 4.0

Fig. 5.1c Reproduced from https://commons.wikimedia.org/wiki/File:Hemangioma.JPG – Author: cbheumircanl under Public Domain

Fig. 5.1d Wang X, Tian C, Duan X *et al.* (2014) A medical manipulator system with lasers in photodynamic therapy of port wine stains. *BioMed Research International*, vol. 2014, Article ID 384646. https://doi.org/10.1155/2014/384646 – under CC 4.0

Fig. 5.1g Reproduced from https://commons.wikimedia.org/wiki/File:Congenital_melanocytic_naveus_new_pic.jpg. Author: Mohammad2018 – own work, under CC 4.0

Fig. 5.2 Reproduced from https://commons.wikimedia.org/w/index.php?curid=534054. Author: AMH Sheikh – own work, under CC 4.0

Fig. 5.3 Reproduced from https://commons.wikimedia.org/wiki/File:X-ray_of_infant_respiratory_distress_syndrome_(IRDS).png. User: Michael Haggstrom under Public Domain.

Fig. 5.4 Arora K *et al.* (2014) Primary spontaneous bilateral pneumothorax in a neonate. APSP Journal of Case Reports, [S.I.], 5(3). Available at: www.apspjcaserep.com/ojs/index.php/ajcr/article/view/211/236. doi:http://dx.doi.org/10.21699/ajcr.v5i3.211. – Open access under CC 4.0

Fig. 5.5 Reproduced from https://commons.wikimedia.org/wiki/File:DuodAtres.png. Author: Kinderradiologie Olgahospital Klinikum Stuttgart

Fig. 5.6 Reproduced from Centers for Disease Prevention: www.cdc.gov/ncbddd/birthdefects/omphalocele.html – Public domain

Fig. 5.7 Agbara K, Moulot M, Ehua A. *et al.* (2019) Gastroschisis associated with cleft lip and palate: report of three cases. *Open Journal of Pediatrics*, 9, 1–6. doi: 10.4236/ojped.2019.91001. – Open access under CC 4.0

Fig. 5.8 Reproduced from https://commons.wikimedia.org/wiki/File:Cleft_Lip_%26_Cleft_Palate_Repair.png - Blausen.com staff "Medical gallery of Blausen Medical"

Fig. 5.9 Reproduced from https://pressbooks.bccampus.ca/thescienceofhumanpotential/chapter/the-medical-model-of-behavioral-disorders/ (Figure 11.1) original by Vanellus Foto – under CC BY-SA 3.0

Fig. 5.11 Reproduced from https://cnx.org/contents/57cfLKUe@7.2:jZnM0LLx@3/Images-of-Memorable-Cases-Case-143 – Open Access

Fig. 5.12 Reproduced from Mata-Machado NA (2019) Everolimus for treatment tuberous sclerosis complex with refractory epilepsy: management and out comes. A case report. *Mathews J Cytol Histol*, 3(2): 13. (Figure 1). Open Access under CC 4.0

Fig. 5.13 Reproduced from Haveri FTTS & Inamadar, AC (2014) A cross-sectional prospective study of cutaneous lesions in newborn. *International Scholarly Research Notices*, vol. 2014, Article ID 360590. https://doi.org/10.1155/2014/360590 under CC 4.0

Fig. 5.14 Murthy AS & McGraw M (2014) M to T rearrangement: an approach to correct webbed neck deformity. *Case Reports in Medicine*. Article ID 682806. https://doi.org/10.1155/2014/682806 – Open access under the Creative Commons Attribution License.

Fig. 5.15 Reproduced from https://commons.wikimedia.org/wiki/File:Fragile_x_syndrom.png Under Free Art Licence

Fig. 5.16 Reproduced from Cortés F, Alliende MA, Barrios A, *et al.* (2005) Clinical, genetic and molecular features in 45 patients with Prader-Willi syndrome. *Revista médica de Chile*, v. 133 n. 1. www.scielo.cl/scielo.php?script=sci_arttext&pid=S0034-98872005000100005 – under a Creative Commons License

Fig. 5.17 Reproduced from Yokoyama-Rebollar E, Ruiz-Herrera A, Lieberman-Hernández E (2015) Angelman syndrome due to familial translocation: unexpected additional results characterized by microarray-based comparative genomic hybridization. *Mol Cytogenet* (Open Access)

Fig. 5.18 Reproduced from https://commons.wikimedia.org/wiki/File:Figura_1-_Fisionomia_de_um_portador_da_S%C3%ADndrome_de_Williams.jpg – Author: Gisele Monteiro Araújo – under CC 4.0

Fig. 5.19 Reproduced from Makrariya A & Adlakha N (2016) Thermal patterns in peripheral regions of breast during different stages of development. *Biology and Medicine* (Open Access)

Fig. 5.22 Reproduced from Marrani E, Burns JC & Cimaz, R (2018) How should we classify Kawasaki disease? *Frontiers in Immunology*, 9, p. 2974. doi: 10.3389/fimmu.2018.02974. – under CC 4.0

Fig. 5.23 Reproduced from Ed Uthman Flickr 'Target cells, Peripheral blood smear' at www.flickr.com/photos/euthman/with/39144139915/ – under CC2.0

Fig. 5.24 Reproduced from https://commons.wikimedia.org/wiki/File:Blood_film_of_Hemoglobin_SC_disease.jpg – Author: Spicy under CC 3.0

Fig. 5.25 Reproduced from https://commons.wikimedia.org/wiki/File:Coagulation_simple.svg – Author: Joe D under CC 3.0

Fig. 5.26 Reproduced from https://commons.wikimedia.org/wiki/File:Acute_leukemia-ALL.jpg – Author: VashiDonsk under CC 3.0.

Fig. 5.27 Reproduced from National Cancer Institute – Reed-Sternberg Cell – AV number: CDR576466 (Public domain)

Fig. 5.28 Reproduced from National Cancer Institute – Retinoblastoma – AV number: CDR800189 (Public domain)

Fig. 5.29 Reproduced from Murányi M, Salah MA, Benyó M & Flaskó T (2012) Serious contracted bladder and vesicoureteral reflux after intravesical Mitomycin-C treatment. *International Journal of Case Reports and Images*, 3(3):27–9. (Open Access)

Fig. 5.30 Reproduced from https://commons.wikimedia.org/wiki/File:Purpuraschoenleinhennoch2.JPG – Author: Peter Rammstein under CC 3.0

Fig. 5.31 Reproduced from https://commons.wikimedia.org/wiki/File:Neonatal_Heart_Circulation.png – Author: Blausen Medical

Fig. 5.32 Reproduced from Centers for Disease Control and Prevention: https://commons.wikimedia.org/wiki/File:Asd-web.jpg (Public domain)

Fig. 5.33 Reproduced from Centers for Disease Control and Prevention: https://commons.wikimedia.org/wiki/File:Vsd_simple-lg.jpg (Public domain)

Fig. 5.34 Reproduced from Centers for Disease Control and Prevention www.cdc.gov/ncbddd/heartdefects/coarctationofaorta.html (Public domain)

Fig. 5.35 Reproduced from Centers for Disease Control and Prevention www.cdc.gov/ncbddd/heartdefects/tetralogyoffallot.html (Public domain)

Fig. 5.36 Reproduced from Centers for Disease Control and Prevention https://commons.wikimedia.org/w/index.php?curid=29525842 (Public domain)

Fig. 5.37 Reproduced from https://commons.wikimedia.org/wiki/File:SVT_Lead_II-2.JPG – Author or original: Displaced, Derivative: James Heilman – under public domain

Fig. 5.38 Based on BTS-NICE Guidelines

Fig. 5.39 Reproduced from https://commons.wikimedia.org/wiki/File:Hypsarrhythmia.png – Author: Ralphelg under CC 3.0

Fig. 5.41 Reproduced from https://commons.wikimedia.org/wiki/File:Charcot-marie-tooth_foot.jpg – Author: Benefros under CC 3.0

Fig. 5.42 Reproduced from Church A & Peterson F (1908) *Nervous and Mental Diseases*. Public Domain

Fig. 5.43 Reproduced from https://es.wikipedia.org/wiki/
Archivo:Pied_bot,_varus_%C3%A9quin_(bilateral).jpg – Author:
Brachet Youri under CC 3.0

Fig. 5.44 Reproduced from https://commons.wikimedia.org/
wiki/File:HipdisX.png – Author: James Heilman under CC 3.0

Fig. 5.45 Reproduced from https://commons.wikimedia.org/
wiki/File:Roe-perthes.jpg – Author: Praxis Dr. Lengerke (Public
Domain)

Fig. 5.46 Reproduced from Meiling JB, Bowman WP & Mayfield
ME (2018) A comparison of varus and valgus slipped capital
femoral epiphysis: a case series. *J Case Rep Images Orthop Rheum*,
3:100011Z14JM2018 (Open Access)

Fig. 5.47 Reproduced from https://commons.wikimedia.org/
wiki/File:Buckle_fracture_of_the_Radius.svg – Author: RouDhi
under CC 4.0

Fig. 5.48 Public domain

Fig. 5.49 Reproduced from Chavda V, Henderson L, Chavda R
et al. (2017) Intussusception following rotavirus vaccination: a
reminder for practitioners. *BJGP Open*, 1(1): bjgpopen17X100629.
DOI: 10.3399/bjgpopen17X100629 under CC BY 4.0.

Fig. 5.50 Reproduced from https://commons.wikimedia.org/
wiki/File:Sigmoidvolvulus.jpg – Author: Mont4nha under Public
Domain

Fig. 5.51 Reproduced from https://commons.wikimedia.org/
wiki/File:Hypospadias.jpg – Author: Peter Thanos under Public
Domain

CHAPTER 6

Fig. 6.3 Reproduced from https://commons.wikimedia.org/wiki/
File:Brain_bulbar_region.svg Patrick J. Lynch, medical illustrator;
C. Carl Jaffe, MD, cardiologist. CC 2.5 License 2006

CHAPTER 7

Fig. 7.1 Reproduced from Pixabay – Stock Image, Psoriasis –
https://pixabay.com/photos/psoriasis-skin-disease-
inflammation-5996424/

Fig. 7.2 Reproduced from https://commons.wikimedia.org/
wiki/File:Acne_vulgaris_on_a_very_oily_skin.jpg – User: Roshu
Bangal under CC 4.0

Fig. 7.3 Reproduced from https://commons.wikimedia.org/wiki/
File:Atopic_dermatitis_child_3.jpg – Author: GZZ under CC 4.0

Fig. 7.4 Reproduced from https://commons.wikimedia.org/
wiki/File:Scabies_hand_and_fingers_1.jpg – Author: Gzzz under
CC 4.0

Fig. 7.5 Reproduced from https://commons.wikimedia.org/wiki/
File:Impetigo2020.jpg – Author: James Heilman, MD - Own work,
CC BY-SA 4.0

Fig. 7.6 Reproduced from https://commons.wikimedia.org/wiki/
File:HotTubFolliculitis.jpg – Author: Lsupellmel in public domain

Fig. 7.7 Reproduced from Haasnoot PJ & de Vries A (2018)
Staphylococcal scalded skin syndrome in a 4-year-old child: a
case report. *J Med Case Reports*, 12, 20. https://doi.org/10.1186/
s13256-017-1533-7 – Figure 1 (Open Access under CC 4.0)

Fig. 7.8 Reproduced from de Carvalho, HT *et al.* (2019) Diagnosis
and treatment of streptococcal toxic shock syndrome in the
pediatric intensive care unit: a case report. *Rev. bras. ter. intensiva*
[online], 31(4) – Figure 2 (Open Access under CC 4.0)

Fig. 7.9 Reproduced from https://commons.wikimedia.org/wiki/
File:Recurrent_erysipelas_on_edematous_leg.jpg – Author:
Mikael Häggström

Fig. 7.10 Reproduced from Fujioka M, Fukui K & Ishiyama S
(2016) Necrotizing fasciitis without inflammatory signs
in patients receiving anti-interleukin-6 receptor antibody
(tocilizumab): two cases report. *J Musculoskelet Disord Treat*
2:027. – Figure 1a (Open Access under CC 4.0)

Fig. 7.11 Reproduced from https://en.wikipedia.org/wiki/
File:Cellulitis_Left_Leg.JPG – User: Colm Anderson under CC 3.0

Fig. 7.12 Reproduced from https://commons.wikimedia.org/
wiki/File:Scarlet_fever_2.jpg – Author: Estreya under CC 2.5

Fig. 7.13 Reproduced from Coyle C, Mangar S, Abel P *et al.*
(2015) Erythema nodosum as a result of estrogen patch therapy
for prostate cancer: a case report. *J Med Case Reports*, 9, 285.
https://doi.org/10.1186/s13256-015-0776-4 – Figure 1 (Open
Access under CC 4.0)

Fig. 7.14 Reproduced from https://commons.wikimedia.org/
wiki/File:Vasculitis.JPG – Author: James Heilman under CC 3.0

Fig. 7.15 Reproduced from https://en.wikipedia.org/wiki/
File:Wart_filiform_eyelid.jpg – Author: Schweintechnik under
Public Domain

Fig. 7.16 Reproduced from https://commons.wikimedia.org/
wiki/File:Varicela_Aranzales.jpg – Author: Camiloaranzales under
Public Domain

Fig. 7.17 Reproduced from www.wikidoc.org/index.php/
File:ShinglesDay5_ed.JPG – Original Author: Mariegriffiths under
CC 3.0

Fig. 7.18 Reproduced from https://commons.wikimedia.org/
wiki/File:Herpes_labialis_-_opryszczka_wargowa.jpg – Author:
Jojo under Public Domain

Fig. 7.19 Reproduced from https://commons.wikimedia.org/
wiki/File:Molluscaklein.jpg – Author: Evanherk under CC 3.0

Fig. 7.20 Reproduced from Huey, ANS *Father's Discovery* –
https://fatheringchildren.blogspot.com/2008/08/hand-foot-and-
mouth-disease-preventable.html – under CC 3.0

Fig. 7.21 Reproduced from https://commons.wikimedia.org/
wiki/File:Pityriasisfront.jpg – Author: James Heilman under CC 3.0

Fig. 7.22 Reproduced from Siegfried EC & Hebert AA
(2015) Diagnosis of atopic dermatitis: mimics, overlaps,
and complications. *J Clin Med*, 4(5): 884–917. doi:10.3390/
jcm4050884 – Figure 19 (Open Access under CC 4.0)

CHAPTER 8

Index of conditions